Managing

Information

in Healthcare:

Concepts

and Cases

Managing

Information

in Healthcare:

Concepts

and Cases

John Abbott Worthley

HEALTH ADMINISTRATION PRESS
Chicago, Illinois

04 03 02 01 00   5 4 3 2 1

Library of Congress Cataloging-in-Publication Data

Worthley, John Abbott.
    Managing information in healthcare : concepts and cases / John Abbott Worthley.
        p.   cm.
    Includes bibliographical references and index.
    ISBN 1-56793-131-6 (alk. paper)
    1. Medical informatics.   I. Title.

R858 .W673 2000
362.1'068'4—dc21

00-032299

The paper used in this publication meets the minimum requirements of American National Standard for Information Sciences—Permanence of Paper for Printed Library Materials, ANSI Z39.48–1984. ∞ ™

Health Administration Press
A division of the Foundation
    of the American College of
    Healthcare Executives
One North Franklin Street
Chicago, IL 60606-3491
312/424-2800

Contents

Preface ix

Chapter One: Taming Information Technology 1

Case One: The Best Is None Too Good for St. Serena's 2

Commentary 4

Readings:

Can Computers Cure Health Care?
Erick Schonfeld 18

The Irrepressible Computer: The Brave New World of
Healthcare Information Technology
Steve Heimoff 24

**Chapter Two: Understanding Information
Management Concepts** 35

Case Two: The State of the Art 37

Commentary 38

Readings:

Information Management and the Decisionmaker
Philip H. Hutchens....................................... 50

Towards a Framework for Information Management
Jennifer Rowley.. 56

**Chapter Three: Thinking Systematically About
Information Systems** 73

Case Three: Calling All Drivers 74

Commentary 75

Readings:

The Right Mind-Set for Managing Information Technology
M. Bensaou and Michael Earl 88

Managing the IT Procurement Process
Robert Heckman 102

Chapter Four: Managing Organizational Impacts 121

Case Four: What Hath God Wrought? 122

Commentary 123

Readings:

Basic Principles of Information Technology
Organization in Health Care Institutions
Joyce A. Mitchell 133

The Computer as a Focus of Organizational Change in
the Hospital
Coralie Farlee 150

Chapter Five: Managing User Resistance 165

Case Five: The Retarding Resisters 165

Commentary 168

Readings:

How to Prevent and Cope with Resistance to Change
William Umiker 178

Electronic Medical Records: Are Physicians Ready?
*Kathryn H. Dansky, Larry D. Gamm, Joseph J. Vasey,
and Camille K. Barsukiewicz*. 186

Chapter Six: Maintaining Security 205

Case Six: Phil's Pills 207

Commentary 208

Reading:

Data Security and Patient Confidentiality:
The Manager's Role
Fleur Fisher and Bruce Madge 218

Chapter Seven: Maintaining Information Privacy 225

Case Seven: Protecting Private Parts 225

Commentary 227

Reading:
Driving Toward Guiding Principles: A Goal for Privacy,
Confidentiality, and Security of Health Information
Suzy A. Buckovich, Helga A. Rippen, and
Michael J. Rozen 240

Chapter Eight: Understanding Social Impacts 255

Case Eight: Party or Produce or Else 256

Commentary 257

Reading:
Ethics and Long-Term Care: Some Reflections on
Information Management
Robert E. Brenning 263

**Chapter Nine: Directing the Future of Information
Management** 277

Case Nine: The Jedi of St. Serena's 278

Commentary 279

Reading:
An Organizational Memory Approach to Information
Management
Vikas Anand, Charles C. Manz, and William H. Glick 284

Index 305

About the Author 315

PREFACE

NEARLY TWO decades ago, my book *Managing Computers in Healthcare* appeared in the first of what later became three editions. In those days, computer technology was relatively new in healthcare organizations and was, for most healthcare professionals, a rather intimidating reality that was causing disruption and problems as well as producing great benefits.

Today, computer technology is no longer strange and intimidating to most healthcare workers. It has become a routine part of organizational life with which most healthcare providers and many patients are very comfortable. The challenge now is more focused on using this technology to better respond to the changing environment of healthcare, which now emphasizes managed care, legal compliance, and competition for customers.

This book is a response to both the heightened comfort level with information technology and to the changing environment of the healthcare enterprise. Therefore, rather than focus on managing computers, this book targets the management of information, which now is intertwined with technology. The concepts, while similar to those posed in the *Managing Computers in Healthcare* books, are presented in the context of 21st century reality.

Because years of use in classrooms and healthcare facilities have confirmed the merits of the design of those books, the format of commentary, cases, and readings is retained here but with one adjustment: Instead of appearing at the end of the chapters, the cases are now fully integrated within the chapters. I am grateful to the readers for the feedback that has resulted in this improvement.

The readings are all new and their sources—*Fortune Magazine*, *Harvard Business Review*, and *Academy of Management Review*, to name a few—are indicative of the sophistication that has evolved in the field of information management. The sources also manifest the broad recognition of the importance of information in this century.

My students over the years, at Indiana University, the Chinese University of Hong Kong, University of Illinois at Chicago, and the Beijing University of International Business, deserve credit for the improvements in thinking represented in this book. They have been my teachers as much as I have been theirs.

I want to gratefully acknowledge the staff at Health Administration Press—particularly Renée Anderson and Jane Williams—who have brought this project to fruition. Without the responsive professionalism of Anne Kohler, of the Indiana University Library, the research that supports this book would still not be complete. Thank you, Anne!

Information management in the healthcare industry of the 21st century will be a major challenge for healthcare professionals. I hope this book helps in addressing that responsibility.

TAMING INFORMATION TECHNOLOGY

T HREE REALITIES underlie the focus of this book. The first reality is the general pervasiveness of information technology in managing information in organizations today. Information processed by computer technology is now a standard aspect of organizations in general, of healthcare organizations in particular, and of our society at large. According to Kleinke (1998), in 2000, the healthcare industry will surpass the $25 billion budget it apportions annually in expenditures on information technology. With more than 80 million Americans now using the Internet (Newsweek 1999), healthcare consumers are increasingly armed with healthcare information, which can be downloaded onto their increasingly sophisticated computer systems (Appleby 1999). Computers and the plethora of information they generate are a reality from which today's healthcare managers, providers, and consumers can hardly escape.

The second reality is that this computer-processed information continues to offer wonderful opportunities for significant improvements in organizational and social life, and in healthcare in particular. A Price-WaterhouseCoopers survey of physicians, for example, found that group practices foresee major improvements in billing, scheduling, and medical records (Sandrick 1999). Large facilities are already realizing major improvements in prescription-drug management through use of information technology (Sandrick 1998). Stefl (1999) echoes the consensus in maintaining that "information technology, appropriately chosen to match an organization's culture and behavior patterns, has tremendous capacity to improve performance and enhance value." Clearly, the potential benefits to be derived from sound information management continue to be enormous.

The third reality is that actual experience—as opposed to touted expectations—with managing information technology in organizations and in society often has been disappointing and problem laden, a reality from which healthcare organizations have not been exempt, as Bell (1998) confirms: "The theoretical link between a good information system and the ability of a hospital to achieve organizational success is well documented and understood. However, the reality of the situation does not match the theory." The road from potential benefits to actual improvements continues to be inordinately rocky. The world of healthcare professionals today, thus, continues to be a computerized-information environment characterized by great promise and hope but sobered by struggles, frustration, and disappointment; as Kennedy (1990) suggests: There may be more questions than answers regarding information technology for healthcare as we enter a new century. The following case illustrates the challenges that healthcare managers may face in this regard.

CASE STUDY

Case One: The Best Is None Too Good for St. Serena's

St. Serena's Healthcare System is a comprehensive healthcare organization operating a 300-bed hospital, a long-term care facility for 200 residents, a home care agency with a hospice program, and a rehabilitation center. When Samantha Savage became CEO last year she articulated a vision for making St. Serena's a "state of the art healthcare complex offering comprehensive healthcare services at the cutting edge of medical technology."

Among Samantha's first initiatives was acquisition of the long-term care facility and installation of an integrated information system. From her six years' experience with a major financial institution and ten years with a large suburban hospital Samantha knew first hand the strategic advantages of offering a full range of services and the managerial and operational benefits of modern information technology.

Under her predecessor, St. Serena's had developed a sound information system based on technology of the 1980s and early 1990s. However, knowing the considerable technological advances of information systems in recent years, Samantha envisioned a St. Serena's that reaps the advantages of internal information integration, as well as external Internet capabilities.

To accomplish this goal, she created a new top-level position—vice president of information systems—and hired Stewart Savvy, a Massachusetts Institute of Technology (MIT) MBA graduate, to manage the task. Throughout the hiring process Stewart was told that he would be given, as quickly as possible, all the resources needed to upgrade St. Serena's information system and maintain it to remain at the forefront of the healthcare industry's information systems. Stewart agreed that the benefits in cost efficiencies, marketing, and delivery of quality care would be enormous. Moreover, the new system would exceed JCAHO (Joint Commission on Accreditation of Healthcare Organizations) standards, which St. Serena's had barely met during the last accreditation process.

Stewart was convinced that these would be exciting times at St. Serena's: Samantha was a visionary CEO, necessary resources would be available, and, given St. Serena's committment to mergers and acquisitions, he could be part of the vanguard leading the healthcare industry into the future.

The first thing Stewart did was to hire Hacker Associates, a consulting firm that specializes in computer technology, to evaluate the existing system at St. Serena's and to recommend upgrade options. He also convened a meeting of all department heads to explain the initiative and to request their open and frank cooperation with consultants as they evaluated the system and solicited input on departmental operations and needs.

For three months, Hacker Associates consultants roamed the corridors of St. Serena's. They diagnosed an information system that consisted of what they called "isolated enclaves," some of which were up to date, but only a few were integrated or interconnected. The consultants found limited familiarity with software that could unite disparate operations, such as pharmacy, billing, and medical records, into an efficient, integrated system. Their recommended plan would provide St. Serena's with hardware and software upgrades, which would not only significantly enhance its organizational posture but would improve the operational efficiency of each department.

The Hacker Associates's plan was circulated among all the department heads for review and comment. The responses were sufficiently mixed, which confounded and disappointed Stewart. For example, instead of expressing expected enthusiasm over improvements in nursing services that the new system would offer, the Nursing department head voiced concerns about the impact of the plan on nurses' routine tasks and on the privacy of patient information, which is a concern also echoed by St. Serena's corporate counsel office who favored a "go slow" approach to the upgrade initiative. The Billing head complained that the consultants underappreciated the difficulty of coding standards when trying to integrate their system with others. The medical staff expressed probably the most discomfort with the plan, suggesting that the physicians were unlikely to cooperate.

Stewart spoke with Samantha and called a second meeting with the department heads to discuss their concerns. "It seems that we have too many problem makers and not enough problem solvers at St. Serena's," Stewart quipped as he began the meeting.

Questions for Discussion

1. What is happening at St. Serena's?
2. Why is Stewart so enthusiastic and the department heads so cautious?
3. Following the negative response from department heads, what action should Samantha and Stewart now take regarding St. Serena's information system?
4. How would you begin the second meeting were you in Stewart's shoes?

COMMENTARY

Stewart and St. Serena's experience from optimistic enthusiasm to sobered concern is hardly atypical. Clearly, modern information systems have become ubiquitous because the potential benefits are so significant, and Samantha and Stewart have seen such benefits in their previous organizational positions. Information systems technology can, and has, produced considerable advantages for healthcare organizations so the optimistic enthusiasm is understandable. The causes of our problematic experiences with information systems, however, are not so clear. Typically, the information technology itself is blamed when problems occur, as though technology were people responsible for their own actions. Thanks to computer scientists, information technology today is highly sophisticated, reliable, and affordable. It is a powerful force, but one that still has not been tamed by those who confront it in organizations and society. The technological challenge of computers has been met so well that we now are faced with a powerful tool that poses a major managerial challenge—namely, how to reap the possible benefits and minimize associated problems by using and managing information technology responsibly and wisely. This book is designed to help healthcare professionals tame information technology for better information management. The importance of the subject is suggested by an astute commentator who, in reflecting on information management in the 1990s, suggests that "while health care executives perceive great benefits from new technology, they often have problems managing it" (Boxerman and Gribbins 1990). This appears to be precisely the case with Stewart and St. Serena's.

The emerging trends of managed care competition and JCAHO accreditation standards additionally intensify the importance of effective information management generally and of the situation at St. Serena's specifically. In 1994, JCAHO's *Accreditation Manual for Hospitals*, in identifying information management as one of four critical organizational functions and in setting forth 10 information technology standards, augured a new way of thinking about information and its management.

Indeed, Samantha's vision at St. Serena's seems to reflect this change as articulated in the preamble of the accreditation manual: "Healthcare is . . . highly dependent on information . . . and the need to coordinate and integrate. . . . The organization's leaders have overall responsibility for this activity" (JCAHO 1993). Given the frustrations, disappointments, and fears that are frequently generated by computers, healthcare professionals might prefer to delegate the challenge to someone else or, better yet, to stay away from information technology altogether. However, the ubiquity of information management technology, combined with JCAHO standards, makes avoidance unrealistic.

The Ubiquity of Information Technology

In today's society, computers are used for everything from analyzing football plays in Dallas to sorting political campaign messages in Washington. Microcomputer technology has brought the "black box" into the home where the computer is rapidly becoming as common as a television set. Modern society is thoroughly inundated with information technology, as a survey by the Times-Mirror Center for the People and the Press reported: "Not only have computers entered tens of millions of American homes, but they have become indispensable tools for people who use them" (*USA Today* 1994). Even physicians are now using palm-sized computers for ordering prescriptions (Cabot 2000) as well as for communicating with patients on non-urgent matters (Galewitz 2000). Clearly, the traffic has thickened on the information highway.

Business usage of information technology began in 1954 when a UNIVAC-I was installed in a General Electric plant in Kentucky. Since then, the technology has so expanded that today even small, private businesses depend on information technology for record keeping, payroll, accounting, inventory control, and so forth.

Similarly, public agency use of technology for information management has proliferated since the U.S. Census Bureau used a UNIVAC-I in 1951. Today, all federal, state, and local government agencies are affected by information technology. Healthcare executives, like Stewart and Samantha, have apparently embraced computers as well and view technology as a solution to many healthcare challenges. A 1994 study found that 93 percent of a representative sample of hospitals expected to increase their spending on information systems by an average of 10 percent a year on operations and almost 12 percent on capital projects. One in five respondents said that an average annual jump in capital spending of more than 20 percent was expected (Morrisey 1994). According to Greene (1997) these projections have been far surpassed.

The situation is clear. Information technology is everywhere, and healthcare professionals—like the doctors, nurses, and staff at St. Serena's—must deal with this reality in their organizations. To the long-recognized legal, fiscal, political, and organizational aspects of healthcare administration, the technological has now been added. And, as the St. Serena's case suggests, the management task is not simple.

The Potential of Information Technology

A second reality prompting this managerial challenge is the promised, and proven, benefits of information technology. A basic management challenge is to harness these benefits for healthcare. With the impetus to improve clinical care, connect with outside facilities, and install a financial link to claims processors, combined with the drive for patient information on demand, healthcare executives have awakened to the need to improve their information systems. Accreditation pressures are keeping them awake (Yennie 1999).

A study commissioned by the Healthcare Financial Management Association underscored the potential of information technology. The study projected total net savings of $2.6 billion to $5.2 billion per year from automating and standardizing just the total number of administrative transactions in healthcare (Gardner 1993a).

Propaganda on the potential benefits of information management technology abounds. In fact, computer salespeople have boxes of flashy brochures that tout the glory of their wares. To hear some vendors tell it, installation of their system in your organization will be like a "second coming"—a magic potion with almost limitless capability to improve your organizational systems. In fact, actual benefits often are considerably less than promised, but are substantial nonetheless. Consider the following litany of success stories:

- St. Alphonsus Medical Center in Georgia has integrated more than a million patient records in three rural hospitals (Herrmann 1999).
- The Western New York Health Sciences Consortium and New York Telephone Company have created a high-speed communication network, or superhighways, to improve data sharing among consortium members, which include seven hospitals, a cancer center, and a medical school. The network has enhanced medical education, research, and patient care. "Compared with our current data-sharing capabilities, it's like expanding a highway from one to eight lanes," boasts the CEO of one member hospital (*Hospitals & Health Networks* 1994).
- The Harvard Community Health Plan has patients in about 150 households who use home computers to receive medical advice and general health information. In use for about seven years, the goals of the system are to improve patient education, raise the quality of healthcare, and lower costs by reducing the number of unnecessary visits to the doctor. Ninety percent of the patients who use the system gave it a high rating for usefulness, and participants' visits to the health center dropped by 5 percent (*Hospitals and Health Networks* 1994).
- Lutheran General Health System of Park Ridge, Illinois, spent $7–8 million to install an "enterprise-wide network" as part of a $19 million project to automate all of its clinical data. This enterprise network links the information systems within the entire system, an approach similar to Samantha's vision at St. Serena's (Gardner 1993b).
- Saint Joseph's Hospital and Medical Center of Paterson, New Jersey, has implemented a $25 million computerized patient-records network. This network of 500 personal computers within the hospital and affiliated outpatient centers allows doctors to call up a patient's name to check on everything from the latest lab test results to a running tally of charges. Administrators are able to calculate the exact cost of every variable of cardiac care or any other procedure. Nurses are able to direct lab orders directly to the lab. Everyone, from the cleaners in maintenance to the dietitians in food service, has online access for their departments (*The New York Times* 1994).
- Lakeland Regional Medical Center in Lakeland, Florida, has automated a user-friendly, protocol-based charting

system. By documenting only those times when a care decision departs from the protocol, Lakeland found that charting time dropped dramatically, from 20 to 30 percent of caregivers' time to 6 percent (*Hospitals* 1993).

- Physicians at Boston's Brigham and Women's Hospital can call up a patient's medical history, including a list of previously prescribed medications, by using a computer terminal in the internal medicine clinic. Before the electronic records, physicians would have to locate the patient's medical record from the central files and then search for the necessary information. According to the hospital, the system has made the ambulatory medical record the primary information resource for physicians in the clinics, and has saved money by substantially reducing the need to routinely pull files for the clinics from the medical records department (Bergman 1993). Sound like something St. Serena's would like?
- A family practice clinic in Port Angeles, Washington, has increased revenues 7 percent through an electronic medical record system that has freed staff for direct patient care and facilitated Medicare reporting requirements (Maxwell 1999).

The preceding examples are just a few of the documented benefits from available information technology. In healthcare—as well as in police work, education, transportation, research, and nearly every functional aspect of government and nonprofit organizations and businesses —information technology is providing significant benefits. St. Serena's appears simply to be trying to reap some of the harvest available.

All of these benefits, potential and actual, can be categorized into two: (1) administrative or processing benefits and (2) decision-assisting benefits. Information technology assists in carrying out predetermined operations and it aids decision makers in clarifying and planning because of its enormous capabilities—speed, memory, and storage capacity. The speed facilitates extended calculations and rapid retrieval of stored information, while the memory facilitates the storage and availability of enormous amounts of data.

Healthcare professionals today—like Samantha and Stewart—face the task of harnessing the technology to realize these benefits; it is a prodigious challenge, as Stewart is rapidly learning.

The Problems of Information Technology in Organizations

The most compelling reasons why healthcare professionals must tame information technology are the major problems that have been reported, even sensationalized, with remarkable, if alarming, consistency in the last decades. Indicative of the overall situation is a classic *U.S. News and World Report* (1979) article, "Those Computers Get Temperamental," that reported about computers that swallowed credit cards, delayed commuters and shoppers, raised havoc with bills, and generally disrupted life. "Americans are learning," the article concludes, "that electronic gadgets can be a curse as well as a blessing." Anyone who has tried to correct an erroneous credit card bill, not to mention an automated hospital bill, or to get removed from a mailing list should well appreciate the story. *USA Today* recently reported that "glitches" with information systems cost U.S. companies $100 billion annually (Strauss 1999). And, remember the Y2K bug?

Some healthcare industry reports would be laughable if they were not so alarming. A major survey of hospital information systems by the Meta Group concluded: "Data systems may need some intensive care" (Baldwin 1999). At one Eastern medical center, nurses noticed that electronic patients' records were mysteriously disappearing, and nearly 40 percent of the records were destroyed (*Newsweek* 1988). Is this the kind of report that worries the nurses at St. Serena's? Similarly, hearing some people describe how their drive "crashed" or how they lost everything stored on their computer is not uncommon, as this disquieting report supports: In a newly inaugurated system, the user—an occupational nurse—neglected to back up daily entries on a computer. When the disk on the new computer "crashed," the data could not be salvaged and four months of daily transactions were lost. Moreover, the individual responsible lost her job because the corporate operational quality-assurance criteria mandated frequent software backups (Wolfe 1991). Is this the sort of anecdote that has been discussed in the rehabilitation unit at St. Serena's? Another story reported a person "killed by computer." According to the story, a New Jersey man was informed by Medicare that his medical bills would not be paid because it insisted he had died during a recent hospitalization (*Newsweek Star Ledger* 1988). Are the billing administrators at St. Serena's concerned about this?

Furthermore, the following excerpt from a newspaper article, "Workers Celebrate the Demise of a Balky Computer," exemplifies an attitude toward information technology to which many healthcare managers undoubtedly can relate:

> Ames, Iowa (AP)—When it came time to retire a testy computer, office workers invited guests, dropped it from a cherrypicker and bashed it with sledgehammers. "It was a good feeling," said Cindy Jorgenson, office manager at Professional Property Management. The computer was dropped from 40 feet. Tenants of other buildings managed by the company were invited. Popcorn

and soft drinks were served. "The computer," Jorgenson said, "caused us a lot of grief." Employees first considered hiring a hearse to haul away the old computer, but decided that wasn't enough (*Newark Sunday Star Ledger* 1994).

Some observers note that we, in fact, are being enslaved by technology, rather than harnessing these tools to serve our needs. In a survey that examined the hospital executives' expectations and impressions of how well their current information technology produces the kind of data they need and want, most executives reported they do not receive operational data in a form they can use to make decisions, and, as a result, many rely on personal instincts and experience in their decision making (Johnson 1991). Could this attitude be prevalent at St. Serena's too?

Behind these tales of woe is a stark reality—information technology in healthcare often has proven to be difficult. In particular, fiscal, operational, organizational, psychological, legal, and socio-political problems have emerged as major challenges in this area.

Fiscal

The cost of information technology has often been more than anticipated. Until recently, major investments in hardware have been required; today, with lower hardware prices, the issues are software and personnel costs. The salient problem has been the fiscal return on these investments and the fiscal efficiency with which the computer resource is handled. Reports in the 1990s have crystallized the extent of this problem in healthcare organizations. Research shows that the paradigm shift in healthcare, characterized by changes in financing and delivery, is driving huge increases in spending on information technology (Morrisey 1994). At the same time, the primary concern appears no longer to be information technology's capital cost versus its benefits, as one information systems consultant notes: "It looks like people are spending money because they have no choice . . . people are thinking about spending more money to make themselves more efficient" (Morrisey 1994). The *Wall Street Journal* estimated in 1993 that the total price tag for information technology in healthcare would run into the billions of dollars in the years ahead. Indeed, a Frost and Sullivan study estimates that hospitals will expend $7.1 billion on information systems by 2003 (Greene 1997).

The Crozer-Keystone Health System in Pennsylvania exemplifies this kind of spending. Having installed an $80 million enterprise-wide data system, the CEO of the system revealed that, while it was somewhat difficult to justify to the board of directors such a large capital expenditure, future competitive and cost-containing pressures had forced the company to make such a choice to appear progressive (*The New York Times* 1993). Does this "image" syndrome prompt Samantha's initiative at St. Serena's?

As healthcare institutions continue to invest heavily in technology, however, many run the risk of basing their investment on underestimated costs and overestimated payoffs. As a number of experts assert, there is no guarantee that the investment will pay off, but any institution not making it will not survive in the future U.S. healthcare system (*Wall Street Journal* 1993). Clearly, the fiscal problems are imposing.

Operational

In a 1994 newspaper article "Air Traffic Computer System Still Grounded," a writer for the *Los Angeles Times* described a $5 billion U.S. government state-of-the-art computer system designed to let controllers better handle air traffic in the nation's increasingly crowded skies. The writer reported that the computer project was a disaster—a case of bureaucratic bumbling, corporate failings, repeated delays that have set back the project's completion at least two years, and one of the biggest potential cost-overruns in the U.S. government history: $2 billion and counting (*New Star Ledger* 1994).

This, and other, notorious illustration of an operational problem have become so common that the terms "computer downtime" and "computer error" need little explanation in the modern lexicon. For example, patients are billed incorrectly, or not at all, because of "computer error" or clients become hypertensive while waiting to be issued a medical record number because a computer is "down." Have St. Serena's staff experienced this in past information systems "upgrades"? Does this explain some of their hesitation about Stewart's plan?

Less recognized, but nonetheless common, are two other operational computer problems: data pollution and security breakdowns. While new information technology has given healthcare managers unprecedented opportunity to tap into an organization's raw operational data, it is commonly reported that hospital executives are drowning in data. Take, for example, the case of the University of Chicago Hospitals in 1991. Hospital executives who track trends in patient care had to wade through more than one million computerized records of inpatient stays (Johnson 1991). The sheer volume of information contained in these files is staggering, which made this case a classic example of an organization overwhelmed by "information junk" or literally polluted with data. The information overload syndrome pervades our daily lives.

Anyone with an e-mail address can relate to a story of an employee who returned from vacation to find 1,218 e-mail messages, only seven of which were "actually worth reading." The employee lamented: "I was doomed to spend half my workday just deleting junk" (Leonard 1999).

As healthcare operations have grown in volume and complexity, the extraneous has become common. Information systems that simplify, rather than add to the complexity and confusion, are the exception in healthcare administration, not the rule, as one experienced observer noted: "We still kill too many fleas with elephant hammers" (Kanter 1986). Is something like this being uttered in the halls of St. Serena's?

Accompanying the inundation of data is the issue of security. While modern information systems increase the amount and availability of information, wider access raises concerns about protecting an organization's information resources (Hard 1992). This security concern seems to be reflected in the comments of St. Serena's nurses and legal counsel office. Security problems have become so widespread and serious that a separate chapter of this book—Chapter 6—is devoted to that challenge.

Finally, the ultimate operational problem is the computer that never becomes operational at all. Lurking in the basements of government buildings, hospitals, and clinics are more than a few computers, purchased months or years ago, that have never been uncrated because somehow when they arrived no one knew what to do with them. This occasional occurrence illustrates one fallout from a fairly pervasive operational problem that managers have had—dealing with smooth-talking computer vendors. One might wonder what St. Serena's past experience has been in this regard.

Organizational

Perhaps the greatest problems experienced thus far have been organizational impacts stemming from the introduction of information technology itself. Although changes in organizational structure, such as the establishment of a new department for information systems, were anticipated and recognized, much more unintended and subtle impacts have proven to be the nemesis of many information management projects. Chief among these unanticipated consequences is the underappreciated phenomenon of user resistance to the technology. Inevitably, resistance has emerged as a powerful obstacle to the successful implementation and utilization of technology in healthcare organizations. At St. Serena's, resistance seems to be at the heart of what has unfolded for Stewart, but he is by no means alone.

The effect of resistance is that technically sound information systems do not work. The war of person versus machine has proven to be no contest—the machine may be smart, but a resisting person is clever. Related to the resistance problem are other informal organizational impacts that have tended to disrupt organizational life. Information technology has brought with it shifts in power and changes in informal groups. It has tended to relegate previously important file clerks to less-significant roles, and to raise computer technicians to lofty heights. Antagonism between aloof technicians and intimidated users has been common, while the breakdown of informal organizational networks has disrupted other functions. The organizational impact of information systems in healthcare has been considerable and, more often than not, dysfunctional.

Psychological

Closely connected with organizational difficulties are psychological reactions to information technology. Despite the preponderance of computers in society, widespread computerphobia is still apparent. Larry Rosen, a psychology professor at California State University, who has been studying technophobia for over 10 years, described this fear: "We're talking about a phobia that in its worst form actually causes sweaty palms, heart palpitations and headaches" (*USA Today* 1993).

Such intimidation produces fear and paranoia that, in turn, can contribute to the operational problems of handling vendors and to the organizational difficulties of resistance. How many healthcare managers, doctors, hospital administrators, not to mention clients and patients, harbor a deep-seated uneasiness about the strange devices associated with information technology? And how many of them, consequently, prefer to keep new technology out of their lives? Are some of these technophobes employed at St. Serena's, even in the managerial ranks?

Aggravating these psychological predispositions can be disillusionment and distrust generated by legions of bad experiences with consultants and information systems. Fear and distrust of the technology can be fully exacerbated when the consultants' promises never materialize, when the new software goes down in the middle of a transaction, and when printouts are incorrect. The psychological forces behind these negative attitudes have proven to be powerful obstacles to reaping the potential benefits of information technology in organizations like St. Serena's.

Legal

Two federal legislations, with counterparts in most state and local governments, further complicate the situation of information management in healthcare. Freedom of information, or "sunshine," laws have placed legal responsibilities on organizations to make available to the public information that they hold. On the other hand, privacy laws place legal restrictions on information processing. Healthcare professionals frequently are caught in the middle of these two categories of laws and confront a dilemma. When computers are employed, more data tend to be collected and stored, which means that under sunshine laws, more data must be made available and under privacy laws, more data must be protected. In both cases, "computer error" is considered to be an unacceptable excuse for breaking the law. Providers and payers that operate in more than one state must also comply with a multitude of "often inconsistent laws and regulations that are overly burdensome and costly" (*Hospitals & Health Networks* 1993).

These legal requirements are becoming both more stringent and more applicable. Lawsuits and other legal proceedings under these laws are an increasing burden for healthcare organizations, which is a reality well known to St. Serena's lawyers.

Socio-political

Nearly three decades ago, systems analyst Ida Hoos (1971) issued a caveat about information technology that is as relevant now as it was then: "Insensitivity to the special problems involved, preoccupation with the mechanistic formal model, and ignorance of the stuff and substance of the real-life situation can result . . . in designs for a neatly programmed future fraught with disaster." Her warning points to the social and political implications of the use of information technology, and her incisive words have repeatedly proven to be prescient. In 1992, an article proposed that because of information technology's seductive capability to store and manipulate enormous quantities of data, it would have a tremendous impact on the future economy; hence, technologically savvy users could presumably flourish in the future and were increasingly being looked at as a powerful elite (Brody 1992). While groups such as Computer Professionals for Social Responsibility (CPSR) continue to anticipate that technology will bring much good, they are concerned about technical experts exercising too much control over organizational processes, which could result in insensitivity to human values. Undoubtedly some of this same concern is shared by staff at St. Serena's.

Implications for Healthcare Professionals

Although it may seem remarkable, and ironic, that nearly all of the problems organizations have experienced with information technology are not technical in nature, it is the case. The basis of the problems encountered while seeking the benefits of information systems is managerial—unenlightened use and management of the technology. Clearly, many chief executives of healthcare organizations are less than pleased with their investment in an upgraded information system. The fundamental problem, however, may be that information technology often has been viewed as the answer, rather than as one part of an approach, to problem solving (Ryckman 1991). For practical purposes, the technology is nearly flawless; management and use of that technology, however, are underdeveloped. Even "downtime," which appears to be a technical problem, usually is caused by a user–managerial failure of control over the system. The challenge vis-a-vis computers, therefore, is a user–managerial challenge, and it is considerable, as Roger Spoelman, CEO of Muskegon (Michigan) General Hospital, observed: "Executives should manage their hospital's information as carefully as they oversee its financial results" (Johnson 1991). But what, precisely, is involved in "managing" information? Does Stewart at St. Serena's have a good grasp of this concept, or is his sense of managing information a bit myopic?

Harvard professor Regina Herzlinger (1977) puts Spoelman's sentiment a bit more soberly: "The one factor accounting for most failures of information systems lies directly within the control of the organization: the characteristics and attitudes of top management." Heard unfailingly among academics and practitioners alike is this refrain: Enlightened managerial perspective is vital to effective information management (Boxerman and Gribbins 1990). Similarly, a former graduate student of mine, who now manages a healthcare agency, put the point poetically:

> *Dear Boss:*
> *The Computer is a wondrous thing*
> *A million benefits it can bring.*
> *It can store our files*
> *Eliminate our paper piles*
> *Save hours of calculation*
> *And enable data manipulation.*
> *But if we don't manage this thing*
> *A million headaches, it can bring.*
> *We'll need a well planned approach*

And ensure that our managers we coach.
We'll need a user's point of view
And, boss, the whole thing depends on you.
—Julie Freestone

The key to managing "the whole thing" is prescribed in Thomas Carlyle's often-quoted aphorism: "When a person kens, that person can." Understanding and appreciating information technology and its ramifications and developing managerial perspectives attuned to the realities of information today are needed to enable information systems to facilitate healthcare and societal benefits.

References

Appleby, C. 1999. "Net Gain or Net Loss: Health Care Consumers Become Internet Savvy." *Trustee* 52 (2): 20–3.

Baldwin, G. 1999. "Data Systems May Need Some Intensive Care." *American Medical News* 42 (12): 27.

Bell, R. 1998. "Assessing the Connection Between Information Systems and Hospital Success." *Hospital Topics* 75 (4): 17.

Bergman, R. 1993. "Electronic Medical Records Make Life Simpler for Clinic Physicians." *Hospitals and Health Networks* (July 20): 60.

Boxerman, S., and R. Gribbins. 1990. "Technology Management in the 1990s." *Healthcare Executive* (Jan/Feb): 21–3.

Brody, H. 1992. "Of Bytes and Rights." *Technology Review* (November–December): 23–9.

Cabot, L. 2000. "Tiny Computer Helps Docs Access Approved Drugs." *Business Journal of Portland* 16 (49): 29.

"Corporate Alliance." 1994. *Hospitals & Health Networks* (20 March): 28.

"Computers Are Everywhere." 1994. *USA Today* (24 May): 2D.

"Computers in the Hospital." 1994. *The New York Times* (8 April) 9: B-1.

"Computer Phobia." 1993. *USA Today* (3 August): 2B.

Galewitz, P. 2000. "Take Two Aspirin and E-mail in the Morning." *The Times* (5 May): D4.

Gardner, E. 1993a. "Automating and Standardizing Claims Processing." *Modern Healthcare* (May 17): 42.

———. 1993b. "Hospital on Road to Data Highways." *Modern Healthcare* (June 7): 32.

Goleman, D. 1988. "Why Managers Resist Machines." *The New York Times* (7 February): B-1.

Greene, J. 1997. "Technology." *Hospitals & Health Networks* 71 (19): 27.

Hard, R. 1992. "Keeping Patient Data Secure Within Hospitals." *Hospitals* (October 20): 50.

"Health Care Technology." 1992. *Wall Street Journal* (8 October): B-9.

Herrmann, S. 1999. "Solution Deployed at St. Alphonsus." *PR Newswire* (November 18).

Herzlinger, R. 1977. "Why Data Systems in Nonprofit Organizations Fail." *Harvard Business Review* (January–February): 83.

Hoos, I. 1971. "Information Systems and Public Planning." *Management Science* (June): B-671.

Johnson, J. 1991. "Information Overload: CEOs Seek New Tools for Effective Decisionmaking." *Hospitals* (October 20): 24.

Joint Commission on Accreditation of Healthcare Organizations. 1993. *Accreditation Manual for Hospitals.* Chicago: JCAHO.

Kanter, J. 1986. "The Role of Senior Management in MIS." *Journal of Systems Management* (April): 37–45.

Kennedy, G. 1990. "Info Systems Head Toward Central Decisionmaking." *Modern Healthcare* (July 9): 32.

Kleinke, J. 1998. "Release 0.0: Clinical Information Technology in the Real World." *Health Affairs* 17 (6): 23–38.

Leonard, A. 1999. "We've Got Mail—Always." *Newsweek* (September 20): 58.

Maxwell, M. 1999. "EMR: Successful Productivity Tool for Modern Practice." *Health Management Technology* 20(9): 48–9.

Morrisey, J. 1994. "Spending More on Computers to Help Keep Costs in Line." *Modern Healthcare* (February 14): 63–70.

Newark Star Ledger. 1988. (10 July): 26.

Newark Star Ledger. 1994. (1 May): Sections 8–10.

Newark Sunday Star Ledger. 1994. (27 March): 31.

The New York Times. 1993. (2 May): 8.

"Pioneering Protocols: Hospitals Test Computer Use in Patient Care Decisions." 1993. *Hospitals* (May 5): 18.

Ryckman, D. 1991. "Information Technology Is Not Enough." *Healthcare Executive* (May–June): 39.

Sandrick, K. 1999. "Information Management Systems." *Health Management Technology* 20 (2): 10–11.

———. 1998. "Beyond the RxD2." *Health Management Technology* 19 (12): 26–32.

Stefl, M. 1999. "Editorial." *Frontiers of Health Services Management* 15 (3): 1.

Strauss, G. 1999. "When Computers Fail." *USA Today* (December 7): A-1.

"Technology Alarm." 1988. *Newsweek* (1 February).

"The Dawn of E-Life." 1999. *Newsweek* (September 20): 38.

"Those Computers Get Temperamental!" 1979. *U.S.News and World Report* (20 August): 54.

"Washington Outlook." 1993. *Hospitals & Health Networks* (20 November): 14.

Wolfe, K. 1991. "Getting a Grip on Computerphobia." *American Association of Occupational Health Nurses Journal* (July): 352.

Yennie, H. 1999. "The Technology Costs of Accreditation." *Behavioral Health Management* 19 (4): 8–11.

READINGS

Erick Schonfeld's *Fortune Magazine* article provides a perspective on the tremendous potential of information technology in improving information management and service delivery in healthcare organizations. The article also reveals the enormous investment being made in technology, which suggests, perhaps, an overemphasis on technology and an underemphasis on the management of that technology and the information it is designed to produce.

Steve Heimoff is attuned to this managerial concern, which is evident in his article in the *Healthcare Forum Journal.* While observing the tremendous promise of information technology in healthcare, Heimoff soberly suggests the dimensions of the managerial task involved in harnessing the promise toward better healthcare. Do you think Stewart read the Schonfeld article but missed Heimoff's message? What points in these articles would you most recommend to St. Serena's executives?

Can Computers Cure Health Care?

Erick Schonfeld

Experts still debate whether computers really save time and money. But Dr. Neal Kaforey, emergency room chief at a Kaiser Permanente clinic in Cleveland, says there's no doubt they can save lives. As proof he nods toward a smiling patient sitting up in bed. The man was wheeled in yesterday with a heart attack. One of Kaforey's colleagues was about to give him a heart drug called a beta blocker, but first the doctor checked the man's medical records on a computer terminal in the ER. It revealed he was severely allergic to the drug. If that tidbit had been tucked away in a paper file at a doctor's office instead of instantly popping up on the screen, says Kaforey, "he'd be dead."

For most of us, such seamless delivery of vital statistics isn't an option. Our medical data are buried in bulky paper files that typically require hours or days to be passed from one doctor to another. That contributes to countless hassles, wasted hours, and errors. "Nearly a third of things we do to patients are not needed," says Robert Brook, a health professor at the University of California at Los Angeles. "And a third of things they need they don't get."

Reprinted by permission from Fortune *137:6 (March 30, 1998): 111–6. © 1998 Time Inc. All Rights Reserved. Erick Schonfeld is a staff writer for* Fortune *Magazine.*

Few HMOs have focused heavily on quality issues. "Managed care is a fiction," maintains Dr. Earl Steinberg, a healthcare–quality consultant with Covance, a clinical–research company. "We don't have managed care. We have managed price."

But revolutionary change is afoot. HMOs now cover some 67 million Americans, and their competition for patients is growing ever fiercer. In saturated markets, offering low–cost care is no longer enough to give an HMO an edge—it must also distinguish itself as a provider of high–quality care. That in turn is contributing to major investments in the computerization of medical records—the new systems are essential both to help HMOs provide better care and to compile data to prove it. Hambrecht & Quist analyst Stephen Fitzgibbons estimates that the health–care industry spent $15 billion on information technology last year. By 2001 he expects such spending to nearly double. "The lion's share of that today is in administrative and financial systems, but the clinical area is the fastest–growing," Fitzgibbons says.

Kaiser, the country's largest HMO, is one of the trend's leaders. Over the next five years the not-for-profit organization plans to pour about $1 billion into a national clinical–information system. Kaiser wants to electronically link its 10,000 doctors, as well as nurses and other care providers, in 19 states. It eventually will keep medical records for all nine million of its members in a standard digital format. CEO David Lawrence considers the pioneering computer system to be Kaiser's key national priority: "It will be the central nervous system for bringing together all the elements, needed to take care of patients, and it will do so in ways currently unimaginable."

He'd better hope so. Last year Kaiser lost a staggering $270 million, on revenues of $14.5 billion. Like other HMOs, Kaiser was caught with medical costs that rose much faster than its premiums.

Of course, deploying vast computer systems is risky, as shown by the recent financial meltdown at Oxford Health Plans after a new billing system ran amuck. But many HMOs may soon have little choice. Some of their biggest customers, including General Motors and Xerox, already are ranking health plans by cost and quality, and giving employees financial incentive to choose the best. Within a few years HMOs that can't offer the advantages of systems like Kaiser's will find it more difficult to win favorable rankings. A computer that reminds doctors to prescribe aspirin for cardiac patients, for instance, could avert heart attacks, keeping patients healthier and warding off costly emergencies. Says Bruce Bradley, GM's director of health benefits: "Improved care gives us the best cost at the end of day."

Kaiser hopes to roll out basic elements of its new system to all its regions by 2001. About half of its 13 regional centers already have tinkered with such systems—the ones in Cleveland and Portland, Ore., in particular, provide glimpses of how the national version is likely to work.

Cleveland's project is overseen by Dr. Allan Khoury, a practicing physician who enthuses about his computer system as if it were a breakthrough medical study. When he started cobbling it together in 1991, he faced two main problems: First, he had to link all the pieces of clinical information about patients—laboratory X–ray, pharmacy, and physician dictation data—that were stored in mainframe computers throughout Ohio. Then he had to electronically capture information generated in doctors' offices, which traditionally was recorded only on paper.

The latter problem proved the thorniest. A patient's medical "chart" typically consists of fat folders of paper inscribed with doctors' hieroglyphic scrawls, including notes on everything from vital signs to currently prescribed drugs. Khoury encountered resistance by doctors, who didn't want to take on the data–entry chores needed to maintain charts in digital form. Many doctors also feared that if they were fiddling with computers while interacting with patients, they would wind up paying more attention to the machines than to their sick charges.

So Khoury settled on a compromise: He got rid of paper charts but not of paper. When a patient comes in for a visit, the system automatically prints out a packet summarizing traditional chart information. The doctor writes notes, as usual, on the paper and also checks off items on a computer–readable list to show which procedures were performed—the options include things like common immunizations. After the patient leaves, digital images of his updated paper records are stored in a database. Ironically, notes Khoury, "the paper intermediary has been the key to breaking down physician resistance."

Khoury's system has had clear benefits for patients, partly by helping ensure they don't fall between the cracks. For instance, it asks doctors to rank the risk that each diabetes patient faces of having a leg amputated. Those at elevated risk are automatically referred to Kaiser's podiatry department, where a nurse teaches them how to take care of their feet. Diabetic amputations among Kaiser patients in Cleveland have dropped by about 20%.

Khoury's counterpart in Kaiser's Portland operation, Dr. Homer Chin, says that giving doctors a "total picture of the patient" from all of the HMO's departments is a key to improving the quality of care. Dr. Steve Gordon, an internist at a Kaiser clinic in Portland, says he got hooked on Portland's computer system for just that reason: it lets him get instant updates of everything going on with his patients. "We don't have to wing it anymore," he says. The system also fosters more cooperation among doctors caring for the same patient.

Kaiser's Portland system, like the one in Cleveland, reminds doctors when their patients are due for, say, mammograms. And it helps prevent emergencies. Care manager Denise McKnight, for example, follows up with all Kaiser members whom the system identifies as having recently been released from a local hospital emergency room—a job she describes as "making sure patients don't get lost in the shuffle." On the day after Christmas last year, she phoned an 87–year–old woman at home who was just out of the hospital after a spine injury. McKnight learned that the woman was unable to take her medications properly or look after herself—and that the only person available to help was her sick 92–year–old sister. By the end of the day, McKnight got the woman admitted to a short–term nursing facility.

Such cases have helped win over the approximately 700 doctors who use the system. Barbe West, Chin's boss, says early surveys showed that many of the doctors didn't like it at first, "but now they wouldn't know what to do without it." The effort to change their minds, she adds, required a lot of handholding, as well as getting the doctors heavily involved in refining the system. It doesn't rely on paper as the Cleveland system does—the Portland physicians actually use keyboards and computerized menus. A physician–friendly format enables doctors to quickly enter diagnoses into a database, then type in more detailed notes. Alternatively, doctors can dictate notes that are later transcribed by outside data clerks.

Terminals are usually placed in offices rather than exam rooms, partly because of confidentiality concerns—bored patients waiting by themselves can get nosy. Some of the Portland doctors also have started a pilot program with wireless laptops, which give them access to the system wherever they are in their clinics.

Doctors use the system to help with several chores besides entering and monitoring patient data. To bone up on recent research, they tap into Medline, a massive federal database of medical–journal abstracts available through the Internet. Soon they'll be able to search the entire contents of 28 medical textbooks on subjects ranging from obstetrics and pediatrics to psychiatric disorders. They also can order lab tests, referrals, or medications directly from their keyboards. After appointments with their doctors, patients receive printouts with written instructions detailing the tests or drugs they need. Gordon says some patients have collected their after–visit summaries in binders at home–do–it–yourself medical charts.

The system helps keep doctors mindful of cost–effective treatment guidelines as they make decisions. When a physician enters a prescription for the antidepressant drug Zoloft, a note pops up on his screen informing him that the drug is twice as expensive as similar medicines. He can still prescribe Zoloft, but the number of new prescriptions of it has been halved.

Patients like the system because it saves time. For example, they can send requests for prescription refills to their doctors over the phone or the Internet. Their doctors can then enter the refills into Kaiser's computer system, which automatically conveys the information to the HMO's pharmacy. The drugs are mailed to patients' doorsteps within two working days.

For its national system, Kaiser is combining features from a half dozen or so of the regional ones. "Kaiser nationally wants it all," says Khoury. The rollout is scheduled to begin in October in California, Georgia, and Hawaii. On top of its $1 billion price tag, Kaiser expects to spend more than $500 million to maintain and upgrade the existing regional systems.

With nine million covered lives, Kaiser arguably has the largest repository of patient information in the country, To hold all the data, it will employ two large state–of–the–art data centers. Kaiser also opened a multimillion–dollar Care Management Institute at its Oakland headquarters last year to devise its national treatment guidelines and to coordinate quality–improvement efforts. The clinical information system will help the institute spot and reduce variations in Kaiser's practice patterns and quality of care.

Kaiser recently has come under fire in at least one region for allegedly giving patients substandard care. Lawsuits in Texas charged, among other things, that the HMO denied patients tests that they needed and access to specialists. The company has settled the suits for several million dollars. CEO Lawrence says the problems in Texas have been fixed and represented minor episodes that aren't representative of Kaiser's national pattern of care. The new computer system might be able to prevent such cases in the future by alerting Kaiser to questionable practices.

Kaiser's project is being closely watched in the industry and should help spark medicine's overdue digital revolution. But many smaller HMOs may have trouble keeping pace. Besides its national reach and deep pockets, Kaiser exclusively controls nearly all of its doctors, hospitals, pharmacies, and labs. Thus, it can impose standards across its network of providers—a prerequisite to computerizing medical records. And since all Kaiser's data will be held under a single corporate umbrella, the HMO's project isn't likely to be derailed by one of the main obstacles facing broader efforts to digitize medical records: worries about keeping the information confidential when it exists on electronic networks that link disparate caregivers.

The idea of personal medical information coursing around freely gives most people the creeps. (Imagine if you were denied a job or health insurance because of a past medical condition.) Security concerns are a big reason why the medical world hasn't adopted standards needed to pave the way for the kind of computerization found in most other industries—for instance, there's no widely accepted format for patient identification numbers. To prevent electronic data leaks, Kaiser uses passwords, encryption, and sophisticated audit trails. Employees who breach security, even casually, are fired. Any data used for research or released to outsiders are aggregated and stripped of personal identifiers.

Kaiser's effort could show that the security and other problems that have hindered healthcare computerization are not insoluble. It also could spur investing by other HMOs in competing solutions.

Already, an employer–led consortium called the National Committee for Quality Assurance (NCQA) has devised a barebones set of quality standards that are used to gather statistics for annual assessments of health plans. The standards covet aspects of care such as immunization rates, breast–cancer screenings, and eye exams for diabetics. "An HMO cannot compete" without reporting how it measures up to the standards, says health consultant Steinberg. Most of the information can be derived from existing claims data but the NCQA is expected to add net measures that will be easier to collect for those with electronic medical records.

The NCQA also offers accreditation to health plans. Companies such as GM and Xerox require all their health plans to see the NCQA's seal of approval. GM's ranking of its HMOs for employees is partly based on NCQA accreditation status and on how the health providers perform based on the consortium's quality standards. The plans that rank highest overall are the cheapest for employees to enroll in.

Some other HMOs, such as United HealthCare in Minneapolis, have started their own limited quality-improvement programs based on NCQA standards. Lee Newcomer, United HealthCare's medical director, declares: If I had an electronic medical record, I would start paying physicians based on their performance." Hey docs, welcome to the millennium.

The Irrepressible Computer: The Brave New World of Healthcare Information Technology

Steve Heimoff

Back in 1968, a group of experts got together at Harvard for one of those crystal-gazing sessions where they try to predict the future of their respective disciplines. They cast their gaze at the year 2018, then 50 years distant.

One of the experts was Charles R. DeCarlo, then director of automation research at IBM, who presented a paper on the future of computer technology. At that time, of course, the mainframe still was king (and so, for that matter, was IBM); the invention of the personal computer was more than a decade away, and no one had dreamed of anything as astonishing as the Internet.

Still, viewed retrospectively, DeCarlo's prescience was uncanny. He correctly anticipated that the volume of information able to be stored in computers and made available "to the mind and senses" would "be increased beyond our present imagination." He predicted that room-sized mainframes would be replaced by "small portable storage units" that would permit people to have, for their "individual ownership and use, specific kinds of competencies and experience." And he foresaw the development of better input devices into computers, what he called "stylized writing," that would obviate the need for specialized training.

Finally, in a moment of great clarity, DeCarlo apprehended that "the flood of information generated will force the development of new ways of organizing human knowledge and experience," an epistemological revolution that would literally change how people think and remember.

For all the accuracy of DeCarlo's prognostications, there was one thing he missed. Surveying the human endeavors likely to be impacted by the computer, DeCarlo named office work, government, industry, finance and education. The world of healthcare, of medicine and hospitals and doctors and nurses and patients, even in DeCarlo's fervent imagination, remained computer-free, seemingly locked forever into a Rockwellian *gemutlichkeit* worthy of a *Look* magazine cover.

Today, of course, all that is changing, fast. In retrospect, it's hard to understand why so few saw the computer coming to clinical care. With it, volumes of information; small, portable devices; easy input;

Reprinted by permission from Healthcare Forum Journal *41:1 (January/February 1998): 14–9. Steve Heimoff is a freelance journalist.*

new ways of organizing knowledge, the computer seems tailor–made for what healthcare information technology experts call its "killer app": replacing the paper medical record.

An Advance Outpost

And indeed, whether or not previous generations saw it coming, suddenly, beginning in major medical centers and spreading out and down, information technology is being applied with stunning results. And the best way to appreciate this dramatic change is to visit an advance outpost of the revolution, in which the future can be glimpsed literally in every hallway.

These days, when nurses at the 320-bed John Muir Medical Center (JMMC), in the suburban community of Walnut Creek, just outside San Francisco, want to enter information onto a patient's chart, they no longer have to make their way to the nurses station and write it down on pages stuffed into a clipboard. Instead, they turn to one of 350 wireless personal computers, portable chalkboard–like devices they call "slates," located on wheeled stands scattered throughout the hospital's corridors.

Punching their user ID and password into the 8–pound slates, the nurses—in a glorious example of DeCarlo's "stylized writing"—update the record with a point–and–click stylus, utilizing templates, or menus of options, for predesigned notes. The information is electronically beamed to overhead sensors, which capture and send it to the hospital's mainframe, where it's available to anyone who's authorized to see it, virtually instantly.

DeCarlo would have been delighted with this brave new world, and particularly by the electronic health records that Kris Andresen, R.N., JMMC's clinical projects coordinator and self–described "visionary," calls "the biggest change that has ever happened to nurses and clinicians."

To be sure, electronic records are a giant step toward the paperless organization, with all the advantages that confers. But, Andresen adds pointedly, "computerization is a strategic decision. In order to provide quality care in the future, you have to know what's going on with your patient."

Which can be a challenge. "The average nurse collects 106,000 data points in an eight–hour period on a single patient," explains Roy Simpson, R.N., a specialist in nursing informatics at HBO & Co. (HBOC), an Atlanta–based company that's one of the nation's leading developers of healthcare information technology software. Pulse, glucose, bowel patterns, respiration, temperature, gastrointestinal activity, blood pressure, hematology, renal–urinary function—the data elements pile up, and keeping track of them, much less interpreting them intelligently when they are crammed onto paper, sometimes illegibly, "simply will not work in the future," Andresen declares.

To demonstrate the point, her colleague, Carol Melvin, R.N., support and services coordinator, opens up a patient's electronic record. Pointing out that the screen is capable of displaying data in almost countless ways, Melvin chooses one that, from the point of view of a harried clinician, is of particular interest: Displayed is a week's worth of temperature and blood pressure readings, in graphic form that allows the observer to spot tell–tale trends and patterns. "I could determine that from the paper chart, but then I'd be flipping pages and not being with my patient," Melvin says. The computer frees her from the old physical constraints, or, as Simpson puts it, "lets you evade space and time."

That the JMMC team and Simpson are on the same wavelength is no coincidence; the software that guides JMMC's computers was created by HBOC, and Andresen frequently attends company workshops in Atlanta and Dallas where she learns the skills she then relays to JMMC's nurses and doctors. It hasn't been easy, as she's the first to admit. Anytime there's change of this magnitude, there's resistance" by "orientees" (the somewhat Orwellian term information technology experts use to refer to the rest of us).

But the struggle is not without its rewards. "It's not uncommon for us to see one physician teaching another a trick he's learned," reports Andresen.

How to "Populate the Repository"

JMMC still is in the early stages of its computer revolution. A truer information technology pioneer has been Moses Cone Health System, a nonprofit integrated delivery network based in Greensboro N.C., that began building what Vice President and CIO Michael Lopez calls its centralized "clinical repository" of electronic health records back in 1993 and immediately confronted problems.

It was easy enough, Lopez recalls, to develop a strategic plan that included the idea of a centralized clinical repository, but the reality of transferring all of Moses Cone's existing data into it—how to "populate the repository," in information technology jargon—proved, at first, to be daunting.

The trouble was that each of the hospital's departments—pharmacy, radiology, admissions and so on—had over the years developed its own computerized systems that couldn't communicate with each other. Not only were such "legacy systems" incompatible and archaic, there was also the likelihood they wouldn't be able to interface with the software, created by Sunquest Data Systems of Tucson, Ariz., that formed the brains of Moses Cone's new repository, thus condemning years of data to a kind of cyber–purgatory. The potential result of such a fiasco, says Lopez, would be that, "You'd have a fancy repository and nothing to put in it." The solution was to come up with a computer language that all of Moses Cone's technology, both old and new, could embrace. Efforts at constructing such languages, which are a kind of Esperanto for different computer platforms and software, have been gathering steam since the 1960s and 1970s, although they were concentrated in industries other than healthcare, like banking and government. (The languages and protocols that enable computer users to connect with and browse the Internet and World Wide Web, regardless of what kind of Systems they log on with, are examples of such universal languages.)

The dilemma in applying technology in healthcare is that clinical care requires such exquisitely precise terms and definitions that only healthcare professionals themselves could develop such languages. And until recently, because there was no demand for computerization within the industry, no one stepped forward to develop them.

That began to change in the late 1980s, when healthcare researchers, mainly in academic institutions, began tackling the situation, and to-day there are new languages, as well as associations that oversee their continued development, whose costs are underwritten by dues–paying members such as hospital systems, health insurers and pharmaceutical companies. These new languages and standards allow for the intelligent exchange of clinical and other data among different legacy systems, and they are what enabled Moses Cone to solve its problem.

Once Lopez and his team decided on the specific language to employ, they instructed Sunquest to use it. That meant Sunquest's software designers had to develop something from scratch—an initial difficulty that turned into a later advantage, as it turned out, because the system was customized to meet Moses Cone's precise needs, which off–the–shelf "plug and play" software would not have been able to do.

True; this meant Moses Cone served to some extent as Sunquest's "alpha and beta site," as Lopez puts it, and the resulting reaction from Moses Cone's physicians and nurses was "Missourian," as in: "Show me."

That's hardly surprising: Doctors and nurses, says Lopez, "require a great amount of documented objective evidence as to when something is significant and when it's not." But they soon recognized the project's significance, Lopez says, and, "Now, when we send information across our network, we all know what it means."

The Next Step: Automated Clinical Decisions

Once a system like Moses Cone or JMMC creates a centralized clinical repository for its electronic records, it can take the next step, one that seems almost to come from the pages of a sci–fi thriller, but which is actually a logical extension of the computer's ability to assemble huge databases and then crunch their numbers, in the course of which mere data becomes useful information. In healthcare information technology, this means real medical decisions can be "made" by computers and then ratified by providers.

Explains Michael Knepper, a healthcare information systems analyst at the San Francisco investment firm of Volpe Welty & Co., "Once you have all this data centralized, you can use value-added tools, such as decision support, to provide caregivers with the information they need to make decisions."

At JMMC, they're taking this step with the help of another HBOC software product, which uses preprogrammed protocols to make automated clinical decisions. In such decision–support systems, the software will continuously scan all of JMMC's electronic records, automatically tracking trends and intervening when appropriate. For instance, by utilizing so–called "push technology," it will alert physicians to potentially life–threatening variances in a patient's status that might otherwise be obscured in the avalanche of data.

"This is not automated diagnosis," JMMC's Andresen emphasizes, anticipating fears that computers could undermine the doctor–patient (or nurse–patient) relationship. But it is an early and exceedingly powerful example of how the "flood of information" DeCarlo predicted computers would capture and analyze can bring about "new ways of organizing human knowledge."

"Decision support is really the biggest driver that makes this whole thing worth doing," says Lance Lang, M.D. He's a vice president of The Permanente Co., responsible for designing and implementing a National Clinical Information System for all of Kaiser Permanente. As such, his task, spread over 16 states and the District of Columbia, and involving more than 9,300 physicians and 8.5 million insured patients, is more daunting than Andresen's at JMMC. Instead of creating an Intranet—linking together different departments within a single system, like JMMC—he's got to link together multiple Intranets into a national Extranet. But in terms of the theoretical underpinnings, Lang and Andresen are doing the same thing.

For Lang, decision support occurs when healthcare information technology approaches what he calls "automated intelligence" (although he, like Andresen, is careful to stress he's not talking about cookbook medicine). Lang gives an everyday example in which push technology becomes highly useful. "Say someone comes in with a sore throat, and the physician does a strep culture. But in busy office practice, physicians don't follow up on 10 percent of the positives; they're just not treated. That's been shown in Harvard studies. Now, if all this is in the computer, there's a rule programmed that says if a strep culture comes back positive, the computer checks to see if the doctor has treated it. It will actually check with Kaiser's pharmacy on a national database. If the computer sees no prescription has been written, it will automatically alert the physician, so we can ensure that nothing falls between the cocks."

Once Kaiser has its national "registry" in place, a process Lang expects to take at least three years, the practice of evidence–based medicine" will save both money and lives and vastly improve the quality of healthcare, especially for the chronically ill, who will be tracked more carefully over time. Lang concedes that reaching this idealized state will require enormous investment, and that it won't come about without confusion, disruption and human resistance. But "if a physician can ensure that all patients get exactly the care he or she intends for them to get, it will revolutionize healthcare," Lang says.

Facing the Obstacles

Suppose that day comes, and a Kaiser patient from Rhode Island, vacationing in California, winds up, perhaps unconscious, in a Kaiser facility in Los Angeles. It will be an easy matter for the Kaiser physician in Los Angeles to access that patient's medical records at the Kaiser facility in Rhode Island. (Actually, the records would exist in cyberspace, but that's another story.)

But what happens to that same patient if he or she winds up in, say John Muir Medical Center's emergency room in Walnut Creek? To put it another way, will Kaiser's computers and software (which is being developed by Oracle Corp.) be able to communicate with JMMC's computers and the HBOC software that runs them?

The answer, for the immediate future, is no, for three reasons. First, healthcare information technology has reached its technological limits— in fact, by definition, information technology is always at the limits of its development—and currently there are no easy "turnkey solutions" to the challenge of different systems communicating with each other. (Think how hard it is to translate a word processing document from a Macintosh system to a PC system.)

Also, hospitals and health systems, their mind–set still geared to a competitive era in which companies zealously guarded proprietary information from falling into enemy hands, have so far resisted sharing data with each other.

Finally, setting up and then maintaining and upgrading extranets (or even larger community health information networks, or CHINs, which for years has been the dream of public health officials) takes money. Someone has to pay for developing and maintaining the infrastructure, and so far no one has rushed forward to volunteer.

Nonetheless, with each passing day it becomes clearer that all these obstacles are capable of being overcome. Marketplace forces, known collectively as managed care, are changing the personality of healthcare and will continue to do so. The resulting integrated delivery systems and networks make the sharing of data not only logistically possible but necessary, as former competitors become collaborators. Hospitals, medical groups and IPAs, health plans and other insurers, pharmaceutical companies and other entities, all responsible for different aspects along the continuum of care, will share data whether they want to or not.

As for technological limits, if the computer industry (including software development) has any guiding spirit at all, it lies in the attitude that, if a thing can be imagined, it can be done. But the biggest development in allowing for the creation of Extranets or other CHIN–like structures may turn out to be that 1990s phenomenon, the Internet, which, it must be admitted, caught the healthcare information technology crowd completely off guard.

Internet to the Rescue

The Internet, whose universal language and protocols (like HTML and TCP/IP) are understandable and accessible by all computers, has enabled, for the first time, low–cost (or no–cost) interfacing among all computers—it has, to other words, created the possibility of developing something that looks like a CHIN, sounds like a CHIN and walks like a CHIN. Moreover, no one has to maintain or pay for this CHIN–like structure. And that, in the opinion of some experts, has changed the nature of the game.

Richard F. Gibson, M.D., is medical director of information services at Portland, Ore.'s Providence Health System, where he's in charge of developing Providence's own electronic health record repository. He expresses an increasingly popular viewpoint: "Instead of having a CHIN where you dump all the data into one giant database and then have everyone in the community—doctors, nurses, clinics, from all competing systems—look it up in one place (with all the problems that implies), the easier way is for every hospital to maintain its own database and provide a Web–enabled browser, like Microsoft Explorer or Netscape." That way, providers can access the Internet, and network with whatever other systems are online in cyberspace.

It's an elegant concept whose implications are just now being worked out, but futurists say it can and will happen. Deborah Kohn, principal of Dak Systems Consulting, a San Mateo, Calif. healthcare technology consulting firm, even goes so far as to call the World Wide Web—and not the electronic health record—the "killer app" of health-care information technology. It is the Web, that subset of the Internet characterized by graphic images and sound, that, Kohn maintains, "is allowing the Internet to become the CHIN everyone is waiting for." One way to think of the Internet, Kohn points out, is as a vast Externet of the kind Lang has been constructing for Kaiser Permanente, but potentially involving everybody on Earth. If proper "firewalls" are built to prevent unauthorized access (a big "if" and one that's outside the scope of this article), it's the way to go.

Kohn, as a futurist, is willing to venture where few information technology experts (who often are overly focused on the here and now) dare to go: Decades out in time, where she envisions scenarios that make mere electronic records seem modest by comparison. Complete, up–to–the–minute patient records will be available to anyone who needs them, instantly, around the globe. Should the patient be wheeled into the emergency room, unconscious and without identification, he or she will be identifiable through biometric means: retinal scans, fingerprints, hand geometry, facial image recognition and other unique identifiers. Immediately following ID, medical records will gush forth, whether originally housed in California or Calcutta.

Push technology of the most advanced kind will become routine, she predicts, with caregivers receiving alerts whenever patient health and safety are compromised. Clinical pathways and protocols, which change daily, will likewise be quickly relayed to those who need them. "I believe," Kohn declares with the fervor of a true believer, "that all this is doable."

Unfolding in Bits and Pieces

How might it all come about? For starters, the National Committee on Quality Assurance has recently theorized how a national link–up of electronic health records might occur. They describe a seven–stage process:

1. Standardize the set of data elements collected by all health plans and providers.
2. Link all systems.
3. Standardize the way medical information is defined and coded.
4. Screen and monitor all data constantly.
5. Build protocols that ensure confidentiality and security of patient records.
6. Fully automate patient record keeping.
7. Share data completely among health plans, providers and public agencies in support of performance measurement and improvement.

This is probably a fairly accurate description of the way events will develop. Obviously, the process will occur in bits and pieces, rather than unfold in a smooth way, and partial solutions will erupt from different quarters. For example, on the question of coding medical information, the notorious problem of different systems identifying patients in different ways is already being tracked by the U.S. Department of Health and Human Services, which is developing a unique health identifier (based on the Social Security number) for use by patients, providers, health plans and employers everywhere.

Another piece will fall into place through the simple and irrepressible process of simplifying software and making its inner workings opaque from the point of view of the end–user. Television became universal when turning a set on and off and changing channels, became so easy, "a child could do it."

Information technology software, even in its most sophisticated forms, can still be cumbersome to use: The nurse has to log on, download, search and, more often than anyone would choose, put up with the inevitable iconic hourglass or clock while the computer churns away. Complaints about the laboriousness of the process are common. Still, as technology gets more and more accessible, the complaints should wither away and die.

We are only at the dawn of the healthcare information technology revolution; a degree of grumbling, of stumbling and losing the way, is only to be expected. But the year cannot be far off when a new generation of physicians and nurses finds the one–time existence of and reliance upon paper records as amusingly anachronistic as we today view the medieval physician's casting out of demons.

Four hundred and fifty years ago, the historian Daniel Boorstin tells us, scientists had little use for the newly invented occhialino that evolved to become the microscope. Most distrusted it as a mere conjurer's device that produced optical illusions. It was not until a century later, when Robert Hooke published his groundbreaking "Micrographia," that (in Boorstin's words) "The microscope opened [to scientists] dark continents never before entered and in many ways easy to explore." Among those dark continents have been the germ theory of disease, and an understanding of the structure of matter.

Boorstin likened the greatest of the Age of Enlightenment microscopists, Leeuwenhoek, to the great sea voyagers like Magellan, calling Leeuwenhoek "an irrepressible explorer" who opened vistas into new worlds "where knowledge would be advanced" in immense but unknowable ways. DeCarlo likewise saw the irrepressibility of the computer, albeit not in healthcare, as advancing knowledge to an unprecedented extent. He was right, and one can only wonder what dark continents of clinical care will be discovered in the future.

UNDERSTANDING INFORMATION
MANAGEMENT CONCEPTS

REPORTS OF information system challenges abound, as the following actual cases confirm. A 1,200-bed healthcare complex in San Antonio, Texas, found that despite its large, inhouse "management information system (MIS)" department (see discussion on this concept later in this chapter), and a major computer-service contract with an outside firm, its information system was unreliable. Information provided to managers within the complex was reportedly inconsistent and incomplete, and, in the words of the complex's president, the system "could not respond to the current health care environment, resulting in high cost, duplication and lack of relevant information" (Rockers and Vaughn 1989).

In a related situation some years ago, New York City developed and installed a "match-up" information system designed to detect and reduce welfare fraud. The system was viewed as a godsend and well-worth the considerable investment. It would, after all, detect and eliminate, and hence save the city millions of dollars in, welfare cheating by matching welfare rolls against payrolls and other lists, and also greatly simplify record keeping. Instead, according to an internal report, the system caused "tremendous confusion" because clients identified as fraudulent turned out to be legitimate. Errors in recording and transcribing data seemed to have been aggravated, rather than diminished, by automation.

Ultimately, and typically, the system, not its managers or users, was blamed for the problem (Sherry 1979).

The very same kind of scenario continues to appear in today's healthcare organizations. For example, a physician in the Midwest spent $50,000 on an automated patient accounting information system that, he was told, would tremendously simplify record keeping and billing. Instead, accounts receivable became larger than ever, bills became frequently erroneous, and patient records became more difficult to maintain. He, too, blames the system that he bought.

Each of these cases, and thousands of others like them, illustrate the prevalence of a dangerous myth: The key to better information is technology and, concomitantly, the cause of information technology problems is "computer error." One commentator facetiously suggested that this computer error myth has become so mired that many organizations buy a computer system just to have a credible object on which to blame problems (Johnson 1991).

A second pervasive myth is that the more data available to us, the better off we are. Witness the plethora of data windows that adorn our computer screens, even though most of them are seldom used. Similarly, in healthcare organizations today, many healthcare executives acknowledge that the plethora of data available to and generated by their organizations are often not worth the increasingly inexpensive screens on which they appear. One insightful healthcare executive suggests that "*How* people use the information is much more important than what the computers spit out—if management is given data and those data are not relevant for decision making, then the data are worthless for everybody." Unfortunately, "data proliferation" is a major reality, and many agree that healthcare executives are drowning in it (Johnson 1991).

A third myth is that everyone understands the meaning of "computerese"—basic jargon such as "database," "real time," and certainly the frequently heard "management information system." In truth, the jargon of information systems is often misused and misunderstood, and sometimes altogether unfathomed. Technology, in the guise of jargon, acronyms, incomplete sentences, and codes, often puts the nonexpert user in a position of maximum uncertainty and minimum productivity (Bell and Richter 1986).

These three myths, and others, stem from an underappreciation of information systems as a resource that needs to be managed by its users. The following St. Serena's case illustrates typical situations and suggests important concepts that can provide a foundation for better undertaking the task of information management.

Case Two: The State of the Art

St. Serena's home care subsidiary had grown dramatically in recent years. Its director, Kimba Curtis, was excited when Stewart initially met with her about upgrading the agency's information system to better handle the tremendous expansion of data that accompanied the agency's growth. Together they selected an information system, developed specifically for home care organizations, with broad, fully integrated applications. The system specifically was designed to encompass process management needs, such as centralizing client records; care management needs, such as providing staff with diagnostic expertise and protocols; and health management needs, such as generating medical histories and genetic profiles useful in preventive care.

But soon after the new system went "online" (see discussion on this concept later in this chapter), Kimba regretted ever trying to upgrade the original system. The old system at least had worked reasonably well, albeit at a minimal level. Now, client names were misspelled, numerous identification numbers were incorrect, and patient histories were incomplete and some were missing altogether. Her staff was spending more time at their new computers, correcting information, than with clients. Although all sorts of interesting data were now available, they did not seem to be helping the agency become more efficient, and certainly not more caregiving.

A bit frustrated, Kimba met with Stewart. He told her that the new hardware and software were "state of the art" and that her staff probably was just adjusting to the new keyboards, data-entry devices, and software procedures. Also, he promised to send a "techie" to provide more training. Two weeks later, Kimba felt the information system situation was worse, not better. More and more information was being accessed by her staff, but less and less seemed to be helping her agency's efficiency and caregiving capability. More alarming to her was the sudden rise in incidents of erroneous billings and missing patient records. She knew that she had to act and that Stewart's technical people did not seem to have the answers. She decided to gather her supervisors to begin remedial measures.

Questions for Discussion

1. What kinds of questions should Kimba raise at the meeting with her supervisors?

2. Is the problem technical or managerial?
3. Were you consulting, what would you recommend to Kimba and her staff?

COMMENTARY

St. Serena's home care agency seems to have embraced technology as the key to effective information management. Reflection on the following basic concepts is useful in analyzing the wisdom of that approach as well as in suggesting alternative approaches.

Data Versus Information

The phone directory is a collection of names, addresses, and phone numbers. Does it contain data or information? Many healthcare professionals daily view terminal screens that contain words and numbers in large, color images. Do these screens present data or information? Is St. Serena's home care agency getting data or information from its new system? The answer is probably both.

Data are the raw material from which information can be generated. Information is the relevant, usable commodity needed by the phone caller, the manager, the healthcare provider—the user. If I need to call someone, the phone book may very well be a source of information for me if, from among those thousands of words and numbers (data), I am able to derive the one correct number (information) I need within the time period in which I need it so that I can effectively accomplish the task of contacting the person whose number I am seeking.

Similarly, a window on my screen may be intended to contain a needed piece of information. If the data are there and I am able to derive them, then the screen has been a source of information for me. If the data are not there, or if I am unable to decipher them, then the window contains a mere collection of data. Does the system at St. Serena's appear to be providing information or data?

There are three important points to note from these examples. First, information is something that a user can effectively employ in a required task; words and numbers are merely data unless we can effectively use them. Second, users need information to do their jobs; data that cannot be effectively used are not needed. Third, most professionals today seem to receive a lot of data and not nearly enough information. They are deluged with reams of printed sheets and rays of bright computer screens, which, at best, waste time and, at worst, may conceal needed information. Anyone can produce data, but only the user can produce information.

Today's healthcare professionals receive more data than their predecessors and are probably much too patient with the situation. If information is what is needed, then healthcare workers should demand more information and less data, which appears to be at the heart of Kimba's concerns. Studies, such as the one conducted by Mendlen, Goss, and Heist (1996), found many long-term care providers moving into the managed care arena without the information they need "to set rates, negotiate contracts, and generally make their managed care business successful." What, then, distinguishes information from data?

Characteristics of Information

Every information user has *particular* substantive information needs; that is, a nurse manager needs data concerning patients on the floor; a hospital supervisor needs data concerning worker performance; and a food services manager needs data concerning food prices and availability. However, in addition to such particular substantive information needs, all users also have *generic* information needs.

Generic information needs are the characteristics that distinguish data from information. Substantive words and numbers that bear on a user's job remain mere data if they lack distinguishing characteristics such as accuracy, timeliness, completeness, conciseness, and relevancy. These characteristics are precisely what JCAHO emphasized in its information management standards (see Figure 2.1).

Accuracy

Have you ever gotten a wrong number from a phone book? When that happens, what would otherwise be a good piece of information becomes mere data—a row of digits—because it lacks accuracy. What commonly occurs in healthcare organizations is screens display inaccurate accounting numbers or patient files contain incorrect words. St. Serena's home care agency seems to be experiencing such an accuracy problem. JCAHO's information management standard number 5 highlights accuracy.

Timeliness

Several years ago, a stockbroker I know sent her client a report about a healthcare company that financial analysts projected to be a prime takeover prospect. Immediately after receiving the report on Thursday, the client called the broker to place a buy order. The client was informed,

Figure 2.1 Characteristics of Information

>Accuracy
>
>Timeliness
>
>Completeness
>
>Conciseness
>
>Relevancy

however, that a takeover had been announced on Wednesday, and that the stock price had doubled. As a result, the client lost a chance to invest profitably because the report was not timely and, therefore, could not be effectively used. Because the tip failed to meet the timeliness need, it remained merely interesting, and potentially profitable, data. Similarly, finance reports can be useful to help you manage finances, but not if they are received weeks after decisions need to be made. St. Serena's information system seems to be designed to provide timeliness, such as in diagnosis decisions, but is it delivering on the promise? JCAHO's information management standard number 5 decrees that it should be.

Completeness

I once discovered that the phone book I was using had a corner of a page missing, so that the number I needed was missing its last digit. Although the six-digit number was accurate and timely, it was unable to effectively meet my need because it was incomplete. I had to try the ten possibilities for the seventh digit before I could complete my call! Patient files that have a thorough medical history but lack the most recent laboratory test results make decision making difficult, if not impossible. Incomplete, the files are mere collections of data, instead of useful sources of information. We might ask whether St. Serena's home care's information system includes lab test results in the patient medical history reports.

Conciseness

Professional reports are too often unnecessarily lengthy. Although they frequently contain important information, the reports require so much of the reader's time that the information is difficult to absorb. St. Serena's home care staff appears to be receiving lots of lengthy information on its screens, but is all of it useful or is it rather making recognition of needed information more difficult to achieve?

Medical records, whether electronic or manual, often are similarly flawed. For example, records with years of notes that are unindexed are unwieldy, and lacking conciseness, which can remain unread and unused data.

Relevancy

A report, printout, or screen display must be relevant to a user's needs or interests for it to be considered information. Equally important is that although the report may be substantively relevant, it is irrelevant if presented in a disorganized format; that is, if it contains meaningless codes and symbols that are not understandable. The phone book, for example, would be irrelevant if the thousands of names and numbers were not formatted alphabetically. Similarly, St. Serena's home care staff needs reports that help them do their jobs. The data contained on their screens need to be organized in format and understandable in content if they are to be relevant to the work of the agency. From what we have read in the case, a relevancy problem may well be central to Kimba's frustration.

While sometimes other required characteristics of information exist, such as confidentiality in sensitive areas, the absence of the generic characteristics that distinguish information from data often is a major reason why healthcare professionals are inundated with data and starved for information. A significant task of information management is to ensure that these distinguishing characteristics are provided, as Bradley (1995) stressed, "information is a resource and must be actively managed." Kimba and her staff would do well to address their problem with the help of this simple concept.

Information Systems

Every healthcare administrator has heard of an information system. But just what, exactly, is an information system?

An information system is a network, or series, of steps taken to collect and transform available data—words and numbers—into needed and usable information. Many so-called information systems actually are merely data systems, which are collected data transformed into more data. Too many healthcare administrators tolerate data systems when information systems are what they need to do their jobs well.

At least nine basic steps, identified below, are followed to form an information system network (see Figure 2.2). Understanding what is involved in each step is necessary for effective information management.

Figure 2.2 Information System Analysis

Step	Key Characteristic	Technology Role
1. Identifying	Relevance	None
2. Collecting	Completeness	Limited
3. Recording	Accuracy	Limited
4. Sorting	Conciseness	Tremendous
5. Calculating	Relevance	Tremendous
6. Storing	Completeness	Tremendous
7. Retrieving	Timeliness	Tremendous
8. Reproducing	Relevance	Extensive
9. Communicating	Relevance	Limited

Identifying

The essential first step in forming an information system is identifying, as precisely as possible, information needs and the format or classifications of data that would generate that information (Britt and Miller 1997). For example, in a public health clinic hypertension program, we may need to know (a) blood pressure readings so that patient progress can be evaluated, (b) how to contact clients for follow-up visits, and (c) medications prescribed to clients so that tracking can be conducted. To meet these information needs it would probably be necessary for us to have data on periodic blood pressures, on addresses and phone numbers, and on prescriptions written, and to have all of the data in a certain understandable format. For the public health clinic, we have identified information needed and several classifications of data for getting it, as well as the format in which we need them. Note carefully that identifying is a thinking step, not a mechanical one, because it first forms in the minds of the people needing information. Has St. Serena's home care spent too little time developing this step?

Collecting

Armed with specifics on what is needed, we can then collect the data identified, which is the next step in the process. To collect the data, we might design a form and use clinicians, clerks, or both, and we might retrieve the data from the medical record or patient registration form if they have already been collected. If available, we might collect data from the internet or through some kind of verbal exchange.

Recording

A third step in forming an information system is the actual recording of the data collected. It might involve pencil-and-paper note taking techniques, tape recording, use of codes, or scanning or keying a series of hand-written records or forms, such as an original patient chart. Anyone, from doctors and nurses to clerks and temporary help, might participate in data recording. At St. Serena's home care agency we might wonder who is recording, or entering, data onto the "state of the art" information system.

Sorting

The recorded data frequently are sorted or organized, which is the fourth step, to facilitate processing. For example, we could sort the hypertension clinic data by day collected, by alphabetical order of pa-tients' last names, or by range of blood pressure readings. Similarly, St. Serena's home care agency could sort patient data by geographic area, by diagnosis, by staff providers, etc.

Calculating

The recorded and sorted data can be further organized, summarized, or analyzed by the fifth step—calculating. For example, we might want to count the number of blood pressure readings in each range, the number of patients who live in each town, the number of patients taking a certain prescribed drug, or simply the number of patients.

Storing   *day —› week —› or monthly basis*

Information systems usually have some kind of storage capability. We might use folders and file drawers, a card file, a disc, or a computer hard drive to store information, which are all tools in this sixth step.

Retrieving

Retrieval, the seventh step, might involve writing notations on the tab of a folder or labels on file drawers or assigning a designated name to a computer directory. Whatever is required to be able to find information when we need it is the principle of retrieval.

Reproducing

The eighth step—reproduction—might involve carbon paper, copier machines, printouts, or terminal screens.

Communicating

The ninth, and final, step is delivering output to the information user. This might involve a routing slip, a distribution list, or a terminal placed at the proper desk.

Understanding these nine steps can facilitate the construction and diagnosis of an information system (see Table 2.2). If we ask which step is the most important, we can convincingly argue that communicating is critical because failure in this area means the system fails in its ultimate purpose of providing information to the staff person in need. We could also argue, however, that identifying is the key because even the most sophisticated system will fail if information needs are not well specified. Actually, an information system is only as good as its weakest link. An otherwise perfect system will fail if one element fails. For example, if the retrieval step is faulty or data collection is incomplete, reproducing the information is ineffective. Each step in the chain must be carefully managed for an information system to produce information and not just data. Do any of the steps at St. Serena's home care agency appear to be weak and good targets for managerial attention?

We could also analyze each step in terms of its effect on the generic characteristics of information. Where is accuracy most likely to be lost or gained? Given St. Serena's home care accuracy problem, where might Kimba and her staff look to remedy the problem? If timeliness is missing in an information system, at which step would you look for the probable source of the problem?

Relevance is certainly affected at the identifying stage. If the user is not involved in determining information needs, the selected classifications may not be relevant to his or her needs. If the collecting stage is done through an interview and the collector forgets to ask about a relevant item, the resulting data may be incomplete. Or if a form is used and the data provider does not understand it or resists providing information, the resulting data may be incomplete or inaccurate.

If a form and a pencil are used for recording, any number of disruptive contingencies could occur. If the recording is done illegibly, accuracy could be completely lost. Conciseness can be promoted at the sorting and calculating stages. A faulty retrieval step could cause delay and reduce timeliness, and blurred reproduction can impede accuracy and completeness.

Of course, each of the generic characteristics of information can be affected to some degree at nearly every step in forming an information system; but in designing or diagnosing an information system focusing on certain steps for certain information characteristics can help. For example, an accuracy problem might suggest that a verifying mechanism should be built into the recording stage; a relevancy problem might mean more user involvement is required; or a timeliness loss might be remedied by improvements in the retrieval or collection steps. Kimba could benefit well from a similar analytical approach that employs such simple concepts.

Finally, we can ask at which steps in an information system a computer might be helpful. Without doubt, a computer can sort large amounts of data; conduct complex, error-free calculations; and store more data than a warehouse full of file cabinets. However, a computer cannot determine our information needs or collect needed data. Those steps are performed by a human being, unless the data have already been collected and stored in machine-readable form. Can a computer communicate the output to the user? It certainly can hasten retrieval and greatly facilitate reproduction, but a person is needed to decide where, when, and how it will occur.

In other words, a "computerized information system" does not exist; what exist are only partially computerized information systems. A computer is useful at only some of the steps in an information system. Placing a million-dollar computer in an information system, therefore, can improve parts of the information system, but the overall system will still be only as strong as its weakest link. Did Stewart adequately understand this concept? Does Kimba?

Management Information System

Few terms are more bandied about in organizations today than "management information system," better known under the acronym MIS. Some sort of MIS seem to exist for nearly everything. We have HISs (hospital information systems), WMISs (welfare management information systems), SSISs (social service information systems), LISs (library information systems), and so on.

But just what is an MIS? The term is so overused and misused that its lack of conceptual clarity contributes to the problems of dealing with MISs in organizations.

First, important to remember is that an MIS is supposed to be an information system; that is, it is supposed to produce information, not merely data. Therefore, it is a network of steps, which is similar to the concept described earlier.

Second, an MIS is supposed to be management oriented; that is, it is intended to meet managerial information needs, more particularly, decision-making needs. Most information systems are designed to meet clerical information needs. A system to develop and maintain a roster, for example, is routine oriented. A payroll system and a billing system are usually intended for specific, routine purposes of concern to clerks and many others. MISs, on the other hand, are intended to assist the decision-making functions of professionals (Simpson 1994). According to Alter (1976), electronic data processing (EDP) is geared toward reporting and consistency needs (routine), while decision support systems (DSS) takes care of ad hoc and flexibility needs (decision making).

Third, because of its decisions-assisting purpose, the concept of MIS is information unity. It is intended to bring together in one system various data that are relevant to managerial-level functions. The administrator of a family practice, for example, needs information on finances, staff, patients, doctors, and so on when planning next year's activity. Without an MIS the administrator must pull vital information from various sources and places and then try to interrelate the data. With an MIS the data are standardized and interrelated so that required information can be easily and quickly retrieved and integrated. This intergration is clearly what Kimba wants and what Stewart intends for St. Serena's home care agency.

Fourth, to facilitate the kind of data integration described above, the concept of MIS nearly always entails computerization.

Two major kinds of management information systems exist: (1) special purpose, or limited, systems and (2) database management, or fully integrated, systems.

Special Purpose Systems

Special purpose systems are information systems that integrate some files into one system to facilitate well-defined, repetitive decision-making tasks. This system in a healthcare organization might integrate patient medical history data with administrative data to facilitate admissions processing, much like airlines use the same system to facilitate flight reservation decisions. Some commonly used, and misused, jargon stems from this kind of MIS. Since these systems usually are geared toward quick feedback for quick decisions, they are almost always "online." To say that a system is online means that a user can directly and immediately access a file. In practice, online means a user can key or browse at a terminal and a screen will display the requested file. For example, airline clerks can call up a flight number on a screen and immediately determine whether or not seats are available.

A "batch" system does not provide direct access to a file. Many modern libraries, for example, have computerized periodical research services; typically, the most recent years are online. The researcher can go to the terminal in the library, type in the subject of research interest, and see on the screen a list of relevant articles. However, the researcher might have to fill out a form to request older articles and return the next day for a printout that lists the relevant articles. The researcher must wait overnight because those older files are in batch mode.

The term batch can have two meanings—(1) the method of sorting or (2) the method of recording data. In the example above, data on older articles are stored in batch mode—data on tapes or disks that are "batched" or stored on shelves "offline" until a request arrives at the data center for information from those batched files; the tape or disk, then, is placed on a machine and the resulting printout is sent to the library. On many e-mail systems, "old mail" is available only offline.

The term batch is also used to describe the method of recording data. Many credit card sales, for example, are still not recorded immediately on our computerized bill file. Instead, after we sign a credit card slip, it is sent to the central billing office, where it is placed in a pile of other slips. When this batch of sales slips reaches a certain size, or at a certain time of day, the data are then recorded and the transactions appear on our monthly statement.

Note that an online system, then, must have online storage, but it might also reflect a batch recording mode; that is, in an online system the user has direct access to the file, but the file might not be up to date if the data in it are entered through a batch mode. Patient records, for example, in the St. Serena's system might be electronically online, but that does not necessarily mean that they are current. A "real-time" system does not have this limitation. It provides not only the online capability of immediately viewing a file, but also the capability of making immediate entries or recordings in the file. A typical example of this capability is the airline reservations system. The reservations clerk uses a real-time capability to book a seat so that every person who accesses that file now knows that one less seat is available. A real-time patient record system, for example, would entail electronic charts in which all notations, diagnoses, prescriptions, etc., are entered immediately in computer mode rather than transcribed at some later time from a hand-written chart.

Batch systems are still widely employed because they are less expensive and because they are adequate for many purposes. Waiting overnight for a printout or for computer entry is perfectly fine for all sorts of functions. For patient records, managers would need to decide what was adequate. Most MISs today are online because decision making frequently requires quick information. Online systems are considerably more expensive than batch systems, though not nearly as costly as real-time systems, which require special software and hardware as well as security and privacy protections. However, online systems without real-time capability might well be sufficient in many cases for health-care organizations. Airlines, clearly, need real-time systems to manage their reservations function because they require instant updating, but relatively few other functions are sufficiently improved by a real-time capability to warrant the additional cost. What would suit the needs of St. Serena's home care agency? A state-of-the-art system or a system that adequately meets its needs?

Fully Integrated Systems

Until recently, fully integrated systems have proven to be very difficult to realize. However, healthcare reform has increased awareness about the importance of information sharing among the organizations' finan-cial, clinical, and administrative components to the future viability of healthcare organizations. Concomitantly, as St. Serena's Stewart ex-emplifies, an expanding interest in implementing these systems, which are sometimes called integrated database systems (DBS) or enterprise-wide systems, was reported in 1992 (Binius). An integrated system is a profound step beyond a "distributed" system. Whereas a distributed system provides for separate, independent systems to be linked or net-worked, a fully integrated system provides for complete integration and standardization so that, in effect, the entire organization works out of one file cabinet. In government, a fully integrated system would mean that if the health department collected your name and address, that data would then be available to the motor vehicle department so when you apply for a license, you would not have to fill out another address form because it would already be entered in the government's total system. If you changed addresses, the change would only have to be reported and recorded once; every user would then have the change. At a healthcare facility like St. Serena's, the system would mean that a patient's file would appear the same whether that patient was in the hospital one day or on the home care's rolls the next.

A hypothetical example can illustrate both the concept and problems with implementing a fully integrated system. It is technically possible today to automate all writing in the world, through personal computers (PCs), and to link them all through the Internet. Since most of the data in the world today pass through a PC at some stage in their generation, it is technically possible to have most of the world's data available in one common system. Of course, to make this workable, everyone would have to use compatible systems. A number of healthcare organizations were on the road to having one total system in which any and all data collected anywhere in the organization would be available to everyone (*The New York Times* 1993). A 1994 report suggested that hospitals, healthcare systems, and healthcare organizations were steering toward integrating disparate systems in their organization to speed the flow of data (Bergman).

While few fully integrated systems exist now, many partially integrated systems do exist; they are commonly called "database systems." A database system builds one file by drawing data from other files. Managers may need financial data from the accounting department, staffing data from the personnel department, and client data from various operating departments. A database system draws the needed data into one file so that the managers can access and interrelate the various data for decision-assisting purposes.

Of course, a database system might also be called a special purpose system, except that database systems are designed to be contingent and flexible to respond to ad hoc managerial information needs. Although, as the *Wall Street Journal* noted in 1993, the healthcare industry is becoming increasingly "data driven," database systems, online systems, and other technological devices are still merely resources at a manager's disposal to help in the task of information management. Alone, these tools can cause more confusion than clarity, as St. Serena's home care's case illustrates (*The Economist* 1986). When used to implement the concepts discussed above, these systems can indeed be an ally of healthcare professionals.

References

Alter, S. L. 1976. "How Effective Managers Use Information Systems." *Harvard Business Review* (November–December): 98.

Bell, J., and W. Richter. 1986. "Needed: Better Communication from Data Processors." *Personnel* (May): 20–6.

Bergman, R. 1994. "Integrated Information Paves the Way to Better Decisionmaking on Patient Care." *Hospitals & Health Networks* (January 5): 56.

Binius, T. 1992. "Conference Report: Executive Forum on Information Management." *Healthcare Executive* (September–October): 38–9.

Bradley, J. 1995. "Management of Information: Analysis of the Joint Commission's Standards for Information Management." *Topics in Health Information Management* 16 (2): 57.

Britt, H., and G. Miller. 1997. "Recent Developments in Information Management for Primary and Community Health Services." *Health Information Management* 26 (4): 193–7.

"Databases Learn to Hop, Skip, and Jump." 1986. *The Economist* (February 22): 76–7.

"Health Care Technology." 1993. *Wall Street Journal* (8 October): B-11.

Johnson, J. 1991. "Information Overload: CEOs Seek New Tools for Effective Decisionmaking." *Hospitals* (October 20): 24–7.

Joint Commission on Accreditation of Healthcare Organizations. 1994. *Accreditation Manual.* Chicago: JCAHO.

Mendlen, J., S. Goss, and K. Heist. 1996. "Managing Data for Managed Care." *Provider* 22 (7): 66.

The New York Times. 1993. (2 May): F-8.

Rockers, T. H., and L. R. Vaughn. 1989. "Audit Helps Transform Inefficient Information Systems." *Health Care Financial Management* (June): 127.

Sherry, M. 1979. "Making Computers the Goat for All Our Woes." *Newsday* (December 2): 41.

Simpson, R. 1994. "Benchmarking MIS Performance." *Nursing Management* (January): 20–1.

READINGS

The first article that follows is a classic in information literature. First published in 1981, it was recently republished because its concepts are timeless. Note specifically Philip Hutchens's emphasis on applying fundamental resource management principles to information as an aid to productivity. St. Serena's home care agency might find his 10 steps for improving information management to be germane to its problems.

Jennifer Rowley, on the other hand, provides a refreshingly clear perspective on the nature of information management. Using a conceptual, rather than mechanistic, approach she wonderfully expands understanding of the nature of information and retrieval of information specifically. Her emphasis on "instilling a structure into electronic information" might be relevant to Kimba's situation at St. Serena's home care agency.

Information Management and the Decisionmaker
Philip H. Hutchens

Abstract
This article addresses the impact of information management on decision makers and productivity and the causes of increased information and

Reprinted with permission from Records Management Quarterly *32 (4), October 1998: 28–30. Philip Hutchens was chief of the information management branch of the Food and Nutrition Service of the U.S. Department of Agriculture.*

information costs. Valuable guidelines are provided for records administrators in the form of 10 points which can be used to control and to better manage information.

Business and government information is normally stored in one or more of the following four mediums: (1) in someone's head, (2) on paper, (3) on microfilm, (4) in a computer. Peter Drucker has argued that the information in someone's head, or intuition, is a common ingredient of management decision making. However Drucker also notes the importance of informed judgment in decision making. Yehezkel Dror, on the other hand, argues for the importance of rational decision making. By rational, Dror means decision making that draws on as much information and facts about the decision as are possible to collect. Dror too notes the importance of informed judgment because it is not always possible to gather all the facts.

Decision makers normally use intuition, but the proportion of decision making based purely on intuition seems to be declining. Rather, paper, computer, and film records are being used more frequently to support decisions. In fact, the more important the decision, the more apt the decision maker is to collect additional background information.

As the volume of records grows, the medium tends to change. The proportion of information maintained on paper declines in relation to film and computer generated records. In many cases paperless records are less costly and of greater utility to the decision maker. Microfilm is frequently made directly from a computer–generated magnetic tape (COM). Video screens also are frequently used to display computer stored and generated information.

Although records may be used to provide information to decision makers, they also may be kept primarily for historical or archival purposes. A bank, for example, will make a microfilm copy of personal checks. The main purpose is to have a record for settling potential disputes. Data used in preparing personal account statements are entered into a separate computer system. Computerized data systems may also provide a summary printout for the decision maker, and the supporting data is stored for future documentation. These non–decision making records are of course expensive to maintain. They must be created, filed, housed, perhaps used, and then eventually discarded.

While non–decision making records are growing in number and are expensive, records used in the decision–making process may be even more costly. The costs for filing, storage, retrieval, and disposal apply to decision making records; but in addition, these records are used. Policymakers refer to them. Line employees use them in everyday work.

If these records systems are not properly designed, they can lead to poorer decision making and lowered productivity. For example, the time line employees spend in reading and responding to information requests, amounts to lost production time. Decision making also will be adversely affected by either too little or too much information. If there is too little information, errors made in ignorance of the facts are more likely. If there is too much information, the decision maker is apt to miss key points, or the decisionmaker may give up entirely on trying to use the information and decide key issues based on intuition.

Information therefore is an important organizational resource which if properly managed can lead to improved decision making and increased productivity. Poorly managed, it will have just the opposite effect. There are many steps that might be taken to improve management of information as a key resource in an organization. Following a brief discussion of the need for, and costs of increased information, 10 points are offered for improving information resources management.

Information Increase

There are two fundamental causes of increased information. The first is modernity. Modernity has brought about a reduction in the number of "mom–and–pop" businesses and an increase in more complex organizations with larger work forces. Employees in modern organizations have a greater need for communication, documentation, reporting, etc. In addition, modern organizational decision–makers and policy developers may need substantial written information supporting their policies and decisions.

The second cause of increased information is modern democratic government. Democratic government frequently requires monitoring of program expenditures and operations, and it regularly requests records from the business community.

Some business and government information is of course necessary; much of it is unnecessary. Program officials in both public and private organizations tend to be overzealous when collecting data about their programs. Modern reproduction equipment and computer processing make data collection easier and more tempting. However, the cost of information collection, storage, and disposal is very high.

Information Costs

The capability to produce information is growing. The printing and publishing industry remains one of the largest in the U.S. Paper mills often are not able to keep up with rising demands. Quick–copy, duplicating, microfilm and computer related industries also are producing at all time peaks.

The cost of information usage also is growing. Increased information costs exist in almost every modern business or governmental organization. Knowledge about these costs can be a road map for locating unnecessary expenditures. Therefore, if information costs are not known, they should be ascertained. If the costs prove to be unnecessarily high, they are worth controlling through improved management. Paperwork costs alone, for example, are estimated in a recent Congressional study to be $25 to $32 billion per year for business and $43 billion per year for the Federal Government.

10 Steps for Improving Information Management

1. *Establish control over the creation and use of new information.* One firm plastered the walls of its halls and offices with large colorful posters depicting tigers. The aim was to eliminate paperwork "underbrush." The results of this "cleanup campaign" were largely ineffectual. During the time in which small amounts of data were being purged from old systems, new data collection requirements were established which exceeded total old requirements. In most organizations, requests for new information arrive regularly. In fact, it seems reasonable to suggest that the pressure for new information is greater in more dynamic organizations.

   To successfully control information, an analyst (independent of program areas) should assist in all policymaking decisions involving establishment or revision of data collection systems. Also, an information analyst should be involved in designing the actual steps or procedures (including forms) for all data collection efforts. Without the initial involvement of an independent analytical source, the temptation to collect unnecessary information will be too great for most program specialists to resist. From a narrow perspective of a program specialist, collection of data frequently appears justified. From the organizational perspective of an information analyst, such data collections are frequently unnecessary.

   The press for information tends to unfairly make the information analyst appear as a hindrance to the program. The analyst must check all the details of all collection efforts, insisting upon, for example, use of scientifically designed, analyzed, and controlled data collection forms. A single unnecessary item on a form can be costly and distracting to the decision maker, and this is the detail level that information analysts are concerned with. Top management must insist upon having such analysis.

2. *Treat information management as a management function.* Pilots use checklists when operating airplanes. Items on that checklist, or absence of items, reflect policy decisions about how a particular plane is to be operated. Too limited a checklist may cause the plane to be operated unsafely. Too broad a checklist may cause unnecessary delays.

   As seen in this example of the airplane pilot, information managers can help determine policy by limiting the establishment of data collection systems to those which are needed for sound policy decisions. They also contribute to efficient operating procedures by including only those information requirements absolutely necessary to perform the task at hand. Information management is not limited to administrative functions such as merely maintaining a forms inventory.

3. *Eliminate unnecessary records.* Several years ago a large English chain store eliminated much of their recordkeeping, resulting in the destruction of 26 million copies of forms weighing over 120 tons. The results were reported to contribute significantly to profit as prices were cut, wages were upped and sales zoomed. This is a bold step, but it illustrates the fact that a lot of recordkeeping is unnecessary.

4. *Insure systematic maintenance and disposal of information.* If we could burn one Federal record a second, we would still be burning them over 2,000 years from now and we would not have started on all new records created while we were burning the old ones. Records must be destroyed according to a predetermined and legal schedule. This includes records on paper, film, magnetic tape, etc. In fact, court cases suggest the wisdom of early but legal destruction. Companies are finding through adverse court action that old records may cause considerable harm by unnecessarily permitting a look into past operations; court orders not to destroy existing old records also can lead to expensive maintenance. See the *Federal Register Guide to Record Retention Requirements,* available from the Government Printing Office, Washington, D.C., for a complete review of legal time frames for maintaining records.

5. *Provide for the proper selection, effective utilization and control of office equipment; conduct in–depth studies of duplicating and quick–copy requirements and costs.* It is estimated that quick–copy machines now produce 50 billion pages annually. Quick–copy and duplicating output is clearly a major contributor to the spread of unnecessary information. These machines may also contribute to effective operations, but

unless closely controlled they will lead to a paperwork blizzard. Analysis must be made of what is being copied on these machines, and why.

6. *Control computer output; solve paperwork problems with computers.* The nation's computers churn out some 10,000 miles of paper daily. Managers are frequently deluged with more data than they need or can use, and at a cost that often is much higher than frequently realized. Corrective attention can be focused on elimination of reports; reducing the size of reports by delivering only summaries; preparing only deviations from prescribed norms, etc.

   Other paperwork problems can be simplified by the computer. For example, where it might previously have taken years to gather bits of data for a publication (such as catalogs or listings), the same information might quickly be handled on a computer and also might include use of a photo typesetting process. The amount of file space needed to store hardcopy records also may be reduced through use of microfilm or computer output microfilm (COM).

7. *Instruct staff to filter or combine related paperwork.* Staff assistants, managers, and secretaries can reduce the amount of paper passed up the line if they are specifically told what to eliminate. By filtering out the unnecessary, these people reduce executive paperwork harassment and help streamline the decision–making process.

8. *Control promotional propaganda paperwork.* Propaganda printing usually involves a change of program, system, budget, or policy etc. It is usually one-sided. It is frequently unnecessary in terms of overall organizational needs. The Federal Government prohibits it within government. Companies need a strict policy on who may approve propaganda printing, and printing managers need to be instructed on how to recognize it.

9. *Contact public officials.* The business community and private citizens should not hesitate to contact public officials to voice their complaint over unreasonable information collection. Legislatures pass many laws requiring public agencies to collect information. Both legislatures and implementing governmental agencies often are over–zealous in interpreting how much data should be collected. Complain to your legislators or to the requesting agency if you are receiving unnecessary requests. In the Federal Government, many agencies are not allowed to collect information from the public without approval of the Office of Management and Budget (OMB) associated with the White House. When

dealing with agencies subject to OMB approval of public–use forms you may refuse to complete Federal forms if the data collection is not authorized by OMB. OMB is therefore an excellent source of protest regarding Federal information collection requirements.

10. *Don't review information just because you might be asked about it.* Many of us feel we must read and respond to whatever crosses our desk. Don't, and use your own judgment as to when and how you should write a note back and tell someone that you haven't reviewed a particular package because on the surface it does not appear to involve you in a direct way.

Summary

Intuition is declining proportionally as a basis for decision making. There is a greater reliance on hardcopy mediums. Increased use also is being made of film and computer generated records. There is, of course, a need for information in a modern business or government organizational environment. However, much of the information that is collected is unnecessary.

There are ways to improve management of information. Once information resources are under control, responses to government or court requests for data will be more efficient and less costly, and a clearer basis will exist for challenging unnecessary government requests for information. Decision making will improve as managers have more time to concentrate on essential information. Productivity will improve for all employees as they eliminate unnecessary information from their daily schedules and have more output time. Information costs are alarmingly high, but if controlled, information can become a good and faithful resource instead of a drag on productivity and a disrupter to sound decision making.

Towards a Framework for Information Management

Jennifer Rowley

Abstract

This article proposes a framework for information management which has four different levels: information retrieval, information systems, informa-

Reprinted from International Journal of Information Management, *18 (5),* Jennifer Rowley, *"Towards a Framework . . ."* 1998, with permission from Elsevier Science. Jennifer Rowley is head of the School of Management and Social Science at Edge Hill University, Ormskirk, UK.

tion contexts, and information environments. The first two of these levels, information retrieval and information systems, focus on the individual and their use of information and the systems that are designed to facilitate such use, and constitute the subdiscipline microinformatics. The second two of these levels, information contexts and information environments comprise the subdiscipline macroinformatics. Effective information needs to address issues at all of these levels and the relationship between these issues. An analysis of perspectives on information management demonstrates the relationship between the proposed framework and earlier contributions on the nature of information management. Further debate on a general information theory, leading to a core terminology, an understanding of the relationships between these terms, coupled with some models that can be applied to information processing, might facilitate a more complete understanding of information management at all of the levels within the framework.

Introduction

Information is not merely a necessary adjunct to personal, social and organizational functioning, a body of facts and knowledge to be applied to the solution of problems or to support actions. Rather it is a central and defining characteristic of all life forms manifested in genetic transfer, in stimulus response mechanisms in the communication of signals and messages and, in the case of humans, in the intelligent acquisition of understanding and wisdom. [1]

"Without an uninterrupted flow of the vital resource, society as we know it would quickly run into difficulties, with business and industry, education, leisure, travel, and communications, national and international affairs all vulnerable to disruption. In more advanced societies this vulnerability is heightened by an increasing dependence on the enabling powers of information and communications technologies." [2] (p. 18)

Information is an essential but elusive concept. It is all around us. At a very fundamental level information colours our perceptions of the world around us and thereby influences attitudes, emotions and actions. The central significance of information has led many authors to seek to define the concept of 'information', and to better understand how information is, and might be processed and managed. This, in turn, has led to attempts to refine the concept of information management, or more recently, knowledge management.[3] Contributions to this debate are to be found in the literature of a wide range of disciplines, including: communication theory, library and information science, information systems, other professional disciplines, cognitive science, organization science and policy making. These contributions offer a variety of different perspectives which can be summarised as four distinct definitions:

- information as subjective knowledge; [4–6]
- information as useful data, or as a thing; [7–9]
- information as a resource; [10, 11]
- information as a commodity; [3, 12–14] and
- information as a constitutive force in society. [14]

These different perspectives on the nature of information must be embedded in any robust framework that seeks to understand the nature of information management. This article proposes a framework for information management which recognizes that it is possible and necessary to manage information at the level of the individual, the system, the context and the environment.

What is information management?

Given the difficulty that appears to surround the concept of information, it would not be surprising if there were to be some difficulty in reaching agreement as to the nature of a discipline that is described as 'information management'. Nevertheless, although the various disciplinary perspectives do not yield a unified view of the nature of information, they are all consistent in one respect. No professional or disciplinary perspective appears to be able to avoid the consideration of the processing of information, when seeking to define information. The next step must be to examine information processing, and the associated concept information management, in more detail.

Information processing might be viewed as doing something to information to make it into something else, e.g. subjective knowledge, differently arranged information or summary information. Curtis, [15] for example, identifies the following as types of information processing:

- classification of data,
- rearranging/sorting data,
- summarizing/aggregating data,
- performing calculations on data,
- selection of data.

Information processing might then be viewed as an activity common to all information users. Information management, on the other hand, is viewed as the province of the professional, although the precise boundaries of the professional group remain to be defined.

Ever since the early days of the birth of courses in information science and information management and the creation of bodies such as the

Institute of Information, Scientists and Aslib the Association for Information Management, educators and professional bodies have sought to identify the ideal curriculum for information management and to specify the core competencies and knowledge base of professional information managers. In general terms, information management can be viewed as a response to, and a search for new and improved means of controlling the information explosion and the resultant increasing complexity of decision making by improving the flow, the control, the analysis and the synthesis of information for decision makers. Nevertheless, it has to be acknowledged that the term information management has as many definitions as the authors who have attempted to define it. [16] It is, however, significant that a number of leading management thinkers have emphasized the need for managers to take managing information seriously. [17–19]

The following definitions of information management are useful: [20]

> The aim of information management is to promote organizational effectiveness by enhancing the capabilities of the organization to cope with the demands of its internal and external environments in dynamic as well as stable conditions.
>
> Information management includes organization wide information policy planning, the development and maintenance of integrated systems and services, the optimization of information flows and the harnessing of leading edge technologies to the functional requirements of end-users, whatever their status or role in the parent organization.
>
> Information management has two dimensions, the management of the information process and the management of data resources.

Information management is then a practice-based discipline that has both technical, most broadly in the sense of systems based, and behavioral dimensions. For example, the *International Journal of Information Management* asserts that the journal:

> "provides a focus and source of up-to-date information on the developing field of information management. Papers are welcomed in the areas of information systems, organizations, management decision-making, long-term planning, information overload, computer and telecommunications technologies, human communications, and people in systems and organizations."

This can be further defined through an understanding of the role of the information manager. The information manager will have a central role in:

- Managing and coordinating the mechanisms for keeping a business team aware of market developments and taking some responsibility for wider environmental scanning.

- Designing, implementing, and when necessary, monitoring and updating information systems, and the exploitation of information in information systems in appropriate decision making.

A more holistic perspective, which returns to the relationship between information processing and information management, is proposed by Cronin and Davenport,[10] who state that in a sense all of us are information managers. We all manage information on the personal level which is formal and structured, as well as informal and less structured. Davenport [21] places personal information management in an organizational context. She notes that it may be viewed as a higher management function since it contributes to strategy, but that, on the other hand, it may be equally argued that it applies right down the line. Fairer-Wessels [22] attempts to integrate the personal and organization perspective with the following definition:

> Information management is viewed as the planning, organizing, directing and controlling of information within an open system (i.e. organization). Information management is viewed as using technology (e.g. computers, information systems, IT) and techniques (e.g. information auditing/mapping) effectively and efficiently to manage information resources and assets from internal and external sources for meaningful dialogue and understanding to enhance proactive decision making and problem solving to achieve aims and objectives on a personal, operational, organizational and strategic level of the organization for the competitive advantage and to improve the performance of the system and to raise the quality of life of the individual (by teaching him/her information skills, of which information management is one, to become a global citizen).

Another perspective is offered by Taylor and Farrell, [23] who propose some possible components of an information management construct, as in Figure 1. This figure shows the disciplinary influences on information management and the possible subdisciplines within information management.

The boundaries of information management will be influenced by the mix of disciplinary components. The business perspective, for example, uses technology to produce results. In information science the accent is on information retrieval, and the use, testing, evaluation and characterizing of information systems; and in engineering, it is on the architecture. Marchand,[24] also, proposes a multidisciplinary perspective and argues that the sciences of information include: information science, library science, computer science, informatics mathematical theory of communication, systems theory and systems analysis, operations research, cognitive psychology, artificial intelligence, robotics, cybernetics, decision sciences, semiotics and cognitive science.

Figure 1 Typology of IM Components

Contributing disciplines	*Sub-disciplines*
Business principles	
Management science	
Information systems	Information services
Office automation	Knowledge management
End-user computing	Information resource management
Information science	Information policy
Information technology	Information economics
Systems analysis	Social intelligence
Computing science	
Cybernetics	
Engineering	

Cronin and Davenport [10] point out that information management involves systems. They remind us that technologically information management relies on codified knowledge to produce formal representation of information entities which allow the automation of transaction processing, decision making and information retrieval. An information manager uses appropriate modeling techniques to support the exploitation of information to achieve organizational objectives. As such information management has generated, evaluated and refined a number of systems which facilitate effective information processing. New opportunities posed by technological advances in the telecommunications and computer hardware and software industries have changed the nature of those systems, and much of the emphasis in the discipline over the past 20 years has concerned itself with the adaptation of established systems, so that they might exploit the opportunities posed by these technological advances. Thus, publishers are preoccupied with the transition from the print journal to the electronic journal, electronic ordering systems speed commercial transactions, and organizations find themselves with huge databases that demand the development of techniques such as data warehousing and data mining in order to be able to extract information from this plethora of data.

In conclusion, there has been extended and continuing debate about the nature of information management. This debate clearly illustrates that information management draws on a variety of different disciplines and that from those disciplines, there are a number of stakeholders who will compete for the high ground. This article proposes an approach to the definition of information management which recognizes the need to consider the individual, the organization and systems in information management. The framework for information management that is proposed in this article seeks, instead, to examine the different levels on which information processing, and therefore management, take place.

Introducing the framework for information management

The framework in Figure 2 is intended to present a structure of the knowledge, research and practice in the area of information management. The terms used to label the levels in Figure 2 can be defined thus.

Information environment—The environment that surrounds information contexts; it consists of political, legal, regulatory, societal, economic and technological forces.

Information context—The context in which information systems are encountered. The context influences systems design, and encompasses the user. Organizations and businesses are an important category of context, but other contexts are also possible, including education, home and the community.

Information systems—The systems designed to enter information, store it and facilitate effective retrieval. Facilities to support efficient and accurate data entry must be coupled with adequate physical storage capacity and appropriate logical database structures. Systems include hardware and software, and data, and, in some models, users.

Information retrieval—Information retrieval is concerned with the individual interfacing with a system or range of systems or sources with a view to meeting specific conscious or unconscious information requirements. It concerns the actions, methods, and procedures for recovering information from stored data.

It may be helpful to embellish each of the above definitions. *Information retrieval* commences with an individual's explicit or implicit need for information. Typically, the individual will then select one or more sources, that on the basis of previous experience they might expect to offer access to the required information. Once an appropriate source has been selected the user interacts with the source. This may involve conversation or a telephone call, but for most recorded knowledge involves consultation of a printed or electronic information source or range of sources. In order to achieve successful retrieval in this source the user needs to make effective use of indexing and search languages, and, in the case of electronic information sources needs to be able to interact with the system through the human computer interface. Increasingly human computer interface designers strive to make interfaces self-explanatory, so that the user can learn as they use the system. Nevertheless, whether a user learns through use or through a training course, an understanding of the processes associated with learning to use information systems is necessary. Information retrieval

Figure 2 A Framework for Information Management Information Environments

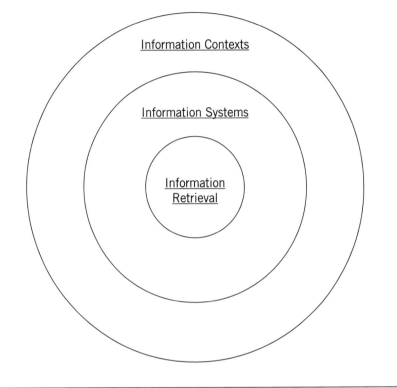

might then be viewed as having three main components: indexing and search languages, interfaces, and learning and cognitive frameworks.

One level in the framework is labeled *information systems*. An alternative perspective might be that the entire framework is concerned with information systems. An individual or an organization can be regarded as an information system, or perhaps more explicitly an information processing system. However, the conventional use of the term information system carries connotations of technology, probably in terms of hardware, software and telecommunications networks. Information systems should be the invisible tools that support the information processing of individuals or organizations. The impact of such systems on information processing and developments in information processing in recent years have been so significant that it is appropriate to consider this level in the framework explicitly. Whether developments in information management are viewed as technologically led or technologically constrained there is no doubt that they are technologically facilitated.

Accordingly, the categories of information systems reveal the need for organizations to, for example, create basic data from their transactions, retrieve information about their environment and channel this into their strategic planning process and distill and summarize information for different groups of workers and managers within their organization.

Information contexts are the contexts in which information processing and management take place. The context in which a specific system operates determines the functions that the system can be expected to perform. On the other hand, the ability to perform or record transactions and achieve more flexible communication of information may change the context such that the functions that need to be performed change. Thus, those opportunities offered by enhanced electronic information and communications systems have affected the way in which businesses operate and are impacting both on internal communication and communication with suppliers and customers. In general, the impact of systems on organizations is to provoke change, coupled with a growing emphasis on quality and customer focus. Information context is not, however, restricted to formal organizations. Information processing may also occur in public places, in the home and within informal groups. Also, it is important to recognize that libraries and other organizations in the information industry are an important category of information context. Whilst, in other organizations effective information management may be a means to an end, or an internal product that supports staff in achieving organizational objectives, the primary product of most of the players in the information industry is information management, either in the form of a service, such as information management consultancy or library services or as a product which provides packaged information as in a database or printed directory.

In the same way that business or marketing systems exist in a wider environment, so the contexts in which information management occurs can be placed in a wider context. Whilst sociological, technological and political forces are important in the information environment, those factors which transcend national and international boundaries, with all of the associated social and political ramifications, are those of the information marketplace. These include matters of pricing, intellectual property, international data transfer, social inclusion and exclusion, security and data protection and archiving and bibliographic control, all of which will remain topical as the electronic information marketplace develops further.

These levels can be broadly grouped into two sub-disciplines of information management: microinformatics, and macroinformatics, which are defined thus:

Microinformatics is concerned with the individual and their use of information, and the systems that are designed to facilitate such use. It focuses on information retrieval and information systems.

Macroinformatics is concerned more generally with the relationship between information and society and its organizations; this is a two-way symbiotic relationship. Many economic, political, technological and social factors affect an individual's access to information, yet, taking the opposing perspective, information is an important political, moral and economic force, or tool. It focuses on information contexts and the information environment.

This framework can be further developed to identify the information processing agent at each level, as in Figure 3. Information processing is not normally the same process or performed by the same agent as information management, although the relationship between these two is growing closer. Information managers are, in general, information professionals who act as agents on behalf of information processors to create and continuously improve systems, so that information processors are better able to meet their objectives. Information managers need to be able to understand and interpret these objectives in the context of the resources available to them.

The framework shows the different levels at which information management must be studied. This paper seeks to clearly identify these levels and to label them. At the same time it provides an important link between the levels and the differing perspectives on the definition of information. It is important to remember that there is an interface between each of the levels of the system, and that this can only be drawn categorically in a specific situation, and also that the inner systems are subsystems within the broader systems. So, for example, the systems designer must accommodate the perspectives of strategic managers, on the one hand, and trainers, users and indexers, on the other. Further, each of the inner subsystems are part of the system within which they are contained and are both influenced by and influence the systems of which they are part. Thus, the information systems level is seen to include the information retrieval level. The effectiveness of systems at one level impacts on the effectiveness of systems at the other levels. The nature of this impact changes over time. Compared with, say an individual 20 years ago, organizations and society experience:

- more information, communicated from
- a greater range of sources, through
- a wider range of channels, many of which have
- faster response and turnaround times.

Figure 3 Level Definitions of Information Processing and Management

Level	Information processor	Information managers	Definition
Information retrieval	Individual	Database designers, HCI designers, indexers, users	Information as subjective knowledge
Information systems	System	Systems analysts and designers	Information as useful data/information as thing
Information contexts	Organisation	Strategic information managers, strategic managers, organisational scientists	Information as a resource
Information environments	Society	Governments, multinational corporations, educational institutions	Information as a commodity/information as a constitutive force in society

- competitiveness and effectiveness of individuals, organizations and societies is increasingly dependent on their information processing and knowledge creation capacity, which means that
- there is a greater focus on individual, organizational and societal competencies in relation to communication, information processing and knowledge creation.

The need to structure information which was always present has become more pressing. Koniger and Janowitz [25] remind us that "Information is only valuable to the extent that it is structured. Because of a lack of structure in the creation, distribution and reception of information, the information often does not arrive where it is needed and, therefore, is useless."(p. 6)

In a non-electronic age, information structure was achieved through the presentation and production processes associated with paper documents, such as newspapers and encyclopedias, but the separation of content from medium has denuded information of this structure. Agents are needed who will take responsibility on behalf of individuals, organizations and societies for the creation of a structure, which addresses issues of selection, time, hierarchy and sequence. This process of instilling a structure into electronic information is information management's role for the future. The really interesting challenge is the determination of an appropriate structure, which must depend on individual cognition, systems design, context and environments.

Knowledge creation and information management

The above debate concerning the nature of information management has perhaps slipped into an instrumental view of information. In order to keep alive the debate on the different approaches to the nature of information a brief excursion into the process of knowledge or information creation, otherwise described as research, is a useful reminder that it is necessary to consider both knowledge creation and information management. Definitions of research immediately reveal the close relationship between research and knowledge. For example, Howard and Sharp [26] define research as: "Seeking through methodical processes to add to one's own body of knowledge and hopefully, to that of others, by the discovery of nontrivial facts and insights". (p. 6)

The Shorter Oxford Dictionary defines research as:

"1. The act of searching (closely and carefully) for or after a specific thing or person.

2. An investigation directed to the discovery of some fact by careful study of a subject, course of scientific inquiry."

The central stages of the activities that together comprise research, are then: searching by means of careful critical investigation, in order to discover something specific. The specific thing that is sought in the research process is information. A further common stance is that the purpose of research is to make an original contribution to knowledge. [27, 28] Thus, it can be deduced that information, knowledge and information are tightly interwoven.

"The transformation of information into knowledge and knowledge into information, forms the basis for all human communication; it allows ideas to spread across space and time and links past and present in a network that embraces generations and cultures over millennia". [29]

Having made this link between information, knowledge and communication, Orna [29] goes on to point out that there are close parallels between what information professionals do, and what researchers need to do. She argues that researchers, like information professionals need to

- define their information needs,
- locate sources of potentially useful information,
- transform the useful information into internal knowledge,
- store the physical objects that embody useful information,

- manage the store of useful information, so that they can get into it easily, move around it quickly and find what they need whenever they need it.

This link between information, knowledge and research is consistent with a positivist approach to research, in which a researcher starts with the definition of research objectives for a specific research project. These objectives are usually centered upon the answer to an everyday problem. The Post Office, for instance may seek the answer to the question: 'How do we increase the percentage of letters that carry postcodes?' Many manufacturing businesses may be concerned with the question: 'How do we reduce the percentage of defective products?' The researcher then formulates some hypothesis and collects data to confirm or discredit the hypothesis. Data collection methods assume that the researcher strives for objectivity, validity and reliability. This approach is consistent with the project-based approach to research that is implicit in many research funding models, where the funding agency, for practical reasons to do with satisfying the public interest or the trustees of the fund, needs to demonstrate an outcome from a project to which resources have been allocated. It is important to acknowledge, however, that there is a school of thought, described broadly as the phenomenological approach, that expresses reservations with the concept of researcher's objectivity. Typically, the emphasis is on constructivist approaches where there is no clear cut objectivity or reality. Morgan,[30] for instance, reviews a range of different approaches for engaging and understanding social life. The evaluation of these different approaches has been viewed as hinging on the problem of objectivity, emphasizing the importance of disciplined observation and value-free inquiry as a means of generating 'objective' knowledge. Morgan seeks to challenge the notion of objectivity, and to emphasize the link between the observer and the observed. This perspective argues that scientists engage a subject of study by interacting with it through means of a particular frame of reference and what is observed and discovered in the object (i.e. its objectivity) is as much a product of the situation and the protocol and technique through which it is operationalized as it is of the object itself. This leads to a view of research as engagement which emphasizes that researcher and researched must be seen as part of the whole. Cassel and Symon [31] point out that these two distinct approaches to research, the positivist and the phenomenological, have significant implications for what constitute warrantable knowledge, and for the establishment of criteria by which the outputs of research can be evaluated, and lead back to further debates concerning the nature of knowledge. Such debates are beyond the scope of this paper, but they do have important implications for any model of information management that involves the evaluation of information.

Defining a general information theory

Information access depends on crucial factors such as the ability to pay (environment), appropriate technological infrastructures (systems), and the compilation of appropriate databanks to meet individual and organizational needs. It also depends upon individual cognitive frameworks at the interface, including ability to use the system to execute effective information retrieval. This is dependent upon training and support, the interface design and the availability of and the user's ability to use, appropriate retrieval facilities.

In summary, the definition of a general information theory has much in common with the definition of general systems theory. It needs to draw on many different disciplines, and then to give back to those disciplines a broad conceptual framework and a terminology which contributes to the conceptual framework of those disciplines, which offers a foundation for the exchange and communication between researchers and professionals with different education and disciplinary cultures which is necessary to an advanced information society in which information acts as a major driver for change and disciplinary and professional boundaries are being eroded. This is indeed a significant challenge, and one which information theorists have only begun to address. It would seem that much progress might be made by

1. an agreement on a limited, but core terminology,
2. an understanding of the relationships between these terms,
3. some models, preferably graphical and simple, that can be applied to information processing.

Consensus on the first two of these has yet to be achieved. The models referred to in the third point, probably already exist and are somewhere to be found in the tools used by the various information systems methodologies in systems analysis and design. Such tools, e.g. data flow diagrams, entity life histories, rich pictures and entity relationship diagrams, are valuable in offering a perspective on information processing. There is more work to be done in exploring their wider applicability to information processing beyond the boundaries of specific technologically defined systems.

This paper has proposed a framework which defines and links the terms information retrieval, information systems, information contexts and information environments, and has identified the roles of information processor and information manager at each of these distinct levels in the framework. The paper demonstrates how this framework can be used to draw together perspectives on information and information management, and the relationship between the framework and the literature of information management. Effective information management requires attention at individual, systems, contextual and societal levels. Equally important is the potential for using information, information processing and information management as a window through which to view individual, organizational and social change.

Notes

1. Kaye D. The Nature of information. *Library Review*, 1995, 44(8), 37–48.
2. Martin, W. J., *The Global Information Society*. Aslib/Gower, Aldershot, 1995.
3. Choo, C. W., The Knowing organization: how organizations use information to construct meaning, create knowledge and make decisions. *International Journal of Information Management*, 1996, 16(5), 329–340.
4. Ingerwesen, P., Cognitive perspectives of information retrieval interaction: elements of a cognitive IR theory. *Journal of Documentation* 1996, 52(1) 3–50.
5. Court, A. W., The relationship between information and personal knowledge in new product development. *International Journal of Information Management*, 1997, 17(2) 123–138.
6. Brier, S., A philosophy of science perspective on the idea of a unifying information science. In *Conceptions of Library and Information Science*, eds P. Vakkari and B. Cronin. Taylor Graham, London, 1992, pp. 97–108.
7. Buckland, M., Information as a thing. *Journal of the American Society for Information Science*, 1991, 42(5), 351–360.
8. Lester, G., *Business Information Systems*. Pitman, London 1992.
9. Senn, J. A., *Information Systems in Management*, 4th ed. Wadsworth, Belmont, CA, 1990.
10. Cronin, B. and Davenport, E., *Elements of Information Management*. Scarecrow Press, 1991.
11. Eaton, J. J. and Bawden, D., What kind of resource is information? *International Journal of Information Management*, 1991, 11, 156–165.
12. Lord, R. G. and Maher, K. J., Alternative information processing models and their implications for theory, research and practice. *Academy of Management Review*. 1990, 15, 9–28.
13. Drucker, P. F., *PostCapitalist Society*. Harper Collins, New York 1993.
14. Braman, S. Defining information: an approach for policymakers. *Telecommunications Policy*, 1989,13(3), 233–242.
15. Curtis G., *Business Information Systems: Analysis, Design and Practice*. Addison-Wesley, Wokingham 1989.
16. Lewis, D. A. and Martin, W. J., Information management: state of the art in the United Kingdom. *Aslib Proceedings*, 1989 41(7/8), 225–25Q.

17. Drucker, P. F., Hints on handling the 1990's. *The Independent on Sunday*, 17 June, 1990 26.

18. Porter M. E. and Millar V. E., How information gives you competitive advantage. *Harvard Business Review*, 1985, 149.

19. Peters, T. J. and Waterman, R. H., *In Search of Excellence*. Harper & Row, New York, 1982.

20. Rowley, J. E., *The Basics of Information Technology*. Bingley, London 1988.

21. Davenport, E. Information management: a perspective. *International Journal of Information Management*, 1988, 8, 255–263.

22. Fairer-Wessels, F. A., information management education: towards a holistic perspective. *South African Journal of Library and Information Science*, 1997, 65(2), 93–102.

23. Taylor, A. and Farrel, S., Information management in context. *Aslib Proceedings*, 1992, 44(9), 319–322.

24. Marchand, D. A., Information management in public organizations: defining a new resource management function. In *Information Management in Public Administration*, eds F. W. Horton and D. A. Marchand. Information Resources Press Arlington, VA: 1982, pp. 61–63.

25. Koniger, P. and Janowitz, K., Drowning in information, but thirsty for knowledge. *International Journal of Information Management*, 1995,15(1), 5–16.

26. Howard, K. and Sharp, J. A., *The Management of a Student Research Project*. Gower, Aldershot, 1996.

27. Ghauri, P., Gronhaug, K. and Kristianslund, L., *Research Methods in Business Studies*. Prentice Hall, New York, London, 1995.

28. Phillips, E. M. and Pugh, D., *How to Get a PhD: A Handbook for Students and their Supervisors*. 2nd ed. Open University Press, Buckingham, 1994.

29. Orna, E. and Stevens, G., *Managing Information for Research*. Open University, Milton Keynes, 1995.

30. Morgan, G. (ed.), *Beyond Method: Strategies for Social Research*. Sage, London, 1983.

31. Cassel, C. and Symon, G. (eds), *Qualitative Methods in Organizational Research: A Practical Guide*. Sage, London, 1994.

THINKING SYSTEMATICALLY ABOUT INFORMATION SYSTEMS

HE TYPICAL life cycle of modern information systems has been described by some experienced observers as a remarkably consistent progression in several stages (Burch 1986). Stage one of the cycle begins with "wild euphoria" when decision makers hear about how much an information system has done for other organizations and want to acquire one for their own. Visions of instant information and more efficient processes excite beleaguered program heads. Stage two emerges almost immediately after the new system arrives, and is marked by "mild concern" when the anticipated payoffs fail to appear or when "bugs" crop up.

"Broad disillusionment" arises in stage three when users realize that the system fails to meet expectations or, instead, causes new problems. Employee unrest with using the "confounded machines" is a common symptom in this stage. The culminating stage four is marked by "unmitigated disaster." Such disasters include the failure of the automated billing system to get out the bills or mismanagement or inappropriate use of an electronic patient record, which results in either a privacy lawsuit or a "crash" that erases a disk with no backup.

Stage four, of course, is rapidly succeeded by a search for a perpetrator, punishment of the progressive innocent, and promotion of the obstructionary who had been against the new system all along. In hospitals, in government health offices, and in small and large healthcare facilities this scenario has been constantly repeated and, from what we have seen so far, St. Serena's appears to have experienced the early stages. These pitfalls are so common that a professional technology consultant for McKinsey & Co. has, after his name and from his experience, coined the phrase "Golub's Laws of Computerdom," which initially states: "No major computer project is ever installed on time, within budget, with the same staff that started it, nor does the project do what it is supposed to. . . . It is highly unlikely that yours is going to be the first" (Groobe 1972). Golub does proffer a caveat to this enduring tenet—his laws are not always true, just most of the time.

Evidential stories of this strange cycle abound. A recent *USA Today* cover story, for example, reported as follows: "Clearly, technology provides incalculable productivity and efficiency gains. But industry experts contend that commonplace glitch costs are staggering; up to $100 billion annually in lost productivity" (Strauss 1999). The story goes on to suggest that a major cause of these glitches is "executives too naive to challenge outside consultants or in-house specialists." Many organizations embrace information technology with little in the way of long-range plans—they have no formula for development, but are focused on having state-of-the-art systems (Smith 1991). The consequences of this shortsightedness is that many managers find themselves in the unenviable position of having an advanced information system that fails to address the needs of the organization and, perhaps even worse, impedes the efforts of those seeking useful information.

Why is this so? The major reason is a lack of enlightened analysis—a lack of systematic thinking about the entire project, an absence of user involvement and control, and failure to ask the right questions. In brief, this cycle dominates because no one "in the know" focuses on what needs to be done to make an information management project work. Technicians, who frequently are put in charge, are experts about what technically needs to be done, but only user–managers are in a position to know the organizational situation and to have the overall responsibility to make the system work. Let's see where St. Serena's is at this point.

CASE STUDY

Case Three: Calling All Drivers

Because of the apparent difficulties experienced with the new information system, Stewart decided to convene a "steering committee" of department heads to discuss the problems and determine corrective actions. He brought in the vendors from whom the system was procured, his staff of computer technicians, and an outside consultant who specializes in healthcare information systems.

Stewart started the meeting by summarizing all the complaints and problems of which he had been made aware. Almost all the department heads were nodding their heads in agreement as he went through the litany. In response, Terry Tech voiced the technicians' concerns about how many staff were very uncooperative, despite the technicians' consistent efforts to assist them; about how the departments were not using the new system properly, despite the technicians' patient efforts to instruct them; and about how staff and heads were not attending training sessions, despite the technicians' efforts to schedule them at staffs' convenience. Terry asked the department heads to please tell their staff to "get with the program." Vinny Valdez, the vendor representative, chimed in about how customizing the software would help alleviate many of the problems presented, while Chris Chan, the consultant, offered to provide special training in team building, privacy protection, and other areas of concern.

After a half hour of listening to ideas from the three camps, two physicians announced they had to go to appointments. Stewart then stated that his staff would develop a plan to address everyone's concerns and asked for everyone's cooperation. The steering committee would meet again in a week to review the plan to be drafted. The new system, Stewart reiterated, would make St. Serena's the envy of other healthcare organizations in the region, "so we must make it work."

Questions for Discussion

1. Who and what seems to be "driving" the development-and-implementation process described?
2. What should Stewart now do?
3. What should the department heads do?
4. What approach to information management is evident here?
5. Do you think the meeting, and the plan to be developed by Stewart's staff, is a step in the right direction? Why? What else would you recommend?
6. Are you optimistic about things working out at St. Serena's? Why or why not?

COMMENTARY

Establishing the new information system at St. Serena's appears to be a bit more challenging than first anticipated. This situation is not uncommon in all types of organizations. One might wonder why managers have so often failed to exert the same kind of control over information operations that they exercise over other aspects of their organization. One reason is that the technical aura of modern information systems has tended to conceal its broader ramifications. It has, thus, been difficult for managers to learn how to think about information management.[1] What should Stewart and St. Serena's managers be doing about the information resource?

The Role of Managers and Users

Managers and information users have tended to abrogate their proper, and necessary, role in systematic thinking by falling into traps. The three most common traps are the vendor trap, the hardware trap, and the technician trap, all of which appears to be present at St. Serena's.

The vendor trap entails leaving the thinking to the technology manufacturer in the mistaken belief that the experts know what needs to be done to make its system work well in a particular organization. In reality, however, employees of the manufacturer seldom have managerial insight and expertise about the organizations that buy their products. Stewart needs to be careful with his vendors; he needs to control them instead of be controlled by them.

The hardware trap assumes that computer use and integration into the organization immediately follow acquisition. This trap, consequently, leads a manager to focus on purchasing technology, instead of on meeting organizational needs and figuring out how to meld the organization with the new capability.

The technician trap places unfair responsibility on and unfounded confidence in the data-processing technician or "system analyst" to do the careful thinking needed to make the technology productive. In truth, while a technician can well think through technical needs and implications, only a user–manager can steer a technically sound system toward organizational effectiveness. So, to whom is Stewart turning to deal with the effectiveness problems of the new system? Neumann, Blouin, and Byrne (1999) maintain that "the success of an information system investment must be evaluated from the perspective of those who require the information, those who interact with the technology, and those affected by it." Is St. Serena's appreciating this advice adequately?

Succumbing to these traps is seductively simple. Many managers routinely delegate technology decisions to the "techies"; Stewart, for example, made sure they were fully represented at the steering committee meeting. But, the development of modern information systems affects an entire organization, from strategy to structure. Delegating to wizards does not ensure that the information technology effort will work. In fact, it practically guarantees that it won't. The technical experts seldom have a deep enough understanding of the organization, its culture, and its mission (Davenport, Hammer, and Metsisto 1989). *Healthcare Executive* magazine even suggests that the "top techie"— the chief information officer (CIO) of an organization—needs to be carefully managed by nontechnical executives (Griswold 1998).

The healthcare professional's role in developing a useful information system requires involvement, planning, and communication. Managers and system users should be thoroughly involved in the development of information systems from beginning to end. Instead, they seem to have been on the periphery at St. Serena's. Technology use requires careful planning and an investment of time as well as attention to the problems that inevitably arise. Perhaps St. Serena's, in a rush to get to the vanguard, did not invest sufficient time. Managers should ensure that technicians and system users frequently interact so that problems are quickly discovered and resolved (Spence 1998). We can wonder whether Samantha met this standard in her commission to Stewart. As one veteran of this process puts it: "My best advice is to start planning as soon as you can" (Lumsdon 1993).

But what specifically constitutes "managerial involvement?" How do managers wisely "plan" the application of information technology to their activities? Stewart, it can be argued, tried. How is communication between technician and user really accomplished? How, in short, can managers exercise control over the task of employing information technology?

One practical answer is to ensure that proper systematic analysis takes place before, during, and after the introduction of new technology. This analysis involves identifying objectives, gathering information on meeting them, formulating alternatives, deciding and implementing the most suitable alternatives, and monitoring what happens. Good systematic analysis is asking all the right questions and getting the best answers possible, while good management is ensuring that all the right questions are asked and that the best answers are sought. At St. Serena's, a focus on answers, not on questions, appears to be the case.

Most information technology challenges can be anticipated if the relevant questions are posed; most obstacles can be recognized if the development process is systematically monitored; and most difficulties can be handled if users and managers systematically observe and learn from actual organizational experience. Systematic thinking is one way healthcare managers can anticipate, recognize, and address barriers to the successful use of information technology.

Systematic thinking in managing information entails attention to the process, as well as to the substance, of planning, designing, and implementing modern information systems. Substance is the series of questions and tentative answers that guide the effort to employ information technology. Process involves developing the information system effort in systematic phases, carefully monitoring the actual experience as it evolves, and modifying the effort as important new questions are discovered and better tentative answers are learned.

The Substance of Systematic Thinking

In terms of substance, most healthcare organizations have, historically, employed a kind of systematic analysis for technology applications. They have generally raised questions about and addressed matters of system objectives, alternatives, impacts, and development. However, because user–managers, historically, have not been intimately involved in the analysis, critical nontechnical questions have received cursory treatment at best (Lohman 1999). Cursory treatment of the concerns of St. Serena's department heads may be at the core of the situation there. In particular, impact analyses have typically been limited to fiscal and technical considerations. The impact of a new information system on personnel and clients, the likelihood of resistance, and the implications for data security and privacy have often been neglected in planning and analysis. However, problems in these areas have frequently been the key impediments to effective use of information technology. Clearly, systematic thinking on these matters is needed.

The substance of systematic thinking is asking the following types of questions, the posing of which alone is a great tool for eliciting user involvement, and analyzing the answers:

Specification of Problem
- What is the problem that might benefit from a new information?
- How is the problem area currently handled?
- Why does the problem exist?
- Who is involved in the problem area?
- How severe is the problem for the organization?
- What priority does the problem have in relation to other organizational problems?

Definition of Objectives
- What do we want to accomplish?
- To what extent can we accomplish the objective?
- By when do we want to achieve the objective?

Development of Alternatives

- How could we accomplish the objective?
- Are there options other than new information technology?
- What technology alternatives exist?
- How have other organizations pursued similar objectives?
- What are the pros and cons of each alternative?

Impact Analysis

Fiscal Impact

- What will the project cost?
- How much will hardware and software cost?
- How much will personnel cost?
- How much will training cost?
- How much will development and implementation cost?
- How much will operating and maintenance cost?
- What savings can be expected?
- What nonquantifiable benefits can be expected?
- What are the cost-benefit implications of the project?

Technical Impact

- What technical expertise will be needed to develop and operate the system? Do we have that expertise? If not, where can we get it? How long will it take to get it?
- How will the system affect other technical systems in the organization? Can they be made mutually supportive?
- What is state of the art? Are pertinent technical developments likely in the near future?

Organizational Impact

- How will the system affect organization structures? Will it change the information flow? In what ways? Will any reorganization be necessary or desirable?
- Will the system increase or decrease anyone's power?
- How might it affect informal structures, such as social groups, within the organization?
- Will the system be used? How do we know?
- How might resistance to the system be expressed?
- Who might be threatened by and resistant to the system?
- How would system failure affect organizational operation?
- What could be done to minimize or overcome resistance?
- What could be done to minimize the undesired organizational impacts?

Personnel Impact

- Will some existing staff no longer be needed?
- How can unneeded staff be prepared for other work in the organization or be placed in another organization?
- What training will be needed? Who will do it? When will it be provided? How much will it cost?
- What new staff will be needed? Can they be recruited? How long will it take to recruit them?

Legal Impact

- What do current privacy and freedom of information laws require?
- Can the system meet these requirements? What will this cost?
- What new privacy laws are likely, and how would they impact the system?
- What legal protection can be built into contracts with vendors?

Security Impact

- What security risks are inherent in the system?
- What security problems have other organizations experienced with similar systems?
- What security protections are available to minimize the risk? How much would they cost?

Social Impact

- How will the system affect the organization's clients?
- How might it affect professional or healthcare system values?
- What can be done to minimize negative social impacts and maximize positive impacts?

System Development/Implementation Plan

- In view of the above questions and answers, what activities are required to develop and implement the system?
- Who will do them?
- When will they be accomplished?
- How do they interrelate, and who will coordinate them?
- What resources will be needed, and when will they be needed?

Additional specific questions should be raised to suit the particular applications and organization. Because finding answers can require a good deal of time and money, the extent of efforts employed in finding answers should be determined by the importance of and investment in the project (Morrissey 1999).

Important to remember is that effective management of technology and information systems requires that a broad array of questions be raised and systematically addressed. Management's job is to ensure that the right questions are asked and that satisfactory answers are available. Does Stewart appear to have focused on raising questions or on getting technical answers? Management must also ensure that questions are continually posed and answers are updated as more insight surfaces; that is, managers should ensure that a systematic process for developing the substance of systematic thinking is in place. As Neumann, Blouin, and Byrne (1999) maintain: "(T)here can and should be several points at which the feasibility 'go, no-go' decision is revisited when planning, selecting, and implementing an information system; all risk factors should be continually monitored and managed." Does St. Serena's appear to have such a process in place?

The Process of Systematic Thinking

A critical aspect of systematic analysis is the timing and frequency of posing the kinds of questions suggested above. The questions are typically asked, and answers are developed, once at the beginning of an information system project. This analysis is done through a so-called system study, which is usually conducted by technicians, consultants, or both. Afterward technology resources are acquired and a system is implemented in accordance with the system study. Undoubtedly St. Serena's did something like this.

Two serious problems are involved with the system study approach. First, even an extraordinary system study can neither anticipate all the problems that might impede a particular information system effort nor be expected to provide sufficient answers. Some problems will occur unexpectedly or in a different form than initially predicted and, inevitably, some answers will prove to be inadequate. Second, the approach permits only marginal user–managerial control in that once a user-manager commissions a full-scale system study, the project can easily proceed to implementation and use untempered by a practical, nontechnical, user-oriented perspective.

For these reasons, systematic thinking should also entail a phased process of monitoring developments and modifying the project as an information technology application is being developed. Systematic thinking depends on not only using existing knowledge and insight, but also using the knowledge and insight you gained from your actual experience with the project. Many information systems are failures because their development is guided solely by a pre-project system study. The failure occurs because management made no provisions for learning the intricacies involved as the project unfolded or for using the knowledge gained to modify the system study plan. In effect, the system study tends to be "written in concrete" with no serious review process brought to bear on it.

In contrast, a controlled process of systematic thinking recognizes that a system study is just a guess at what might and should happen and continually monitors that guess and adjusts it as new facts emerge. Such a process can be established and controlled by organizing information systems projects into distinct stages or phases, which are provided for conscious user–manager's review and to help with decision making.

For example, an information systems project can be organized into the following eight phases:

1. **Project Initiation Phase**. This stage focuses on initial clarification of the problem, objectives, and alternatives; obtains quick answers to basic questions; and involves a few people and little money.

2. **Preliminary Study Phase**. This stage probes objectives and feasibility of technological options for the organization; involves more people and money in a more-detailed examination of questions.

3. **System Study Phase**. This is the stage in which the substance of systematic thinking would be thoroughly developed; involves a significant investment of resources in an in-depth analysis of information needs and the formulation of a specific plan of system development.

4. **System Design Phase**. This is the stage in which the measures planned in the system study phase are actually designed; specialists, for example, design training programs and users and technicians design output forms.

5. **System Development/Selection Phase**. This stage is when hardware for implementing the design is tentatively selected—software is developed or identified.

6. **Testing Phase**. This is a key stage in controlling the project; plans and design are tried to ascertain what really happens when they are implemented; and focus is on correcting any inadequate pretest answers and discovering questions not previously asked.

7. **System Installation**. This is the stage in which the major financial investment is made.

8. **System Evaluation Phase**. This is the stage of ongoing series of reviews to see if new questions or problems have arisen, if old answers need updating, and if the system requires modification to meet organizational objectives.

The most important aspect of a controlled process is that at the completion of each phase the user–manager intervenes; reviews the outcome of the phase; and provides direction to either proceed to the next phase, halt the project, or return to a previous stage for additional answers. As Neumann, Blouin, and Byrne (1999) state: "While we advocate the importance of developing a plan, it must be a document or 'road map' that is routinely revisited, revised, and challenged." For example, a preliminary study might be reviewed by a manager who finds that questions on privacy impact and personnel resistance were not raised. The manager could then, at an early stage before development work is begun, direct that the system study address these questions before a decision is made to proceed with system design; important modifications could result.

Figures 3.1 and 3.2 depict such a process in flowchart forms,[2] which are intended as tools for implementing words of wisdom, such as Austin's, that supports requiring continued refinement of plans through the life cycle of information systems projects (Neumann, Blouin, and Byrne 1999). The flowcharts show the inherently iterative nature of the process and how the various stages interrelate. The flowcharts stress two important characteristics of such a systematic process: (1) the clear and unambiguous involvement of user–managers in the process and (2) the continual review and decision making by the user–managers. Notice that at the completion of each stage a manager makes a decision to continue, to stop the project, or to modify a previous phase.

This kind of a controlled, systematic process is, in effect, a process of asking questions and trying to get better answers as needed. The test phase, for example, can uncover impacts that were not anticipated in the preliminary study or system study phases. That impact, having been identified and addressed, can prevent serious problems from occurring when the system is fully installed. Specifically, a manager might direct expansion of the system study to explore a problem, such as user resistance, discovered in the test and to conduct a second test before full implementation.[3]

Similarly, the evaluation phase can disclose problems that were not recognized in the system study or test phases and can point to modifications that might improve the system's effectiveness. More than a few unproductive uses of information technology remain in healthcare organizations because of a lack of periodic systematic evaluation.

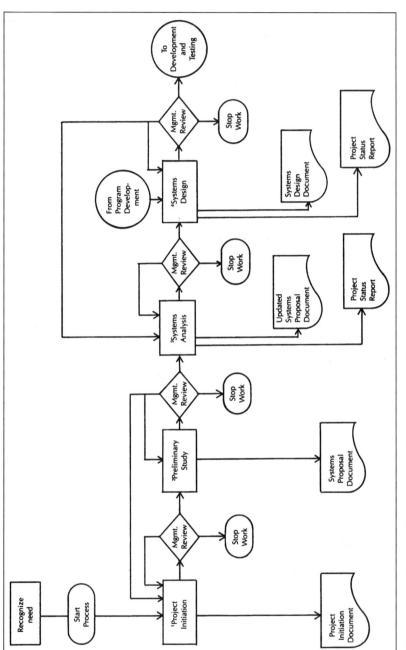

Figure 3.1 Process Flowchart—Study and Design

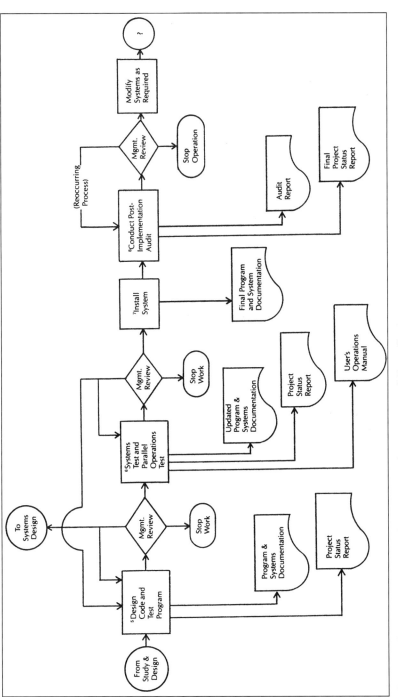

Figure 3.2 Process Flowchart—Development and Installation

In sum, a process of systematic thinking about information systems can prevent the cycle from starting with "wild euphoria" to ending up as an "unmitigated disaster." Systematic thinking can provide a framework for information management, for avoiding an uncontrolled rush to expensive installation of technology, and for steadfastly focusing information systems projects on organizational realities and needs. Such a process might have helped Stewart both anticipate the problems he now confronts and address them in a more systematic way.

The substance and process of systematic thinking can, and should, be applied by healthcare professionals to the development of new information systems and to the improvement of existing ones. It provides a fundamental framework for managing the technology and information systems that organizations need. The following chapters discuss some of the most important and difficult questions of the substance of systematic thinking—questions concerning organizational impacts, personnel resistance, security, privacy, and social ramifications—that appear to be confounding St. Serena's.

Notes

1. The chapter is intended as a framework. It does not get into details of systems design that are important for managers directly in charge of information systems projects. Many books are available for insight on these details, most notably *Information Systems for Health Services Administration*, 4th Ed, by Charles J. Austin and Stuart Boxerman (Chicago: Health Administration Press, 1997).

2. I am indebted to Harry Smith of the University of Calgary for his work on these flowcharts.

3. For an excellent discussion of testing, see "Pilot Projects: A Way to Get Started in Office Automation," by N. D. Meyer and T. M. Lodahl. *Administrative Management* (February 1980): 36–44.

References

Burch, J. G. 1986. "Designing Information Systems for People." *Journal of Systems Management* (October): 30–4.

Davenport, T. H., M. Hammer, and T. J. Metsisto. 1989. "How Executives Can Shape Their Company's Information Systems." *Harvard Business Review* (March–April): 130–4.

Griswold, C. 1998. "To Invest or Not To Invest: Guidelines for Evaluating Investments in New Technology." *Healthcare Executive* (May/June): 21–6.

Groobe, J. A. 1972. "Maximizing Return on EDP investments." *Data Management* (September): 28–32.

Lohman, P. 1999. "Information Systems for IDSs: Meeting the Challenges." *Healthcare Financial Management* 53(3): 29–34.

Lumsdon, K. 1993. "The Clinical Connection: Hospitals Work to Design Information Systems that Physicians Will Use." *Hospitals* (5 May): 16.

Morrissey, J. 199. "Slow Decisionmaking Drains Resources." *Modern Healthcare* 29 (35): 62.

Neumann, C., A. Blouin, and E. Byrne. 1999. "Achieving Success: Assessing the Role of and Building a Business Case for Technology in Healthcare: Reply." *Frontiers of Health Services Management* 15 (3): 46.

Smith, M. 1991. "Adventures in Dysfunctional Computer Land." *Nonprofit World* (July–August): 6.

Spence, J. W. 1988. "End User Computing: The Human Interface." *Journal of Systems Management* (February): 15–23.

Strauss, G. 1999. "When Computers Fail." *USA Today* (7 December): 1A–2A.

READINGS

The following superb articles reinforce the systematic thinking concept of this chapter and provide tangible advice for St. Serena's and all healthcare organizations that face information management challenges. The first article comes from *Harvard Business Review*. It articulates major information management problems that we have seen at St. Serena's, such as a tendency to get technology for technology's sake and rough relations between information users and information system specialists. Authors M. Bensaou and Michael Earl then offer five principles for guiding situations, such as that at St. Serena's, which are strategic instinct, performance improvement, appropriate technology, organizational bonding, and human design. They conclude with advice that managers at St. Serena's would do well to hear: "It's time for senior managers to regain control of technology in their companies: to abandon the dangerous idea that IT [information technology] requires special technocratic means of management."

Robert Heckman's more detailed article applies the notion of managerial control specifically to the information technology procurement process. He provides a management model that consists of six processes: requirements determination, acquisition, contract fulfillment, supplier management, asset management, and quality management. The model is most useful to executives like Stewart because it includes a series of questions for managers to pose as a tool to control information systems development. In the end, Heckman imparts wisdom to all healthcare managers when he stresses that the overarching task in information management is "managing a portfolio of relationships rather than a portfolio of technologies." While this article may provide more in-depth analysis than Stewart is ready to embrace, the emphasis on systematic management of relationships over technology is probably at the core of the situation at St. Serena's and most healthcare organizations.

The Right Mind-Set for Managing Information Technology

M. Bensaou and Michael Earl

Although most executives in the West recognize the importance of information technology, their experience with it as a strategic business tool is often frustrating. Invite any group of senior executives in the United States or Europe to list their complaints about IT and they will typically identify five problems:

- IT investments are unrelated to business strategy.
- Payoff from IT investments is inadequate.
- There's too much "technology for technology's sake."
- Relations between IT users and IT specialists are poor.
- System designers do not consider users' preferences and work habits.

These problems are not new. Such lists have been circulating for the past 15 years, and companies have spent millions of dollars on consulting fees trying to resolve the problems—with little to show for their money. The problems are now so entrenched that top managers are adopting extreme attitudes and deploying extreme policies. Some outsource as many IT activities as possible, in the often mistaken belief that outsiders can manage the function better. Others cling to the vain hope that a new generation of "power users" will come to the rescue by developing creative software built around laptops and Internet browser software. We've even heard one executive declare that somebody should "just go ahead and blow up the IT function."

Why is there such confusion? Because information technology is at once exalted and feared. On the one hand, managers insist on elevating IT to the level of strategy; on the other, they recognize that integrating

Reprinted by permission of Harvard Business Review *76:5. From "The Right Mind-Set . . ." by M. Bensaou and Michael Earl, September/October 1998. Copyright © 1998 by the President and Fellows of Harvard College; all rights reserved. M. Bensaou is an associate professor of technology management and Asian business at INSEAD in Fontainebleau, France. Michael Earl is a professor at London Business School and the director of its Centre for Research in Information Management.*

IT with business goals is only marginally easier than reaching the summit of Everest. It can be done, but it's difficult—and the cost of failure is high.

We believe that Western managers should back away from the immediate problems. They need to reflect on how they are framing the underlying IT management issues. Too many executives in the West are intimidated by the task of managing technology. They tiptoe around it, supposing that it needs special tools, special strategies, and a special mind–set. Well, it doesn't. Technology should be managed—controlled, even—like any other competitive weapon in a manager's arsenal.

We revamped our own thinking in the course of a research project designed to compare Western and Japanese IT management. We were startled to discover that Japanese companies rarely experience the IT problems so common in the United States and Europe. In fact, their senior executives didn't recognize the problems when we described them. When we dug deeper into 20 leading companies that the Japanese themselves consider exemplary IT users, we found that the Japanese see IT as just one competitive lever among many. Its purpose, very simply, is to help the organization achieve its operational goals.

Where a Western CIO might spend time trying, often fruitlessly, to develop an IT strategy that perfectly mirrors the company's business strategy, a Japanese executive would skip that step entirely and base IT investment decisions on simple and easily quantified performance–improvement goals. Where a Western manager might go for a leading-edge application in the almost mystical belief that it would deliver competitive advantage, a Japanese manager would look at performance goals and choose the technology—whether old or new—that would help him achieve those goals (See the exhibit "How Japanese and Western Managers Frame IT Management.")

By now, some CEOs and CIOs may be shaking their heads in disbelief. In visits to Japan, they have found anything but a model to copy. After all, Japanese companies' expenditures on IT are perhaps half that of Western companies. Adoption of many modern technologies has been slow. The ratio of personal computers per capita in Japan compared with the United States, for example, is one to six, and computer use in offices is patchy. In short, the prevailing wisdom is that Japanese companies lag behind the West in IT and that Japanese managers could learn from U.S. and European practices. Some Japanese executives believe that themselves.

A second look reveals that the prevailing wisdom is wrong. In fact, we found five principles of IT management in Japan that struck us as powerful, important, and universal.

From Strategic Alignment to Strategic Instinct

The concept of strategic alignment arose in the West because many organizations discovered they were developing information systems that did not support their business strategies. Development projects were often given priority according to technical criteria rather than business imperatives, and funding commonly went to projects sponsored by groups with the most clout—often the finance function—rather than to projects with the most strategic importance. The solution to these evils was to develop an IT strategy. Thus IT vendors, consultants, and academics invented and sold planning techniques that aimed first at discovering a company's competitive strategy and second at suggesting an IS portfolio to support it. Strategic alignment would then be assured.

Unfortunately, the goal remained elusive. Business strategies were rarely as clear as expected; IT opportunities were poorly understood; the organization's parts had different priorities; and the IT strategies that were eventually drawn up often seemed devoid of common sense. So strategic alignment still heads CIO agendas—and the consulting gravy train still makes frequent runs.

The Japanese executives we interviewed had never considered developing a special IT strategy. They are far more comfortable thinking instead about operational goals. Information technology, seen in that context, is just a competitive lever that helps them reach those goals; it is not fundamentally different from quality, customer service, or new product development.

Consider the case of Seven–Eleven Japan, a company that has invested aggressively and successfully in IT for many years. One could argue that the company's strong performance rests on its IT investments. Yet when we asked executives for the strategic logic underlying those investments, all we got was a long list of incremental improvements dating back to 1974. In each case, an operational objective that reflected a customer need had driven the improvement. Executives, looking back, could describe with great specificity how those customer needs were met. Thus the company has spent more than 20 years learning how to satisfy its customers better; we can label that process "strategic" after the fact, but that's not a term the company's managers would volunteer.

Since Seven–Eleven Japan's inception, founder Toshifumi Suzuki has been obsessed with convenience, quality, service, and the continual application of IT to capture customers' needs better. The company has built an information system that rivals any in the West for just–in–time logistics excellence and deep knowledge of the company's customers. Japanese consumers place a high premium on freshness, for example, and the company started making multiple daily deliveries as early as 1978, modeling itself on Toyota's groundbreaking just–in–time system. Now stores receive four batches of fresh inventory each day. The stores' fresh food changes over entirely three times per day, which allows managers to change their physical layout throughout the day, as the flow of customers shifts from housewives to students to salary men.

This just–in–time system allows the stores to be extraordinarily responsive to consumers' shifting tastes. If a particular kind of *bento* (take–out lunch box) sells out by noon, for example, extra stock can be in the stores by early afternoon. If it's raining, bentos won't be in high demand, so the number delivered will go down—but the system will remind operators to put umbrellas on sale next to the cash register. This level of responsiveness is made possible by a sophisticated point–of–sale data–collection system and an electronic ordering system that links individual stores to a central distribution area.

Seven–Eleven Japan's early investment in those systems, and its constant additions to them, have paid off handsomely. The company is now the largest and most profitable retailer in Japan. Since its creation in the early 1970s, it has continually increased the number of stores, as well as each store's average profit margin and average daily sales, and it has reduced the average turnover time of its stock. Seven–Eleven Japan has been so successful that it recently took over its troubled parent, the Southland Corporation, owner of the U.S. 7–Eleven chain.

What is striking about this example is that investment in IT follows a logic of strategic instinct rather than strategic alignment—although in hindsight, alignment appears to be there. Seven–Eleven Japan's focus on customer satisfaction, product quality, and service makes sense to customers, suppliers, and store managers. These focal points drive not only IT investment but also logistics, sales, store management, and relationships with suppliers and wholesalers. Furthermore, the strategic instinct driving the investments legitimizes a process of ongoing learning in which a small initiative can evolve into an ever bigger one: bolder and better ideas emerge and are developed in a process of learning by doing; that is, by making strategy in small steps.

As we're framing it, strategic instinct almost always reflects a fundamental, down–to–earth source of competitiveness (usually related, in Japan, to operational excellence or customer knowledge). It combines the "what" and the "how" of competitive strategy—both defining strategic intent and envisioning its implementation. That source of competitiveness is the determining actor in decisions made throughout the company. It drives business development even when—as is often the case—there is no formal business strategy in place at all. And it is why IT is seen not as something special, different, and problematic, but rather as part of a fully integrated picture.

From Value for Money to Performance Improvement

Appraising the return on IT investments has never been simple in the West. Both costs and benefits can seem uncertain. Many companies have introduced investment management processes akin to capital budgeting hoping to legitimize IT projects and ensure management commitment to them. In other companies, CEOs and CFOs periodically demand audits of projects, investigations into how much value IT investments have delivered, and one–off accounting of the total corporate expenditure on IT. Such concerns about affordability and return on IT investment are neither irrational nor improper. After all, information technology should not be exempt from the pursuit of shareholder value, and in some industries the cost of IT is so high that it is, properly, a strategic question. However, the cumulative and pervasive value–for–money mind–set can be destructive. It can bias investment decisions toward cost–saving automation projects; it can deter ideas for revenue–generating IT applications; and it can lead to the dangerously late adoption of IT infrastructure improvements. It also carries an implicit message that IT is something to be exploited only when benefits are obvious and certain.

In Japanese corporations, IT projects are not assessed primarily by financial metrics; audits and formal approval for investments are rare. Instead, because operational performance goals drive most IT investments, the traditional metric is performance improvement, not value for money.

We recall an IT investment decision in a large Japanese food and drink company. Retailers were demanding the ever speedier replenishment of stock, so the company had to improve its supply chain management. In the course of reexamining their logistics, group managers concluded that they couldn't solve the problem without a new information system. Once they'd reached that conclusion, the next steps were never in doubt. The managers involved—the directors of logistics, supply and purchasing, IT, and planning—simply developed new system requirements and approved the expenditure. There was no concern about whether the new project had been part of a capital budget or IT plan, or whether it met a threshold rate of return. If supply chain improvement was vital, so was the system: end of story.

The fact that investment decisions are not financially based doesn't mean they're fuzzy. In many companies, the operational performance goals are articulated with fine–grained specificity. Seven–Eleven Japan has translated its focus on convenience, quality, and service into five areas of special concern: item selection, item–by–item control, new product development, quality or freshness of products, and value–added services. If an IT investment supports improvement in one of those areas, it not only justifies itself but also can be validated easily by operational efficiency measures.

The Japanese preference for continuous improvement and incremental advances means that a lot of IT spending comes in small steps. However, major investments are also driven by broad operational–performance goals. Matsushita, for example has been pursuing order–of–magnitude reductions in the lead times for product development and for order taking and fulfillment. Those operational goals recently drove an investment by the company of 32 billion yen in a telecommunications network that will link 140 overseas production sites and sales offices by 1999. The goals also include financial targets that the networked businesses are expected to achieve.

What underpins this performance–improvement principle is the idea of *gemba*, or support for people on the front line, whether they are in manufacturing, supply, or sales. The front line is where investment can be made most effectively—investment in IT or training or simply in the tools to do the job. Such a core value makes the justification of systems intuitive. Very often a business case is never explicitly documented or argued: a gemba case is obvious. Only one sort of audit follows: Are we improving performance as targeted and, if not, what must we do?

The principle of performance improvement is not so easily applied in the domain of organizational computing. But, as we shall see, another Japanese principle comes into play there.

From Technology Solutions to Appropriate Technology

Executives in the West often complain about the phenomenon of "technology for technology's sake." Indeed, some IT vendors and consultants pride themselves on offering "technology solutions." But most would–be customers want to know what the problem or opportunity is first.

The dynamics of the technology–solutions philosophy are clear. Vendors need to create markets for new technologies. IT specialists want to try out the latest and greatest technology toys. Users can't necessarily judge what's possible until they use a new technology, so they depend on the judgment of IT specialists. And sometimes, especially in the United States, people are proud of adopting new technologies ahead of the rest of the world. That bias can lead to wonderful results: the growth of the Internet and the World Wide Web, for example. But it has a dark side, too. Most executives can recall more than one system that was too advanced for the needs of the company and other systems that were redesigned even though they were still perfectly adequate.

So on the one hand, we see IT pioneers in the West introducing and adopting leading–edge technology that often yields early–mover advantages. On the other hand, we see unnecessary investments and many new developments in technology that promise a lot but deliver little. It is a curious mix but may be the inevitable outcome of a society devoted to technological advancement.

Japan has an equally curious mix. The Japanese run some of the best–designed, most technologically advanced factories in the world. Managers and scholars from around the world visit these factories to observe legendary uses of advanced manufacturing technology, robotics, computer–integrated manufacturing, and flexible manufacturing systems. And, as we have seen, some Japanese retail companies are extremely sophisticated in their collection and use of data on customer needs and habits. Increasingly, manufacturing companies are, too. Kao, the leading Japanese cosmetics and soap company, stores all customer complaints (and the advice the customers received) in a database; that database is a major source of ideas for engineers in the new product–development group.

Most Japanese offices, on the other hand, are low tech. PCs are scarce, and they're outnumbered by "dumb" terminals; decision—support and executive—information systems are mostly alien concepts; and e–mail and groupware adoption is slow. There are some readily apparent explanations for those absences. Until recently, computers have not coped well with the kanji characters of the Japanese writing system. Most managers are not used to keyboards. And the IT vendor marketplace has not been open to international competition. We would argue, however, that there is a more important underlying reason.

The Western bias is toward technology for technology's sake. The Japanese bias, in contrast, is toward adopting appropriate technology. Managers identify the task to be accomplished and the desired level of performance; then they select a technology that will help the company achieve that level in a way that suits the people doing the work. Once again, the operational goal drives the choice of technology. Three cases demonstrate the point.

In factories, operational goals can often be achieved best through the aggressive use of advanced manufacturing technologies—often, but not always. A typical Japanese factory has a lot of high tech areas alongside a few low–tech islands where human judgment is still needed.

NSK, one of the world's leading bearings and auto components manufacturers, is a good example. It has highly integrated technology systems, but certain areas are still low tech. For simulation and analysis in component design, engineers use the company's flexible—engineering information—control system and an array of databases and expert systems. But the engineers themselves develop and approve final designs. Similarly, the company's salespeople can search a database and narrow the range of products that they might suggest to a customer, but they make the final judgment about what to offer. (Once they've made that decision, they can immediately obtain a blueprint of the appropriate product design from a fax machine connected to the expert system.) And quality engineers use handheld terminals to monitor quality data, which is automatically recorded from in–line sensors and inspection machines. Although they are well supported technically, they are still walking around the factory, using their eyes and ears to assess progress. A high–tech solution would have been to place the engineers in a separate room, monitoring quality data remotely. All these IT systems are linked to a budgetary control system; during board meetings, senior executives can access the various databases from on-line terminals.

In nonfactory settings, the Japanese use advanced or even conventional technologies more tentatively. In a study of IT use in buyer–supplier relations in Japan and the United States, one of the authors of this article found that parties from both countries exchanged order and quotation data in electronic form. However, U.S. companies used electronic data interchange (EDI) extensively, whereas most Japanese companies still relied on tapes, disks, and courier mail. The Japanese companies had judged the use of EDI to be premature. They wanted to construct effective partnerships first, and then consider how IT could help. In other words, they didn't assume that advanced forms of electronic communication were advantageous.

Finally, consider one technology tool that's often used in Western companies—executive information systems—and another that has been advocated for years—decision support systems. In Japanese corporations, few executives use these systems directly. Why? Because they don't fit well with how decisions get made in Japan. Typically, a top manager in Japan will float an initial idea to a broad group of people throughout the company. They will then discuss and analyze the idea until a consensus about its value emerges. Some employees may raise objections, and their criticisms will lead to modifications in the original idea. Other critics may be coopted with promises of future concessions. These informal negotiations are a highly valued, central part of Japanese decision–making culture. The extensive discussion period means that executive—information and decision—support systems have so far not been appropriate technologies in Japan.

Organizational decision making in Japan is starting to change, however. Many office settings have not felt much market pressure to change until recently. World–class competitors could overlook low office productivity because they were growing so quickly and because they faced little competition from imported goods. In practice, the result has been far muddier operational goals in white–collar settings than in factories.

Economic and competitive pressures have focused managers' attention on white–collar productivity As a result, technology is replacing people in some aspects of information processing. And major electronics companies such as Toshiba, Fujitsu, and NEC have introduced electronic networks to speed up decision making. The networks enable managers to share information more efficiently, to send and receive documents and proposals, to schedule meetings, and to vote on proposals. But serious efforts are being made to preserve the face–to–face discussions between key stakeholders.

From IS User Relations to Organizational Bonding

Although the IT function in Western companies is often relatively decentralized, users frequently perceive it as centralized. They think that specialists are remote and have too much control. And they complain that IT people know nothing about the business: "By the time we educate the IT people about the real world, they've left the company," said one line manager we know.

Indeed the labels "user and specialist," while accurate, also help create two cultures. Differences in vocabulary only exacerbate the divide. As one European CIO remarked to us recently, "When an executive says 'Okay, show me how we can use IT strategically,' the IT folks start talking about data architecture."

Western companies have introduced bridging devices to solve these problems, with mixed results. People who serve in liaison roles that are designed to close the gap often end up as middlemen who only keep the two sides apart. Creating hybrid managers—people who are knowledgeable about business and IT—sounds appealing, but the hybrids soon discover they're stuck in a career cul–de–sac.

Once again, a first look at the organization of IT in Japan seems far from promising. The IT function has low status; it is not a place in which to make one's reputation. Career IT specialists tend to be regarded as engineers rather than businesspeople. Often the IT department is run as an "offshore bureau"; that is, it is not structurally integrated with the rest of the organization. And there are few high-profile CIOs.

On closer examination, however, we found four characteristics of Japanese companies that encourage integration, or organizational bonding, between IT and the business.

First, many Japanese managers spend two or three years, usually against their wishes, in an IT department as part of a job rotation scheme. The postings help them develop knowledge that will prove useful in subsequent jobs. They provide managers not only with technological know–how but also with knowledge about how to get things done in IT and about who can help with what. The rotations can be seen as an institutionalized version of Western companies, creation of hybrid managers.

Second, when IT projects are in progress, IT specialists are usually co-located with the users and managers for whom the application is being developed. Co-location improves communication and understanding between users and specialists; it is another way of encouraging bonding.

Third, the senior executives in charge of IT are usually in charge of one or two other functions as well—often finance and planning. This practice prevents IT from being isolated within the company.

We recall the case of a Japanese beverage company that urgently needed a new order–processing system. No elaborate planning study was done, no format capital–expenditure proposals were drawn up, and there was no bargaining between the interested parties about who should pay for what. The directors of IT, finance, and planning sorted it out very quickly. How? They were the same person. Many conflicts between departments can be avoided when senior managers have overlapping responsibilities; integration and bonding can occur quite naturally.

Finally, Japanese IT departments rely heavily on their vendors for advice. Japanese companies seldom use off–the–shelf packaged software; they usually develop applications in–house, working closely with a dedicated vendor. For example, Seven–Eleven Japan has since its creation entrusted the software and hardware design of its integrated information system to the Nomura Research Institute, the second–largest systems integrator in Japan. Such long–term relationships can constrain experimentation and the adoption of radically new and diverse technologies. But they ensure a committed partnership on large projects, and they help users and specialists develop a mutual understanding of appropriate technologies. The relationships are another means of organizational bonding.

We stress organizational bonding because none of the distinguishing features noted above is structural in nature. That is, they do not depend on setting up committees, creating new liaison roles, or tinkering with the degree of centralization—all devices that are favored in the West. The focus is on proximity, cross training, shared understanding, and relationships. And once again, the Japanese are not treating IT as something that requires special handling.

From Systems Design to Human Design

In the West, system development tends to focus more on the business process being supported or re-designed than on the people who will use the product. Perhaps as a result, people often find new systems difficult to use, counterintuitive, and annoying. Moreover, if you asked people the radical question, How much have IT systems increased job satisfaction? you'd soon learn that IT systems have de–skilled and routinized far more work than they have enriched. Our point is not that job enrichment should be the goal of IT development, but rather that specialists often leave no room in their systems for human judgment or understanding when they become overly focused on technological "solutions."

In Japan, building systems is not an end in itself; enhancing the contribution of people is the higher goal. That's why the principle of "human designer is central to the way the Japanese use IT. If a system automates work that people can do better, it is not considered a good system—and the potential for that result is raised explicitly when an IT project is under consideration.

Consider again the question of whether decision support technologies should be used in organizational decision making. Two aspects of Japanese organizational behavior militate against the practice. The first is the belief that broad participation and consensus not only facilitate commitment but also produce better decisions.

The second is the Japanese reliance on social and experiential processes of knowledge creation.[1] Japanese executives are deeply aware of the importance of tacit knowledge—knowledge that cannot be fully communicated with words and numbers, such as things we don't know we know and things we can't easily explain. Information technology, of course, is much better suited to processing explicit knowledge than tacit knowledge. That's why, when difficult problems arise in development projects, Honda uses brainstorming camps rather than "data mining," computer–aided design, or simulations.

Matsushita's process for developing an automatic bread–making machine illustrates the Japanese awareness of tacit knowledge. The project development team found that when they x–rayed and analyzed dough kneaded by a master baker, they didn't learn much. Rather than continue down an unpromising technological path, team members—led by the head of software development—apprenticed themselves to the best master baker in Osaka. By observing the traditional craft of kneading and twisting dough, and by learning it themselves, they discovered the secret of making good bread.

Because of this very Japanese concern for capturing human knowledge—and also, incidentally, commitment—the process of system design usually involves nonspecialists. When production systems at NSK were being designed, the president announced that the heads of sales, production, and design, as well as the plant managers, would be required to help design and promote the system.

We believe that Seven–Eleven Japan has been so successful not because of its IT systems (though they are world class) but because of its substantial investment in training and supporting front–line workers in the use of those systems. Chairman Suzuki is very clear about the paramount importance of using information intelligently: "It is not enough to exchange information. The information has no value unless it is understood and properly integrated by the franchises and allows them to work better."

Seven–Eleven Japan's franchise operators receive far more training about inputting and interpreting data than do store managers in any other franchise system we know of. In addition, the company has 1,000 operational field counselors who provide the human backup to the distribution system. Each counselor supervises six or seven stores, which he visits two or three times a week to exchange information, criticism, and suggestions. Through this face–to–face contact, franchise operators learn to analyze local data, develop ideas about what they should be ordering, and test their ideas against corporate headquarters' suggestions. The company spends more than $1 million per year on weekly meetings that bring all the field counselors together in Tokyo.

Respect for people also explains why Japanese companies use extensive prototyping and opt for continuous improvement in systems development: Both approaches require the subtleties of human judgment. Both allow systems to be adjusted so that they fit job and work design better. And both are more responsive to user ideas and suggestions than is conventional, formal system development.

It's interesting to remember that Toyota's influential quality circles began as a grassroots movement: factory workers were simply trying to improve the quality of their work life. That their movement was encouraged and co–opted by management suggests how central people are in this incremental approach to system design. Indeed, the subsequent

TQM movement may have influenced Japan's evolutionary approach to systems design.

The philosophy that underpins the principle of valuing people is *chowa*, or harmonization, which is a powerful idea in Japanese culture. In the specific case of managing IT, *chowa* means that technology should fit the people using it rather than the other way around.

Can the West Really Reinvent IT Management?

When considering the five principles outlined here, executives may say, "But we do some of this already. Is this really so different?" We agree that some Western companies are attempting to put into practice some of the ideas we have explored. For example, many companies have thrown out long–term IS planning. And many IT professionals could tell you that their biggest success came at a time when most of the organization's IT resources were focused on a single project that everyone believed was critical to the business. Very often the project started in a small way and grew because of its obvious value. But such experiences have not developed into a principle of strategic instinct. Indeed, many companies still wonder what sort of IT strategy–making process they should adopt.

Some companies do take nonfinancial dimensions into account in IT project appraisals; others admit to unanticipated benefits from some of their IT investments. However, most find it hard to break out of the value–for–money mind–set or to realize that some IT investments have a straightforward support role in business; namely, enabling performance improvement.

Many companies would claim that they avoid leading–edge technologies, stating that "leading edge is bleeding edge." However, the principle of appropriate technology is subtly different: sometimes the most advanced form of IT makes sense, and sometimes simpler, older forms will do. Sometimes high tech should cohabit with low tech.

Other companies continue to experiment with bridge building between the IT function and IT users. What they do not usually recognize is that the integration of IT with the organization has to be from top to bottom and systemic, not structural. In other words, bridges will collapse as long as there's one IT culture and another business culture, but the principle of organizational bonding will keep them strong and stable.

Western companies have tried experimenting with sociotechnical systems development, with ergonomics and "user friendliness," and with less technocratic approaches to information processing. However, those approaches lack a key ingredient: they treat people only as users of systems and do not value them as complements—and even alternatives—to systems.

Another challenge to our ideas is that the Japanese management of IT is culturally specific. Of course, it's not wise—it's probably not possible—simply to overlay practices from one culture onto a very different one. Western managers learned that lesson in the early 1980s, during their first attempt to imitate Japanese manufacturing techniques. However, it is possible to learn from other cultures if it's understood that first some translation is required. Ultimately, Western managers learned a great deal from Japanese manufacturing, but first they needed to differentiate between underlying principles that can be transferred (like lean manufacturing) and culturally specific practices that may or may not work in a different setting like daily quality circles).

Indeed, we believe that the vogue for benchmarking and copying best practices can be dangerous. Business practices are heavily influenced by national culture, industry traditions, and company–level characteristics. It makes more sense to focus instead on best principles. If you understand why a practice works and what distinguishes it fundamentally from conventional practice, you can probably identify the underlying principle involved. That universal idea can then be transported and applied to fit a local context. Certainly the five principles described here can be transferred. There's nothing culturally specific about choosing appropriate technology or about developing an IT system to support well–articulated operational goals.

It's tempting to think about our five IT–management principles at a cultural or national level. "Americans value individualism, so appropriate technology in the United States will support independent decision making," for example. However, we suspect that the principles can best be interpreted, adopted, and customized at the company level, because that's where competitive strategy is developed and played out.

We set out, very simply, to compare Japanese and Western IT–management practices. To our surprise, we found principles—strategic instinct, performance improvement, appropriate technology, organizational bonding, and human design—that we believe are hidden strengths in many Japanese corporations. And these strengths should serve them extremely well as they search for new levels of competitiveness.

At the moment, Western managers are not inclined to think in terms of learning from Japan—or anywhere else. But that could be a grave

---

This concept and the illustrations that follow are drawn from Ikujiro Nonaka and Hirotaka Takeuchi, The Knowledge Creating Company *(Oxford University Press, 1995).*

error. All appearances to the contrary, this may be a more dangerous time for U.S. businesses than it is for Japan's. The Japanese *know* they have to find new ways to compete. U.S. managers, in contrast, are in danger of supposing they'll be on top of the international heap forever.

It's time for senior managers to regain control of technology in their companies: to abandon the dangerous idea that IT requires special, technocratic means of management. As many executives have begun to suspect, the IT management traditions that have evolved over the last 40 years are flawed. Powerful IT vendors, management consultants, and specialists developed those ideas and profited from them. In the end, even those constituencies have begun to doubt their gospels. It is time for Western companies to rethink how they manage technology. The principles underlying Japanese practice provide an excellent foundation.

Managing the IT Procurement Process

Robert Heckman

Abstract

This article presents a process model of IT procurement, which was developed by a group of senior managers who make up the Society for Information Management (SIM) Working Group on IT Procurement. The model systematically describes the processes involved in IT procurement and is a useful tool for bringing managerial discipline to the increasingly important activity of IT procurement.

An IT procurement process, formal or informal, exists in every organization that acquires information technology. As users of information systems increasingly find themselves in roles as customer of multiple technology vendors, this IT procurement process assumes greater management significance. In addition to hardware, operating system software, and telecommunications equipment and services—information resources traditionally acquired in the marketplace—organizations now turn to outside providers for many components of their application systems, application development and integration, and a broad variety of system management services. Yet despite this trend, to date there has been little, if any, research investigating the IT procurement process.

Reprinted with permission from Information Systems Management *16 (1), Winter 1999. Copyright CRC Press, Boca Raton, Florida. Robert Heckman is professor of information studies at Syracuse University.*

Although IS development activities are represented by at least 120 keywords in the keyword classification scheme for IS research literature, market–oriented strategies for information resource acquisition are represented by a single keyword—"Outsourcing of IS."

Several studies of IT procurement issues recently have been commissioned by the Society for Information Management (SIM) Working Group on IT Procurement. These studies are an attempt to begin a systematic investigation of critical IT procurement issues. This article presents a model of the IT procurement process, which was developed by the SIM Working Group to provide a framework for studying IT procurement. This model has provided the conceptual context for the Working Group's empirical research projects and a framework for organizing key issues and questions. The model represents IT procurement as consisting of six major processes. Contained within each major process is a series of subprocesses and a set of key questions.

Background

IT procurement is an interdisciplinary process, typically involving staff members from the IS organization, purchasing, legal, financial/treasury, and end users from all departments and services available. The speed with which new products are introduced to the marketplace make IT procurement an extremely intricate and volatile process. Two relatively recent trends suggest that a disciplined, process-oriented framework might be needed to help users better understand and manage the complex IT procurement activity. The first trend is the evolution of the information resource acquisition process from an internal, unstructured, craft-like activity to a more structured, market-oriented discipline. The second trend is the recent expanded focus on business process analysis and design.

Evolution of the Information Resource Acquisition Process

In 1996, Heckman and Sawyer described an information resource (IR) acquisition model, which characterizes the acquisition process using two dimensions: source and process. Exhibit I shows the model, which illustrates that an IR can be acquired from an internal source throughout the firm. This complex organization structure, the great number of different products (hierarchy) or external (market) source, and the acquisition process can be either structured or unstructured. Exhibit I also shows how the model can be used to illustrate the evolution of information resource acquisition in organizations over time.

EXHIBIT 1   Evolution of the Information Resource Acquisition Process

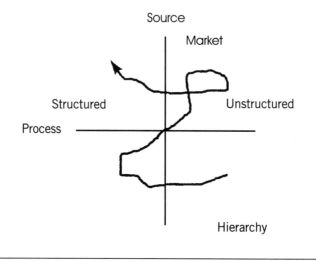

Exhibit I suggests that, in the early years of computing, organizations developed many of their systems internally using relatively
unstructured processes. As experience with system development grew,
more structured methods of analysis, design, and programming were
developed, and software construction began to evolve from a craft–
like activity to an engineering discipline. As information technology
price performance dramatically improved and microcomputers became
available, the era of end user computing began. In this era, organizations
tended to turn outward to the market to meet more of their information
resource needs, but they did so with relatively little structure or discipline
in the process. Finally, in the current era, organizations are recognizing
the need to bring more order to their IR acquisition activities. As
client/server architectures become more complex and interconnected,
the need for more disciplined management of the procurement process
also will grow. The IS literature has begun to address this need indirectly in debates about the appropriate management of IT outsourcing
relationships.

One way to impose discipline or structure on a process is to develop
a framework, which allows the process to be analyzed and managed
in a systematic way. An example of such a framework is the traditional
systems development life cycle (SDLC). The SDLC framework allowed
discipline to be introduced to the process of systems analysis and design and laid the groundwork for the development of methodologies
intended to improve reliability and productivity.[2–5] It enabled not
only the creation of structured analysis and design tools, but also made

possible systems development approaches that transcend the traditional SDLC. It can be argued that the SDLC was an essential evolutionary step, which made possible the more advanced approaches of rapid prototyping, object–oriented analysis, joint application development (JAD), etc. The IT Procurement Process framework might provide a similar evolutionary function.

Business Process Analysis and Design

Business process analysis and redesign has become an important management tool for both American and global businesses. Davenport and Short define a business process as "a set of logically related tasks performed to achieve a defined business outcome."[6] Business processes are generally independent of organizational structure, and this attribute has led to great interest in business process redesign (BPR). In BPR, important business processes are decomposed and reassembled in ways that are intended to be more efficient and effective. Techniques and principles for the analysis and design of business processes have been promulgated widely; however, all have in common the necessity to identify, understand, and measure the components or subprocesses that comprise a critical business process.

The process framework described next attempts to accomplish this objective in the IT procurement domain. It provides a comprehensive description of the processes and subprocesses that are involved in procuring IT products and services. By identifying and describing the process in detail, efforts to analyze, measure, and redesign IT procurement activities can begin from a firm foundation.

Development of the Framework

In January 1994, the Society for Information Management (SM Working Group on Information Technology Procurement) was formed to exchange information on managing IT procurement and to foster collaboration among the different professions participating in the IT procurement process. The IT Procurement Process Framework was developed by a twelve–member subgroup comprised of senior IT procurement executives from large North American companies.

The task of developing the framework took place over the course of several meetings and lasted approximately one year. A modified nominal group process was used in which individual members independently developed frameworks that described the IT procurement process as they understood it.

In a series of several work sessions, these individual models were synthesized and combined to produce the six–process framework presented next. Once the six major procurement processes had been identified, a modified nominal group process was followed once again to elicit the subprocesses to be included under each major process. Finally, a nominal group process was used once again to elicit a set of key issues, which the group felt presented managerial challenges in each of the six processes. The key issues were conceived of as the critical questions that must be addressed successfully to manage each process effectively. Thus they represent the most important issues faced by those executives responsible for the management of the IT procurement function.

The process framework and key issues were reviewed by the Working Group approximately one year later (Summer, 1996), and modifications to definitions, subprocesses, and key issues were made at that time. The key issue content analysis described next was conducted following the most recent Working Group review in early 1997.

The IT Procurement Framework: Processes, Subprocesses, and Key Issues

The IT Procurement Process Framework provides a vehicle to describe systematically the processes and subprocesses involved in IT procurement. Exhibit 2 illustrates six major processes in IT procurement activities. Each of these major processes consists of a number of subprocesses. Exhibits 3 through 8 list the subprocesses included in each of the major processes. These tables also include the key issues identified by the Working Group. Procurement activities can be divided into two distinct types of processes, deployment processes and management processes.

Deployment Processes

Deployment Processes consist of activities that are performed (to a greater or lesser extent) each time an IT product or service is acquired. Each individual procurement can be thought of in terms of a life cycle that begins with requirements determination, proceeds through activities involved in the actual acquisition of a product or service, and is completed as the terms specified in the contract are fulfilled. Each IT product or service that is acquired has its own individual iteration of this deployment life cycle.

Requirements determination: Requirements determination is the process of determining the business justification, requirements, specifications, and approvals to proceed with the procurement process. It includes subprocesses such as organizing project teams, using cost-benefit or other analytic techniques to justify investments, defining alternatives, assessing relative risks and benefits defining specifications,

EXHIBIT 2   The IT Procurement Process

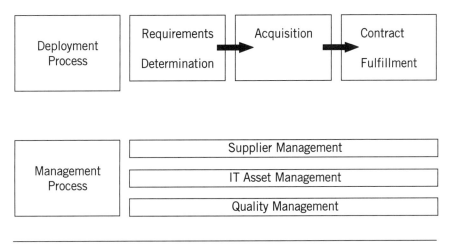

and obtaining necessary approvals to proceed with the procurement process (Exhibit 3).

Acquisition: Acquisition is the process of evaluating and selecting appropriate suppliers and completing procurement arrangements for the required products and services. It includes identification of sourcing alternatives, generating communications (such as RFPs and RFQs) to suppliers, evaluating supplier proposals, and negotiating contracts with suppliers (Exhibit 4).

Contract Fulfillment: Contract fulfillment is the process of managing and coordinating all activities involved in fulfilling contract requirements. It includes expedition of orders, acceptance of products or services, installation of systems, contract administration, management of post-installation services such as warranty and maintenance, and disposal of obsolete assets (Exhibit 5).

Supplier Management: Supplier management is the process of optimizing customer–supplier relationships to add value to the business. It includes activities such as development of a supplier portfolio strategy, development of relationship strategies for key suppliers, assessing and influencing supplier performance, and managing communication with suppliers (Exhibit 6).

Asset Management: Asset management is the process of optimizing the utilization of all IT assets throughout their entire life cycle to meet the needs of the business. It includes activities such as development of asset management strategies and policies, development and maintenance of asset management information systems, evaluation of the life cycle cost of IT asset ownership, and management of asset redeployment and disposal policies (Exhibit 7).

Quality Management: Quality management is the process of assuring continuous improvement in the IT procurement process and in all products and services acquired for IT purposes in an organization. It includes activities such as product testing, statistical process control, acceptance testing, quality reviews with suppliers, and facility audits (Exhibit 8).

EXHIBIT 3   Requirements Determination

Definition

The process of determining the business justification, requirements, specifications, and approvals to proceed with the procurement process.

Subprocesses

- Identify need.
- Put together cross–functional team and identify roles and responsibilities.
- Continuously refine requirements and specifications in accordance with user needs.
- Gather information regarding alternative solutions.
- Perform cost–benefit analysis or other analytic technique to justify expenditure.
- Evaluate alternative solutions (including build/buy, in-house/outsource, etc.) and associated risk and benefits.
- Develop procurement plans that are integrated with project plans.
- Gain approval for the expenditure.
- Develop preliminary negotiation strategies.

Key Issues

- What are the important components of an appropriate procurement plan? [S]
- How much planning (front–end loading) is appropriate or necessary for different types of acquisitions (e.g., commodity purchases versus complex, unique acquisitions)? [S]
- How should project teams be configured for different types of acquisitions (appropriate internal and external resources, project leader, etc.)? [IR]
- How should changes in scope and changes in orders be handled? [P]
- What are the important costs versus budget considerations? [P]
- What are the most effective methods of obtaining executive commitment? [E]

- Can requirements be separated from wants? [P]
- Should performance specifications and other outputs be captured for use in later phases such as quality management? [P]

EXHIBIT 4   Acquisition

Definition

The process of evaluating and selecting appropriate suppliers and completing procurement arrangements for the required products and services

Subprocesses

- Develop sourcing strategy including the short list of suitable suppliers.
- Generate appropriate communication to suppliers (RFP, RFQ, etc.) including financing alternatives.
- Analyze and evaluate supplier responses and proposals.
- Plan formal negotiation strategy.
- Negotiate Contract.
- Review contract terms and conditions.
- Award contract and execute documents.
- Identify value added from the negotiation using appropriate metrics.

Key Issues

- Is these support of corporate purchasing programs, policies, and guidelines (which can be based on technology, financing, accounting, competitive impacts, social impacts, etc.)? [E]
- What tools optimize the procurement process? [P]

  ___ EDI
  ___ Autofax
  ___ Procurement Cards

- What processes in the acquisition phase can be eliminated, automated, or minimized? [P]
- Is it wise to be outsourcing all or part of the procurement process? [IR]
- What are the appropriate roles of users, legal, purchasing, and IS in the procurement process?[IR]

EXHIBIT 5   Contract Fulfillment

Definition

The process of managing and coordinating all activities involved in fulfilling contract requirements

Subprocesses

- Expedite orders and facilitate required changes
- Receive material and supplies, update databases, and reconcile discrepancies
- Acceptance of hardware, software, or services
- Deliver materials and services as required, either direct or to drop–off points
- Handle returns
- Installation of hardware, software, or services
- Contract administration
- Process invoices and issue payment to suppliers
- Resolve payment problems
- Manage post–installation services (e.g., warranty, maintenance, etc.)
- Resolve financial status and physical disposal of excess or obsolete assets
- Maintain quality records

Key Issues

- What are some provisions for early termination and renewals? [L]
- What are the best methods for assessing vendor strategies for ongoing maintenance costs? [ER]
- What interaction between various internal departments aids the processes? [IR]

EXHIBIT 6   Supplier Management

Definition

The process of optimizing customer-supplier relationships to add value to the business

Subprocesses

- Categorize suppliers by value to the organization (e.g., volume, sole source, commodity, strategic alliance). Allocate resources to most important (key) suppliers.
- Develop and maintain a relationship strategy for each category of supplier.
- Establish and communicate performance expectations that are realistic and measurable.
- Monitor, measure, and assess vendor performance.
- Provide vendor feedback on performance metrics.
- Work with suppliers to improve performance continuously. Know when to say when.

- Continuously assess supplier qualifications against requirements (existing and potential suppliers).
- Ensure relationship roles and responsibilities are well defined.
- Participate in industry/technology information sharing with key suppliers.

Key Issues

- How does anyone distinguish between transactional/tactical and strategic relationships? [ER]
- How can expectations on both sides be managed most effectively? Should relationships be based on people–to–people understandings or solely upon the contractual agreement (get it in writing)? What is the right balance? [ER]
- How can discretionary collaborative behavior—cooperation above and beyond the letter of the contract—be encouraged? Are true partnerships with vendors possible, or does it take too long? What defines a partnership? [ER]
- How should multiple vendor relationships be managed? [ER]
- How should communication networks (both internal and external) be structured to optimize effective information exchange? Where are the most important roles and contact points? [IR]
- How formal should a measurement system be? What kind of report card is effective? What are appropriate metrics for delivery and quality? [M]
- What is the best way continuously to assess the ability of a vendor to go forward with new technologies? [M]
- What legal aspects of the relationship are of most concern (e.g., nondisclosure, affirmative action, intellectual property, etc.)? [L]
- What is the best way to keep current with IT vendor practices and trends? What role does maintaining market knowledge play in supplier management? [M]
- What is the optimal supplier–management strategy for a given environment? [S]
- How important is the development of master contract language? [L]
- In some sectors there is an increasing number of suppliers and technologies, although in the others vendor consolidation is occurring. In what circumstances should the number of relationships be expanded or reduced? [ER]
- What are the best ways to get suppliers to buy into master agreements? [L] What are the best ways continuously to judge vendor financial stability? [M]
- Where is the supplier positioned in the product life cycle? [M]
- How should suppliers be categorized (e.g., strategic, key, new, etc.) to allow for prioritization of efforts? [M]
- What are the opportunities and concerns to watch for when one IT supplier is acquired by another? [M]

EXHIBIT 7   Asset Management

Definition

The process the utilization of all IT assets throughout their entire life cycle to meet the needs of the business

Subprocesses

- Develop and maintain asset management strategies and policies. Identify and determine which assets to track; they may include hardware, software licenses, and related services.
- Implement and maintain appropriate asset management databases, systems, and tools.
- Develop a disciplined process to track and control inventory to facilitate such things as budgeting, help desk, life-cycle management, software release distribution, capital accounting, compliance monitoring, configuration planning, procurement leverage, redeployment planning, change management, disaster recovery planning, software maintenance, warranty coverage, lease management, and agreement management.
- Identify the factors that make up the total life cycle cost of ownership.
- Communicate a software license compliance policy throughout the organization.

Key Issues

- What assets are included in IT asset management (e.g., data, human resources, consumables, courseware)? [F]
- How can legal department holdups be reduced? [P]
- What is the best way to communicate corporatewide agreements? [IR]
- How should small ticket assets be handled? [P]
- How does a company move from reactive to proactive contracting? [S]
- Are there ways of dealing with licenses that require counts of users? [L]
- What are the best ways of managing concurrent software licensing? [L]
- Can one be contacting for efficiency using national contracts for purchase, servicing, licensing? [P]
- How can software be managed and tracked as an asset? [F]
- How can the workload in software contracting be reduced? [P]
- Are there ways to encourage contract administration to be handled by the vendor? [P]
- Is it possible to manage all three life cycles simultaneously: technical, functional, and economical? [S]

- How does a company become proactive in risk management? [S]
- What is the appropriate assignment of internal responsibilities (e.g., compliance)? [IR]
- Do all items need to be tracked? [P]
- How much control (a) can the company afford? (b) does the company need? (c) does the company want? [F]
- What are the critical success factors for effective asset management? [S]
- What practices are most effective for the redeployment of assets? [P]
- Are there adequate systems available to track both hard and soft assets? Are there any integrated solutions (support, tracking, and contract management)? [P]
- What are the best ways to handle the rapid increase in volume and rapid changes in technology? [P]
- What is the appropriate reaction to dwindling centralized control of the desktop with nonconformance to guidelines and procedures? [IR]
- Is there a true business understanding of the total cost of ownership over the entire life cycle of an asset? [F]
- What are the impacts on organizational structure? [IR]
- What kind of reporting is most effective? [P]
- How can one manage tax issues-indemnification, payments, and insurance issues? [F]
- What issues should be considered in end-of-lease processes? [P]

EXHIBIT 8   Quality Management

Definition

The process of assuring continuous improvement in all elements of the IT procurement framework

Subprocesses

- Define and track meaningful process metrics on an ongoing basis.
- Conduct periodic quality reviews with suppliers.
    - ___ Provide formal feedback to vendors on their performance.
    - ___ Facilitate open and honest communication in the process.
- Collect and prioritize ideas for process improvement.
- Use formal quality improvement efforts involving the appropriate people.
    - ___ Participants may include both internal resources and vendor personnel.

- Recognize and reward quality improvement results on an ongoing basis.

     ___ Recognize nonperformance/unsatisfactory results.

- Audit vendors' facilities and capabilities.
- Conduct ongoing performance tests against agreed upon standards.

     ___ e.g., acceptance test, stress test, regression test, etc.

- Utilize appropriate industry standards (e.g., ISO 900, SEI Capability Maturity).
- Periodically review vendors' statistical process control data.

Key Issues

- What is the best way to drive supplier quality management systems? [ER]
- What is the appropriate mix of audits (supplier/site/regional, etc.) for quality and procedural conformance?[M]
- What is the importance of relating this process to the earliest stages of the requirement determination process? [P]
- What corrective actions are effective? [P]
- When and how is it appropriate to audit a supplier's financials? [M]
- What is an effective way to audit material or services received? [M]
- What is the best way to build quality assurance into the process, as opposed to inspecting for quality after the fact? [P]
- What metrics are the most meaningful quantitative measures? [M]
- How can one best measure qualitative information, such as client satisfaction? [M]
- When should one use surveys, and how can they be designed effectively? [M]
- How often should measurements be done? [M]
- How does one ensure that the data collected is valid, current, and relevant? [M]
- What is the best medium and format to deliver the data to those who need it? [P]
- What are used performance and quality metrics for the IT procurement function? [M]
- How does one effectively recognize and reward quality improvement? [ER]
- When is it time to reengineer a process rather than just improve it? [P]
- How much communication between vendor and customer is needed to be effective? [ER]

Management Processes

Management Processes consist of those activities involved in the overall governance of IT procurement. These activities are not specific to any particular procurement event, but rather are generalized across all such events. Three general classes of IT procurement management processes are supplier management, asset management, and quality management.

Key IT Procurement Management Issues

Exhibits 3 through 8 contain 76 key IT procurement management issues identified by the members of the Working Group. These issues represent the beliefs of these domain experts concerning the most serious challenges facing managers of the IT Procurement function. To better understand the key issues a content analysis was performed to determine if there were a few main themes underlying these questions. The content analysis identified eight themes, which are shown in Exhibit 9, ranked according to the number of times each theme occurred in the key issue list. (Each theme in Exhibit 9 is labeled by a one—or two—letter code. These codes also appear in Exhibits 3 through 8 to indicate how each key issue was categorized.) The following themes were those that the rankings in Exhibit 9 suggest are most important to the senior procurement managers in the SIM Working Group.

Process Management, Design, and Efficiency

Practicing IT procurement managers are most concerned with the issue of how to make the procurement process more efficient. The questions that reflect this theme address the use of automated tools such as EDI and procurement cards, reducing cycle time in contracting processes, development and use of asset tracking systems and other reporting systems, and the integration of subprocesses at early and later stages of the procurement life cycle. The emergence of process efficiency as the leading issue may indicate that procurement managers are under pressure to demonstrate the economic value of their organizational contribution, and thus to follow the last decade's broad management trend of rigorously managing costs.

Measurement, Assessment, Evaluation

The second most important theme concerns the search for reliable and valid ways to evaluate and assess performance. This search for useful assessment methods and measures is directed both at external suppliers and at the internal procurement process itself. The latter focus

EXHIBIT 9 Ranked Themes in Key Issues

Rank	[Code]	Theme	# Key Issue Containing This Theme
1	[P]	Process management, design, and efficiency	21
2	[M]	Measurement, assessment, evaluation (of vendor and self)	16
3	[ER]	External relationships (with supplier)	9
4	[IR]	Internal relationships (internal teams, roles, communication)	9
5	[S]	Strategy and planning	7
6	[L]	Legal issues	6
7	[F]	Financial, total cost of ownership (TCO) issues	6
8	[E]	Executive support for procurement function	2

is consistent with the notion that procurement managers are looking for objective ways to assess and demonstrate their contribution. The focus on supplier assessment reflects an understanding that successful supplier relationships must be built on a foundation of high quality supplier performance.

Internal and External Relationships

The third and fourth most frequently cited themes deal with the issue of creating effective working relationships. The importance of such relationships is an outgrowth of the cross-functional nature of the IT procurement process within organizations and the general transition from internal to external sources for information resource (IR) acquisition. In 1994, Venkatraman and Loh characterized the IR acquisition process as having evolved from managing a portfolio of technologies to managing a portfolio of relationships, and the results of this analysis suggest that practicing managers agree.

Other Themes

The other issues that concern senior procurement managers are planning to develop an effective procurement strategy, legal problems, financial and total cost of ownership (TCO) concerns, and obtaining executive support for their activities.

A Management Agenda for the IT Procurement Process

The process framework and key issues identified by the SIM IT Procurement Working Group suggest an agenda for future efforts to improve the management of the IT procurement process. The agenda contains five action items that best may be carried out through a collaboration between practicing IT procurement managers and academic researchers. The action items are

1. Develop IT procurement performance metrics and use them to benchmark the IT procurement process.
2. Clarify roles in the procurement process to build effective internal and external relationships.
3. Use the procurement process framework as a tool to assist in reengineering the IT procurement process.
4. Use the framework as a guide for future research.
5. Use the framework to structure IT procurement training and education.

Develop IT procurement performance metrics and use them to benchmark the IT procurement process: Disciplined management of any process requires appropriate performance metrics, and members of the Working Group have noted that good metrics for the IT procurement processes are in short supply. The process framework is currently providing structure to an effort by the Working Group to collect a rich set of performance metrics that can be used to raise the level of IT procurement management. In this effort, four classes of performance metrics have been identified: (1) effectiveness metrics, (2) efficiency metrics, (3) quality metrics, and (4) cycle time metrics. Closely related to the metrics development issue is the need felt by many procurement professionals to benchmark critical procurement processes. The framework provides a guide to the process selection activity in the benchmarking planning stage. For example, the framework has been used by several companies to identify supplier management and asset management subprocesses for benchmarking.

Clarify roles in the procurement process to build effective internal and external relationships: IT procurement will continue to be a cross–functional process that depends on the effective collaboration of many different organizational factors for success. Inside the customer organization, representatives of IS, legal, purchasing, finance, and user departments must work together to buy, install, and use IT products and services. Partnerships and alliances with supplier and other organizations outside the boundaries of one's own firm are more necessary than ever as long–term outsourcing and consortia arrangements become more common. The key question is how these multifaceted relationships should be structured and managed. Internally, organizational structures, roles, standards, policies, and procedures must be developed, which facilitate effective cooperation. Externally, contracts must be crafted that clarify expectations and responsibilities between the parties. Recent research, however, suggests that formal mechanisms are not always the best means to stimulate collaboration. The most useful forms of collaboration are often discretionary—that is, they may be contributed or withheld without concern for formal reward or sanction.[8] Formal job descriptions, procedures, and contracts never will cover all the eventualities that may arise in complex relationships. Therefore, managers must find the cultural and other mechanisms that create environments that elicit discretionary collaboration on both internally and externally.

Use the procurement process framework as a tool to assist in reengineering the IT procurement process: Another exciting use for the framework is to serve as the foundation for efforts to reengineer procurement processes. One firm analyzed the subprocesses involved in the requirements analysis and acquisition stages of the procurement life cycle to reduce procurement and contracting cycle time. Instead of looking at the deployment subprocesses as a linear sequence of activities, this innovative company used the framework to analyze and develop a compression strategy to reduce the cycle time in its IT contracting process by performing a number of subprocesses in parallel.

Use the framework as a guide for future research: The framework has been used by the SIM IT Procurement Working Group to identify topics of greatest interest for empirical research. For example, survey research investigating acquisition (software contracting practices and contracting efficiency), asset management (total life cycle cost of ownership and asset tracking systems), and supplier management (supplier evaluation) has been completed recently. The key issues identified in this article likewise can be used to frame a research agenda that will have practical relevance to practitioners.

Use the framework to structure IT procurement training and education: The framework has been used to provide the underlying structure for a university course covering IT procurement. It also provides the basis for shorter practitioner workshops and can be used by companies developing in–house training in IT procurement for users, technologists, and procurement specialists.

This five–item agenda provides a foundation for the professionalization of the IT procurement discipline. As the acquisition of information resources becomes more market-oriented and less a function of internal development, the role of the IT professional will change necessarily. The IT professional of the future will need fewer technology skills because these skills will be provided by external vendors that specialize in supplying them. The skills that will be critical to the IT organization of the future are those marketplace skills that will be found in IT procurement organizations. The management agenda described in this article provides a first step toward the effective leadership of such organizations.

Notes

1. Barki, H., Rivard, S., and Talbot, J. A keyword classification scheme for IS research literature: An update, *MIS Quarterly*, 17, 209, 1993.
2. Reifer, D., *Software Management*, IEEE Press, Los Alamitos, CA, 1994.
3. Thayer, R., Software engineering project management A top-down view, in IEEE *Proceedings on Project Management*, Thayer, R., Ed., IEEE Press, Los Alamitos, CA, 15.
4. Rook, P. Controlling software projects, *Software Engineering Journal*, 79, 1986.
5. Vaughn, M. and Parkinson, C., *Development Effectiveness*, John Wiley & Sons, New York, 1994.
6. Davenport, T. and Short, J.. The new industrial engineering: information technology and business process redesign, *Sloan Management Review*, Summer, 11, 1990.
7. Venkatraman, N. and Loh, L., The shifting logic of the IS organization: From technical portfolio to relationship portfolio, *Information Strategy: The Executive's Journal*, Winter, 5, 1994.
8. Heckman, R. and Guskey, A., The relationship between university and alumni: Toward a theory of discretionary collaborative behavior, *Journal of Marketing Theory and Practice*, in press.

Recommended Reading

1. Heckman, R. and Sawyer, S. A model of information resource acquisition, *Proceedings of the Second Annual Americas Conference on Information Systems*, 1996.
2. Hammer, M., Reengineering work: Don't automate, obliterate, *Harvard Business Review*, July/August, 104, 1990,
3. Lacity, M. C., Willcocks, L. P. and Feeny, D. F., IT Outsourcing: Maximize Flexibility and Control, *Harvard Business Review*, May–June, 84, 1995.
4. McFarlan, F.W. and Nolan, R. L., How to manage an IT outsourcing alliance, *Sloan Management Review*, 36,1995,9.
5. Sampler, J. and Short, J., An examination of information technology's impact on the value of information and expertise: implications for organizational change, *Journal of Management Information Systems*, 11, 59, 1994.
6. Teng, J., Grover, V, and Fiedler, K., Business process reengineering: Charting a strategic path for the information age, *California Management Review*, Spring, 1994, 9,

MANAGING ORGANIZATIONAL IMPACTS

I N REPORTING about the pervasive presence of information technology in organizations, a *New York Times* article (Wedemeyer 1978) reported that its "effect has for the most part been a subtle one, often unnoticed amid the ballyhoo attending the technical innovations." But, the article concluded, its impact has been considerable: "The look, sound, and sometimes even the shape of the workplace, after computerization, will never be the same."

This insight is prophetic and has since been repeatedly confirmed. For example, in a study that examined the effect of computer technology on the workforce and workplace, Mirvis, Sales, and Hackett (1991) found major organizational impacts that resulted from computerization. In addition, Morris and Brandon (1992) contended that "the ability to analyze the full organizational impact of computerization" will determine the success or failure of reengineering a hospital information system. Most observers agreed that information technology "shakes up the organization for better or worse" (Rogers and Farmanfarmian 1986). Innumerable studies have shown that productivity, organizational structure, and levels of stress in organizations are affected by information technology (Elder, Gardner, and Ruth 1987; Bailey 1986; Ray, Harris, and Dye 1994). Cornell's study (1996), for example, found conflict and disruption to be the norm when technological change enters organizations. He offered that "if we are to respond effectively, we need to understand what factors influence change, how to respond to change, and how to initiate change." With help from St. Serena's, this chapter probes the kind of conceptual understanding that Cornell emphasizes.

CASE STUDY

Case Four: What Hath God Wrought?

St Serena's CEO, Samantha, was becoming increasingly concerned over what was happening in her organization. In her illustrious career she had been accustomed to smooth-running organizations. Recently, however, St. Serena's seemed to be distracted. She could not quite put her finger on the causes, but she was certain that the problem had something to do with the new information management initiative. Stewart seemed to be doing all the right things, but the overall results were confounding. Senior staff meetings, which were usually opportunities for strategic planning, had now become sessions in which low staff morale and operational problems with the new information system were debated.

Samantha shared her concerns with a fellow CEO who had been through a similar information management experience a year ago. The colleague suggested that Samantha was probably just hearing about symptoms and needed to clarify the underlying problem.

Remembering how useful organizational surveys had been in her previous positions, Samantha decided to use her two MBA interns to design and conduct a written survey, which asks a sample of St.' Serena's staff to comment on their reactions to and experience with the information system initiative. The following are some of the more-interesting staff responses received:

> "As a manager I'm delighted that St. Serena's has finally stepped up to the new level of technological developments. The new information system enables me to standardize procedures and to program routine decisions. I can now be much more efficient in my work."

> "Since the new system arrived, the level of 'sick days' requested by my staff has nearly doubled and I have lost some of my best people to other job offers. The amount of my time devoted to helping my people use the new system, and to hiring new people who are comfortable with our system, has been enormous."

> "I'm going to leave as soon as I qualify for early retirement! This new system is giving me headaches and I'm concerned about the health effects of spending more time in front of the computer monitor."

> "I was worried at first about learning how to use the new system, but it was not as difficult as I thought it would be. I feel the new skills it gives me makes me more marketable."

> "I hate this new system! It has me spending more time with this fancy equipment than with my co-workers and clients. The whole atmosphere around here is different and I don't like it!"

"I worry about patient information being so accessible. Can anyone look up my employment history and health record?"

"These new guys from the CIO's staff bother me. I used to feel that I could run my department with confidence; now it seems that they run my operation. This is supposed to be a healthcare place, not a 'techie' place."

"I miss talking with all the people throughout the hospital. I used to spend a good part of my day on the phone with them—getting and giving information. Now, all I seem to do is talk with the screen on my desk, which does seem to have all the information I need. Internal e-mails are all over the place and it takes me hours just to sort them out. Nobody calls me anymore."

Questions for Discussion

1. What is going on at St. Serena's?
2. Sort the comments from the survey. Do some reflect what was anticipated with the new system? Do some reflect unanticipated results?
3. What symptoms of the organizational problems do you see at St. Serena's?
4. Prepare an analysis with recommendations for Samantha.

COMMENTARY

Clearly, the environment and mindset at St. Serena's are different now than before the new information system initiative began. Some of the changes seem to be positive, but others seem to be negative. The survey comments suggest three important lessons in this regard. First, the power of information technology is such that it inevitably has an impact beyond the planned and ostensible area of its application. Second, these organizational impacts have historically been extremely significant to the effectiveness of computer applications in that they often determine the success or failure of the automation effort. Third, the organizational impacts of computers have routinely been neglected, unanticipated, and not understood; that is, they have not been managed. Both the *New York Times* article and the Mirvis, Sales, and Hackett study also support this third lesson. The article discusses the "ballyhoo" focus on the technical aspects, while the study asserts that the impact of information technology on people and the workplace is rarely anticipated. As a result, the technology fails to bring the increase in productivity that the manager expects (First 1990). Moreover, as Stefl (1999) contends, technology is a "driver" that necessitates, as well as instigates, organizational change.

So let's reflect on what can, and usually does, happen in organizations when information technology is introduced or an existing system is changed. How can managers anticipate what the impacts might be? What should St. Serena's have done to avert the current situation, and what can Samantha and Stewart do now? What can healthcare professionals do to minimize any disruptive or undesired organizational impacts of information technology?

A Framework for Organizational Impacts

Impacts on organizational life from information technology run the gamut from the obvious to the sublime. Clearly, as indicated in the survey comments, work methods are often affected, new procedures are established, departments are reorganized, and new employees are hired. The office environment is affected by computer terminals, information system departments are established, clerical work groups are disestablished, and new jargon is heard. Less obviously, the status and power of departments and staff members often change, and work satisfaction and employee morale are affected. How can a manager systematically anticipate and prepare for impacts like these at St. Serena's and in healthcare settings in general?

One way to do so is to use a framework like that developed by Joseph Whorton of the University of Georgia in collaboration with Robert Quinn of the University of Michigan (1978). Whorton and Quinn's framework consists of a simple matrix, which recognizes that a formal and an informal reality exists in every organization, and that for each reality, an individual, a group, and a corporate dimension must be considered. Their matrix, thus, can be depicted as shown in Table 4.1.

The formal reality of agencies consists of organization charts, written rules and procedures, work groups, individual job descriptions, and so forth. The informal reality, often referred to as "organizational culture," is composed of those unwritten, but unmistakable, phenomena of every organization such as "grapevines," power, social groups, individual status, and morale.[1]

The matrix clarifies the six areas of St. Serena's, and all healthcare organizations, that information technology might impact:

1. Formal corporate structure and processes
2. Informal corporate structure and processes
3. Formal group structure and processes
4. Informal group structure and processes
5. Formal individual tasks and processes
6. Informal individual structure and processes

Table 4.1 Whorton-Quinn Matrix

	Corporate	Group	Individual
Formal			
Informal			

Formal Impacts on the Corporate Level

At the formal corporate level, structures and processes might be affected in a variety of ways. Information technology often entails structural reorganization, such as establishment of a chief information office, as was done at St. Serena's, or expansion of a unit to absorb the information system function. A study by Rachid, Combs, and Harper (1990) has found that information technology typically produces consolidation of departments, reduction in the number of hierarchical levels, and decrease in the control span. Indeed, such restructuring is often a logical result of a pursuit of greater efficiency, which is the case at St. Serena's.

Technology usually has a considerable effect on organizational centralization and decentralization. Neumann, Blouin, and Byrne (1999), for example, identify a four-fold spectrum—(1) centralized design, (2) coordinated design, (3) cooperative design, and (4) autonomous design—as evident in healthcare organizations today. The formal impact in the corporate level has been mercurial. During the era of large mainframe computers, information flow was more centralized. With the advent of PCs, distributed processing is having a decentralizing effect by dispersing computers, information system personnel, and decision making throughout an organization.

Overall, system design, not the technology, is what affects centralization and decentralization. For example, even if information processing is centralized in a mainframe computer, decisionmaking authority can be more decentralized through wider access to the information. On the other hand, a decentralized network can be used to reduce decentralized decision making by linking the systems to a central computer with limited access.

In addition, information technology can affect formal procedures. Information flow patterns are the main procedures that can be affected. Typically, modern information systems increase both the speed and volume of data collection, which, in turn, leads to more standardized operating procedures. Patient flow in a clinic, for example, might be changed to accommodate the system. These procedural changes usually entail tighter controls to ensure data input accuracy. Undoubtedly, some of the survey comments reflect this development at St. Serena's. Information technology enables both consolidated information processing and wider access to the processed data.

Finally, information technology can have a significant impact on the operating functions of staff departments, which also seems to have occurred at St. Serena's. The personnel office may find special difficulties in recruiting information specialists [Mazzuckelli 1999]. The legal office may have to deal with privacy legislation. The audit department may find its task complicated by the lack of a written audit trail. In short, information technology may well cause extra work for organizational units.

Informal Impacts on the Corporate Level

The most informal, or unofficial, impact is often on power in the organization. Information technology tends to shift power from line professionals to staff technicians who know the technology and who control information processing. Managers feel this impact when they realize their dependence on the information system over which they may have limited control.

This shift in power, in turn, can exacerbate rivalries and create antagonisms among operating departments that compete for information system services, as well as between information system departments and operating departments. In the same vein, the technical jargon can cause organizational-wide communication difficulties, which can undermine the information system's potential to meet user needs.

On the other hand, information technology can increase the level of cooperation among departments (Mirvis, Sales, and Hackett 1991; Foner et al. 1991). Standardization of procedures often necessitates analyses of missions and consensus, such as developing dialogue to improve organizational harmony.

Formal Impacts on the Group Level

Information technology can affect work groups in several ways. New work groups might be created and old ones changed to accommodate new information systems designs. Group tasks might also be affected, particularly those associated with data collection. Finally, superior—subordinate relationships may be affected. For example, superiors may be required to quantify worker performance for input to an electronic file.

Informal Impacts on the Group Level

In noting the importance of managing change in organizational information systems, Matthews and Smith (1978) assert that "any change in the kinds of tasks, form of technology, reporting relationships, and personalities may have a stressful and disruptive (but perhaps unanticipated) impact on the overall performance of the work group." Their point is that formal, or visible impacts on the formal, or work, group inevitably produce informal, or latent, impacts on the informal, or social, group, which can be serious. In referring to the increased interest in electronic clinical systems, Halseth and Paul (1992) support this point, maintaining that successful information system efforts in an organization require a cooperative "partnership" among technical, management, and professional groups. In all organizations, informal or social groups are a powerful phenomenon. Frequently, these social group realities are the source of considerable satisfaction and are important to work group members. Moreover, they typically control the "grapevine"; that is, they are key communication mechanisms and they establish and maintain work group norms of productivity. The grapevine structure is so important that, in fact, some Total Quality Management and Continuous Quality Improvement approaches empower and formalize the grapevine structure among work groups and quality teams.

These work groups can be affected in a number of ways. First, when work group structure is changed, by removal or addition of members, the social group changes, producing new interactions. This change may seriously affect worker satisfaction and alter group norms, resulting in reduced work group interactions that affect morale. This is likely happening at St. Serena's, given the increased attrition and absenteeism among employees. Group authority and leadership can also be undermined. For example, supervisors who appear to be ignorant about the new systems may discover that their ability to affect the group is impaired. All of these impacts can, in turn, cause resistance to new information systems, which is a problem so critical that the entire next chapter is devoted to it.

Formal Impacts on the Individual Level

At the individual level, the most obvious formal, or visible, impact is on the nature of individual tasks. New forms and procedures might mean less individual discretion and more control over workers; new processes might reduce personal contact and might mean more interaction with an impersonal computer terminal instead of with another worker. Similarly, a decision maker who previously interacted with several colleagues or subordinates to gather information may obtain it directly from a computer, which may enable faster and more informed decisions, but also limits personal contact. On the other hand, the change could ease the individual task and even make the job more fun, as suggested by one of the survey commentators at St. Serena's.

Second, new individuals and new tasks may be added after new information systems are introduced, as well as new layoffs or transfers. Technically competent individuals might replace interpersonally competent individuals, which might, as Austin (1999) suggests, lessen managerial competency in the organization. Might this be the situation with Stewart and CIOs at other healthcare organizations?

Third, actual experience with healthcare information systems indicates that personnel turnover and increased employee absenteeism are fairly common phenomena after information systems changes.[2] Shortages of technical workers have produced a seller's market in which healthcare organizations have difficulty competing with business organizations that offer higher salaries. Not unexpectedly, a 1994 survey from the College of Healthcare Information Management Executives revealed that employee turnover for healthcare CIOs was very high and appeared to be on the rise (Glaser and Hersher). Reasons attributed to this high turnover include ambiguity about the position and its expectations and a poor understanding of the corporate culture by many CIOs. Is Stewart soon to join this trend?

Informal Impacts on the Individual Level

Informal, or latent, impacts at the individual level have proven to be among the more critical, yet underappreciated and unattended, factors that affect information systems. The formal changes and impacts at all levels obviously do not occur in a vacuum—they inalterably affect the feelings and perceptions of the individuals involved. Reorganization can produce fear and stress just as more standardized tasks can create boredom and a perceived loss of autonomy. Changed tasks and processes can reduce the status and power of individuals, particularly those not schooled in the technology. These individuals, in turn, may feel intimidated by the new technicians. All of these feelings and perceptions can produce resistance to and resentment of the information system and can generate negative actions aimed at undermining the system (Reed 1988). On the other hand, as we have seen at St. Serena's, individuals could feel greater job satisfaction if new information systems ease the physical burden of their job, make the job more rewarding, or offer opportunity for skill development.

The above discussion is merely suggestive of the variety of possible organizational impacts. A tool like the Whorton–Quinn matrix can be useful in triggering insight on the possible impacts of information management efforts in your own organization. The impacts discussed above are summarized in Table 4.2.

Table 4.2   Possible Areas of Organizational Impact

Impact	Corporate Level	Group Level	Individual Level
Formal or Visible	• Centralization/ decentralization • Departmental tasks • Operating procedures • Communication network • Monitoring mechanism	• Work group structure • Tasks • Intra-group relationships	• Task content • Autonomy • Recruitment needs • Retention
Informal or Latent	• Power centers • Departmental cooperation or rivalry • Communication effectiveness	• Social group • Structure • Group norms • Attitudes • Authority and leadership • Morale	• Stress • Status and power • Attitudes • Feelings

Managerial Implications

The use of information technology unavoidably involves a variety of possible formal and informal impacts on all levels of an organization. The significance of these impacts for managers is suggested by First (1990), who notes that "new computer systems or software can become symbols of the unwanted, uncontrollable change in employees' work lives, especially in a period of corporate transition." Indeed, experience in healthcare organizations strongly indicates that, left unmanaged, these impacts do derail otherwise viable information system efforts. Successful use of information technology depends on the ability of managers to understand, anticipate, and manage these organizational impacts.

In addition to identifying areas of organizational impact, healthcare managers need to understand how these impacts might arise and develop. Several observations are important. First, a strong interrelationship among impact areas exists. For example, a direct impact on the formal corporate level usually produces indirect impacts on both the formal and informal levels of the group and individuals; a direct impact on the formal individual level will typically cause indirect impacts on the group and corporate levels. To illustrate, a small change in the individual's task, such as moving a secretary from a clerical pool setting to an isolated desk with only a word processor might (1) force the secretarial pool work group to alter its work process, (2) disrupt the secretaries' social group, (3) produce feelings of isolation and boredom in the secretary assigned to the word processor desk, (4) eventually alter organizational operating procedures to accommodate word processing capabilities, and (5) create new power centers of departments staffed with employees who have the required skills for information processing. In other words, managers must anticipate the full spectrum of subtle, as well as obvious, impacts.

The degree of impact will undoubtedly vary depending on the nature of the organization and on the technology application. More-structured organizations in more-stable environments that computerize routine tasks seem to experience less-significant organizational impacts than do more-complex organizations that introduce electronic information systems into more discretionary areas of work. For example, automation of hospital laboratories has produced far milder organizational impacts than has the introduction of electronic patient records (Darnell 1993).

Finally, what can managers do to control or influence the course of these organizational impacts? Two general guidelines for doing so are: (1) be as alert to the human systems as to the technical systems, and (2) adapt and sacrifice machine and structural efficiency in favor of social and personnel concerns.

More specifically, managers can plan and implement precise actions to mitigate, enhance, or otherwise control anticipated impacts in each of the six levels discussed above. At the organizational level, managers can consciously determine the amount of decentralization desired and design the change accordingly. They can involve affected managers and users to facilitate cooperation, determine where they want power to be distributed and act on that determination, and restrain inclinations to unnecessarily tighten operating procedures.

At the group level, managers can train supervisors before new technology is introduced so that the supervisors' authority and status will not be jeopardized; involve group members in discussions of how best to restructure work groups; and intentionally maintain social groups by, for example, not disbanding existing work groups even though that would be more "efficient."

At the individual level, managers need to initiate special recruitment and retention efforts, such as "ego" enticements in place of unavailable financial lures, and provide for ongoing professional development and improvement if they are to acquire and retain good technical people and manage technology resources wisely (O'Connell 1994). Managers can also provide training before new information systems are installed to ease the likelihood of stress or status loss among nontechnical workers, and establish rotating tasks to relieve the boredom of repetitive computer-related tasks. These recommendations, as Stewart would undoubtedly attest, are not always easy to put into practice without the requisite organizational-development skills. Some managers might, in fact, benefit from outside professional assistance to help implement some of these recommendations.

Conclusion

A key lesson for healthcare professionals is that unintended organizational impacts are inevitable and, if unattended, can mean the difference between the success or failure of otherwise well-designed information systems. Management of these organizational impacts requires deliberate anticipation, creative and adaptive responses, and a perspective on human and technical realities. Many organizational impacts are predictable and controllable, others can be recognized and influenced. A strategy for effectively managing the change engendered by information technology efforts is crucial for using modern information systems because organizational impacts can produce resistance that, as the next chapter points out, can result in the failure of the entire information management effort.

Notes

1. For unequaled insight on the informal aspects of organizations, see the classic Harvard Business School background note "Informal Networks—The Keys to Successful Management," by J. R. Fox and P. E. Morrison and *The Ropes to Skip and the Ropes to Know* by R. R. Ritti and G. R. Funkhauser (Columbus, OH: Grid, 1977).

2. For a representative case in point, see "Behavioral Reactions to the Introduction of Management Information System at the U.S. Post Office," by G. W. Dickson, J. K. Simmons, and J. C. Anderson. In *Computers and Management* by D. Sanders (editor). (New York: McGrawHill, 1974), 410–21.

References

Austin, C. 1999. "The Coming of the Information Age to Healthcare." *Frontiers of Health Services Administration* 15 (3): 41.

Bailey, N. 1986. "Why the Computer Is Altering Decentralized Management." *International Management* (June): 79.

Cornell, J. 1996. "Aspects of the Management of Change." *Journal of Management in Medicine* 10 (2): 23.

Darnell, J. 1993. "LIS Technologies Must Grow into the 21st Century." *Computers in Healthcare* (September): 41–2.

Elder, V., E. Gardner, and S. Ruth. 1987. "Gender and Age in Technostress: Effects on White Collar Productivity." *Government Finance Review* (December): 17–26.

First, S. E. 1990. "All Systems Go: How to Manage Technological Change." *Working Woman* (April): 47–54.

Foner, C., M. Noue, X. Luo, and J. Kim. 1991. "The Impact of Computer Usage on the Perceptions of Hospital Secretaries." *Health Care Supervisor* (September): 27–36.

Glaser, J., and B. Hersher. 1994. "Turnover Rate High for Many Healthcare CIOs." *Health Management Technology* (February): 49–52.

Halseth, M., and J. R. Paul. 1992. "The Coming Revolution in Information Systems." *Computers in Healthcare* (November): 43–45.

Matthews, J. R., and R. J. Smith. 1978. "Gauging the Impact of Change." *Datamation* (September): 241.

Mazzuckelli, K. 1994. "Be Creative in Your Approach to Healthcare IT Staffing." *Healthcare Management Technology* (June) 20 (5): 14–17.

Mirvis, P., A. Sales, and E. Hackett. 1991. "The Implementation and Adoption of New Technology in Organizations: The Impact on Work, People and Culture." *Human Resource Management* (Spring): 113–39.

Morris, D., and J. Brandon. 1992. "Reengineering: More Than Meets the Eye." *Computers in Healthcare* (November): 52–4.

Neumann, C., A. Blouin, and E. Byrne. 1999. "Achieving Success: Assessing the Role of and Building a Business Case for Technology in Healthcare." *Frontiers of Health Services Administration* 15 (3): 13.

The New York Times. (23 April): R-1.

O'Connell, S. 1994. "Five Principles for Managing Technology Resources." *Human Resources Magazine* (January): 35–6.

Quinn, R. E., and J. A. Whorton. 1978. "Computers and Public Administration: Predicting Resistance to Change." Unpublished manuscript, Spring 1978.

Rachid, K., L. Combs, and K. Harper. 1990. "Government Workplace Environment: Quality Workplace Environment Program—The Impact of Computers and the Future Environment." *Bureaucrat* (Summer): 17–22.

Ray, C. M., T. M. Harris, and J. L. Dye. 1994. "Small Business Attitudes Toward Computers." *Journal of End User Computing* (Winter): 16–25.

Reed, T. 1988. "The Frustrations of the PreTech Exec." *Industry Week* (21 March): 14.

Rogers, L., and R. Farmanfarmian. 1986. "Technology Shakes Up the Organization— For Better or Worse." *Working Woman* (November): 100–5.

Stefl, M. 1999. "Editorial." *Frontiers of Health Services Management* 15 (3): 2.

READINGS

The following two articles go deeper into organizational impact analysis. Joyce Mitchell's contribution focuses specifically on structural or "architectural" impacts of information systems and management with particular emphasis on the chief information office. Using case analysis of her own organization's experience, she provides practical concepts that would be useful to St. Serena's. Particularly insightful is a question and answer dialogue that she includes at the end of her article. Throughout her analysis note the consistent emphasis on management and people over technology.

Coralie Farley's article, despite its 1978 publication, continues to be among the best of the few analyses of systemic organizational impact of information systems in healthcare organizations. She provides a comprehensive view that includes specific examples of impact, which is a different framework from that presented in the commentary above for analyzing and anticipating organizational impacts, and concrete suggestions of the kinds of accommodations that be made to deal with organizational impact. Her framework uses the concepts of formalization, specialization, standardization, and stratification developed by Hage and Aiken to probe more informal and behavioral impacts on organizations that introduce technological change.

Basic Principles of Information Technology Organization in Health Care Institutions

Joyce A. Mitchell

Abstract

This paper focuses on the basic principles of information technology (IT) organization within health sciences centers. The paper considers the placement of the leader of the IT effort within the health sciences administrative structure and the organization of the IT unit. A case study of the University of Missouri-Columbia Health Sciences Center demonstrates how a role-based organizational model for IT support can be effective for determining the boundary between centralized and decentralized organizations. The conclusions are that the IT leader needs to be positioned with other institutional leaders who are making strategic decisions, and that the internal IT structure needs to be a role-based hybrid of centralized and decentralized units. The IT leader needs to understand the mission of the organization and actively use change-management techniques.

Reprinted with permission from the Journal of the American Medical Informatics Association *4 (2 supp), March/April 1997, S31–40. Joyce Mitchell is associate dean of integrated technology services at the University of Missouri Health Sciences Center, Columbia, Missouri.*

Information technology (IT) organizations have been discussed in the literature of the Integrated Advanced Information Management System (IAIMS) grants since the inception of the IAIMS concept and the initial IAIMS grants.[1] If IAIMS plans are to be truly integrated across an entire health care institution, then the IT organization must be flexible enough to deal with computing cultures that are both centralized and decentralized, both liberal and conservative. This is a large challenge for most health care institutions. This article considers the basic principles of IT organization within the health sciences center, a topic that continues to be timely, although the trends and issues are more clearly defined than they were at the inception of the IAIMS concept.

Lorenzi and Riley [2,3] have written two books about organizational theory and leadership in health care IT. They point out that health care institutions differ from many businesses in several respects, including personnel structure, life-and-death issues, alternative ownership characteristics, shareholders, exploding technologies and knowledge, rising costs and unique payment structure, and regulatory and accreditation requirements. The health care industry has tended to emphasize the uniqueness of its culture and mission, while ignoring its similarities to other large organizations. The result has often been an IT culture that is resistant to innovations and cross-fertilization from other institutions. This is a mistake. The health care industry has many important lessons to learn from the banking industry, the manufacturing industry, and other areas of U.S. business about how to organize IT and how to use it to compete more effectively.

Basic Principles of IT Organization

Two important aspects of IT organization that should be considered include the place of the IT organization in the health care institution and the internal structure of the IT organization. With regard to the first issue, it is my opinion that every health care institution and every integrated delivery system needs a chief information officer (CIO). (The specific titles of CIOs differ in various health science centers, but the title needs to be one that commands respect and is recognized as having top-level authority.) A CIO's responsibilities include 1) leadership of the IT organization and its policies, 2) technical management and services, 3) translation of institutional goals into IT efforts, 4) blending academic and business efforts, and 5) blending developmental efforts with traditional business software acquisition. In a health care institution, the CIO should be charged with bringing information to the point of decision making in all areas of education, research, patient care, and administration. The CIO must organize the existing patchwork quilt of IT groups that have evolved independently in most health centers into a unit that is capable of supporting the central mission of the health sciences center. The CIO's job is to determine how best to use technology to achieve institutional missions such as cutting costs, measuring patient outcomes, attaining research grants, educating students, and operating efficiently.

The questions invariably asked are what the scope of the central IT core group support should be and/or what units should be part of the central IT core group. There is no single correct answer. Each health care institution will have a variety of units supported by the central IT core organization. These units may be academic (e.g., the School of Medicine), business (e.g., the hospitals and clinics), or both. The central IT core organization may extend beyond traditional computing with such units as the telecommunications, printing services, multimedia production, or the health sciences library. The mixture of units supported and central core IT units will depend on the vagaries of each institution, its history, and its politics. The IT core group does not need to encompass all individuals with IT titles in all departments or units, but it must have a well-defined relationship with all IT personnel in all units of the institution. However, to maximize the potential for IT in achieving strategic goals, the IT leader needs to report to the key strategic leaders of the health care enterprise, to be in the meetings and discussions when strategic decisions are made, and to be recognized as setting the direction that must be followed by all other IT individuals and groups.

To turn to the principles of internal IT organization is to revisit the theme of centralized versus decentralized IT organizations. This theme is common across many years of literature, and the pendulum has swung in both extreme directions. The pendulum is now settling down in the middle. The Gartner Group, a national consulting firm specializing in IT issues, has stated, "By 1998, more than 70% of large enterprises will have radically restructured their IT. The result will be a blend of centralized and distributed computing." This is one of the basic tenets of a successful and flexible organization. The blend will depend on the roles and functions of the various types of computing support tasks.

Most importantly, the IT organization should fit the institution's strategic plan for using IT to accomplish its business priorities. In many health care institutions, education and research are business priorities just as much as clinical care is. The internal IT model that is rapidly emerging in the corporate world and the organizational literature in the 1990s is a group that is focused on service to the organization and distinguishes the service needed based on the technology role being delivered. Thus, the emerging model for IT is a blend of centralized and decentralized elements, called a structural hybrid organization.

A Case Study: The University Missouri-Columbia Health Sciences Center

This report stems from a survey of many health sciences centers, many of which have formally received IAIMS grants, but it focuses on how the basic principles are brought to bear upon the IT organization of the University of Missouri-Columbia Health Sciences Center (MU-HSC). At MU-HSC, the IT organization has recently been repositioned in the organizational hierarchy. The primary internal IT groups (academic informatics research and support, hospital and clinics information services, and faculty practice plan data processing) have been merged to form one large IT support entity. The resulting unit, Integrated Technology Services, is headed by a chief information officer with an associate dean title who reports directly to the highest executive of the health sciences center (the dean of the School of Medicine and the director of Clinical Services). Integrated Technology Services provides services to the entire enterprise, including academic departments, hospitals, clinics, the physicians' practice plan, and affiliated providers. The services are those of infrastructure, user support, programming, application selection and support, data analysis, evaluation, architecture, research, and information resources.

The specific example of IT support for workstations, networks, and programmers may clarify the concept of role-based organizations. At the MU-HSC, a 1995 study of IT support showed that 45 people were directly involved in supporting the computer networks and electronic mail, although time wise there were only 12 FTEs supporting networks and 4.5 FTEs supporting electronic mail. However, when the network went down, there was not a single person or group to contact to fix the network, since everyone was responsible but no single group was accountable. On further examination, it was found that many of the same 45 people were performing the roles of work-station support and computer programming. Half of these individuals were employed by individual academics departments and were not connected to the core IT units. There were, of course, some differences between the support and staffing in the hospital and clinics versus the academic school structures. As a result of this situation, the academic department chairs were unhappy because programming tasks were never finished. Even special critical projects remained unfinished. The principal reason was that the same person was responsible for the network and the electronic mail, which always took precedence over the programming projects because so many people needed networks and electronic mail to accomplish their jobs.

The role-based organizational model treats each of these roles separately. At MU, the roles are being separated and treated according to their enterprise-wide functions. The network and electronic mail have been declared mission-critical functions and moved to the top level of the enterprise. A completely centralized group that is responsible and accountable for these components has been created.

Workstation support is managed well as a shared-service hybrid function with joint funding between departments and the central IT group. The individual workstation-support specialists, who are based in the units they support, receive their priorities from their departments, yet are coordinated and named as a group. The departments and the central IT group are jointly accountable for the performance of the individual, with the departmental group determining whether the individual is useful functionally and the central IT group determining whether the person's technical skills are adequate. Figure 1 shows an organizational chart for a shared-service hybrid relationship that was developed according to the model of the Gartner Group.[5]

A coordinated model is used for the role of support for computer programmers (Figure 2). The central IT programming group focuses on computer programming and some core technologies (Oracle, C++, Java Script, World Wide Web, Perl). This group takes on the enterprise-wide tasks as well as the responsibility to allow access to institutional data. This central group also assists all programmers in other units to understand the institutional data models or provides tips on the use of specific supported software or techniques. Direct programming responsibilities and funding remain in the decentralized units with accountability to the department or unit leaders unless the programming task is enterprise-wide or crosses unit or departmental boundaries.

The internal IT organization is hierarchical, but supports the institution as an integrated matrix (Figure 3), with each row in the matrix determining a different method of providing services to the units and departments depending on the specific role, as described above. Overall, the IT organization interacts and connects with every component of the health sciences center, with some roles totally centralized (networks), some roles pulled into shared services (workstation support), and some roles left primarily decentralized but with central coordination (unit programming).

Figure 1 Organizational model for information technology support. This graph represents a shared-services hybrid organization between the central information technology group and departmental persons who are jointly funded to provide workstation support.

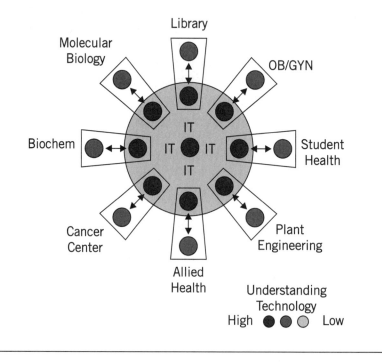

Other Issues

Other major issues are essential to an effective IT organization and are discussed elsewhere in this supplement, but need to be lightly touched upon here. The institution must determine how to fund this essential IT effort. The first step is to determine how much is currently allocated to IT activities. This amount is usually much more than anticipated. Then the leadership needs to determine how best to use this ongoing investment to support the IT plans and the institutional mission. A second major issue is to consider how best to manage change in the organization as it moves to a new organizational and work paradigm. A third challenge is to find an IT leader who understands the dynamics and the mission of the organization. Currently, few educational programs concentrate on IT leadership positions, and thus most leaders emerge from unusual, nontraditional career paths. A fourth major issue concerns

Figure 2 Organizational model for programming support. This graph represents a coordinated hybrid organization between the central information technology (IT) group and departmental programmers. The organizational model is more loosely coupled than the model for workstation support and illustrates the role-based approach to organization of IT.

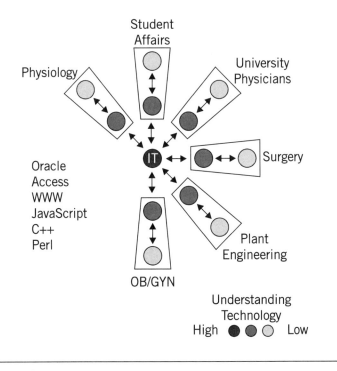

communication both within and beyond the IT organization, since communication is essential but seldom adequate. A fifth issue relates to management across the subcultures that have arisen in health care organizations and how to blend these cultures into a cohesive IT unit. These are all issues identified by previous IAIMS conferences and the current one as "make it or break it" issues with which all institutions must grapple.

Conclusion

The overriding issues of the IT organization are: 1) the importance of IT to the future of a health care institution must be recognized by the institutional leaders; 2) the IT leader must be positioned appropriately in the institution, with each organization being unique in

Figure 3 Matrix organization of information technology (IT) services provided by the central IT group to the operational units of the health sciences center. This chart represents the core services provided (infrastructure, user support, etc) and the components of the support that are provided to all of the health sciences enterprise.

Future Directions

Operational Units	Business Units	Hospitals
		Clinics
		Practice Plan
	Academic Units	Schools of Medicine
		School of Health-Related Professions
		Library
		School of Nursing
IT Services	Infrastructure	Networks (data, video, voice)
		Security
		Disaster Recovery
		Remote Access
		Electronic Mail
		Enterprise Server Operations
	User Support	Help Desk
		Application Training
		Workstation Support and Repair
		End-User Assistance
	Programming	Enterprise Focused Projects
		Coordinate Unit Programmers
		Fee-Based Programming(?)
		Access, Tools
		Database
	Applications	Vendor-Supplied Software
		Installation
		Upgrade
		Maintenance
		Replacement
		Interfaces
		Selection
	Biostat/Epi	Experimental Design
		Data Analysis
		Institutional Research
		Comparison Datasets
	Planning, Evaluation and Dissemination	Strategic Planning
		Plan Evaluation
		Reports
		Publication

IT Services (continued)	System and Data Architecture	Data Dictionary Vocabulary Standards Interface Standards Data Model Data Maps
	Research Services	Informatics Training Telemedicine Electronic Health Care Record Outcomes Research Vocabulary and Integration
	Library	Reference Databases Digital Libraries Information Resources Location

some respects; and 3) the internal IT organization must evolve onto a blend of centralized, decentralized, and cooperative structures based on the specific IT function or role. The IT organization is not an end in and of itself. Rather, it must reflect the organization's mission. The IT leader needs to understand the organization's mission and how to use technology to achieve that mission. The IT leader also needs to manage the organizational changes needed to use technology and information resources as a strategic asset.

References

1. Planning for Integrated Academic Information Management Systems: Proceedings of a symposium sponsored by the National Library of Medicine, October 17, 1984. Bethesda. MD: The Library. 1985.
2. Lorenzi NM, Riley RT. Organizational Aspects of Health Informatics: Managing Technological Change. New York: Springer-Verlag, 1995.
3. Lorenzi NM, Riley RT, Ball, MJ, Douglas JV. Transforming Health Care through Information. New York: Springer-Verlag, 1995.
4. Gartner Group, Research Note, May 1996.
5. Gartner Group, Research Note, August 1996.

Questions and Answers

Moderated by:
W. Edward Hammond, PhD
Duke University, Durham, North Carolina

Panelists:
Mark E. Frisse, MD
Washington University, St. Louis, Missouri
George Hripcsak, MD
Columbia University, New York, New York
Joyce A. Mitchell, PhD
University of Missouri, Columbia, Missouri

John Paton, Yale University—What are the mechanics of introducing an architecture into an institution? How do you actually go about doing that?

George Hripcsak—The technical task of defining the architecture is not the hardest part. The challenges lie in leadership and resource planning. There needs to be someone at the institution who is an information architect, someone who can communicate a vision and redirect millions of dollars. That is done through the processes outlined in Mark's and Joyce's talks. The technical challenges are fairly small. My last diagram may make the architecture appear to be complex. After you get into it and work with it for a little while, it is actually fairly simple.

Joyce Mitchell—The key is organizational. During our planning process, we came up with a view of the architecture that was very similar to that outlined by George. It has been difficult to enforce adherence to the architecture because of our organizational structure. You must have control of the resources that go into the major components of the architecture before you can make the whole thing fit together. It requires a combination of a carrot and a stick. The carrot begins with the vision of the future, the common planning, and making people feel that their voices are heard and that the vision is achievable. But there also comes a time when a stick is needed. You have to look at your investments and ensure that everyone is heading in the right direction.

George Hripcsak—There are two approaches to introducing an architecture—the five-year-plan approach and the free-market approach. The five-year-plan approach requires that you have institutional control. You then outline a plan stating the most efficient way to achieve the organization's goals. The free-market approach is to put into place the network and related infrastructure, set up guidelines, and then wait to see what happens. We experimented with these two approaches at Columbia. The clinical system was a planned approach, and everything else was free-market. As a result, the clinical system came up very quickly and is working very elegantly. This does not mean that the other systems are bad, they just didn't move as quickly. On the other hand, there has been creativity in the free-market systems that we never would have gotten from our central planning office.

David Rodbard, Association of American Medical Colleges—When I was at NIH, we had 23 institutes, each of which had at least one architecture. We used an outside facilitator to help working groups to develop a common strategy. Are others using outside facilitators?

Joyce Mitchell—We have used outside facilitators. Where it helped most was in bringing the hospital information systems group, our hospital CEO, and our hospital CFO into the process. During our planning phase, we identified the electronic medical record as a priority. It was at that point that the hospital team realized the IAIMS was going to impact them. Next, we devoted the time necessary to get them to agree to spend their money to hire facilitators. The facilitators led an intensive four-month planning process, looking at what we should do with all aspects of the hospital information system. The result did not say, "This is how we're going to build an electronic medical record." Instead, it identified our business initiatives and said, "This is how we're going to use IT to focus on addressing those initiatives." The process was time-intensive, but we came out with a plan that everybody understands and supports. We could not have done that without outside facilitators.

Mark Frisse—I would add two comments—one social, one economic. Many of us face situations where doing the right thing offends so many people that it is impossible to lead directly. Sometimes even the act of coordinating is taken as an attempt to seize power. In those instances, there is no substitute for bringing in an outside facilitator. That is the political and social reality. The second comment is economic. Karl Marx said, "The workers will never be able to seize control of the factories because they don't have the capital to do it." That is exactly the state of the health professionals right now. They cannot compete without access to clinical information; the barrier to entry is too great. People are realizing that the only way to succeed is to join forces with someone who is able to provide that information. The person who has the resources (human resources and economic resources) to manage clinical information is going to carry the day.

Ed Hammond—Are CIOs born or created? At a recent NLM training grant directors' meeting, the issue of whether it is appropriate to use NLM training funds to train CIOs was raised. Where do these individuals come from, Joyce?

Joyce Mitchell—At this point, there are no CIOs who were born to that role. They have been cultivated. There are no CIOs who started their professional careers intending to be CIOs, because that title and job description have not existed long enough. The CIOs whom I know came into it from different career paths. When I was in graduate school training to be a geneticist, I never thought I would be concerned with change management and process and role models in IT. That is a long way from where I started.

Ed Hammond—Are CIOs trained, or are they just appointed?

Joyce Mitchell—They have to be trained. If they don't understand the technology, they cannot do the job. They have to be very good at working with people. CIOs can be trained just as we have been trained.

George Hripcsak—A person must have a basic talent to start with, but also training has to be provided. Otherwise, that person is going to end up in another field. If we want individuals to come into medicine, we have to bring them in actively.

Mark Frisse—I don't know how often CIOs are born or are made, but I do know that they are often fired. That speaks to the issue of training, as well as to the issue of the institutions. I was not a part of the NLM discussions, but I think for that institution to do its job, it must take a very broadbased approach with respect to business economics, utility theory, decision analysis, and information technology in health care to provide training for these people.

Bill Stead, Vanderbilt University—What percentage of CIOs understand that they need an architecture, and the fact that they, themselves, have to put the architecture in place because no vendor is prepared to do it?

Joyce Mitchell—All of the CIOs at this meeting certainly understand that concept—many other CIOs do not. What does the title, CIO, mean? There are a number of hospital people with CIO titles who feel that their job is to buy components and to interface them. I doubt that they know what an architecture is. The IAIMS concept makes people think about architecture much more than does traditional data processing.

George Hripcsak—One gauge to measure how the architecture idea has penetrated is to listen to consultants. Five years ago, consultants were not talking about these concepts. Now they want to come and explain the architecture to you. They don't think it should be done internally; they want to do it for you.

Valerie Florance, University of Rochester—What can we do to sustain enthusiasm and interest in planning after the excitement of coming together and participating in the initial planning phase?

Joyce Mitchell—Planning has to be an ongoing process. We identify initial priorities and start to work on them. While that work is in progress, we plan for the next phase. Committee structures are important. The committees may change along the way depending upon what is being done, but there also needs to be a permanent planning office. At Missouri, the position of IAIMS Coordinator is evolving into responsibility for managing an office of planning, evaluation, and dissemination for the IT organization. Vanderbilt is doing the same thing.

George Hripcsak—Columbia University Medical School has about a $300 million budget, and the hospital has about $700 million. There are probably a dozen different offices with the term "planning" in their titles. As frustrating as it may seem, this duplicate effort is necessary to sustain interest in the plan. Everybody rediscovers the plan and thinks it is their own idea. This is healthy, because it has been said that, "The only way to get your idea across is to make it the other people's idea." As individual groups discover IAIMS on their own, they can be herded in. Success then comes from adding incremental value to the collective insights as opposed to starting over every time.

Kevin Johnson, Johns Hopkins University—How has the changing marketplace and your interactions within your region caused each of you to change the scope of your IAIMS?

George Hripcsak—At Columbia Presbyterian Medical Center, we are merging with New York Hospital. We are merging the faculty plans at the two universities and redefining our scope. Thus, we are compelled to redefine our IAIMS completely. We are reaching out to the community more, and most of our new planning focuses outside the hospital.

Joyce Mitchell—We are redefining the IAIMS at Missouri, although the changes in the market place began to occur when we were in the middle of the planning process so it doesn't feel like redefinition. The change is reflected in our telemedicine activities and in other links to the rural and agricultural parts of the state. We have external sites that are part of our organization. It is often difficult to know who is and who is not a part of our system. A problem that we have had to face is, "How do you change what information services are delivered depending upon to whom the service is delivered?" This requires a database of users and a database of roles within our organization in order to implement a role-based security model. Then we can manage what information can be accesses by what people. That is our vision of how to deal with it; all the pieces are not in place yet.

Mark Frisse—Since every part of the enterprise is dependent upon information technology, whether or not it is called IAIMS, you can't be involved in all of it. You have to take the advice of (I think it was)

Jack Welch at General Electric, "If you can't be number 1 or number 2, don't do it." You go where you can see a return, where you think there is something critically important to be accomplished. You have to start with some wins that are immediate and apparent and visible. We are defining the scope of our IAIMS to focus on what we think makes the most difference, the interface between the school of medicine and the hospital. That will not happen without IAIMS; the rest will happen by other means.

Bill Stead, Vanderbilt University—The change in the marketplace is altering the way we at Vanderbilt tackle problems. Our first objective was inreach, trying to solve problems internal to Vanderbilt. We knew at the beginning that we would want people outside Vanderbilt to be able to reach into Vanderbilt to interact with information about patients under our care. We now understand that we need to go a step further. If we are going to be information producers, and if we are going to be experts in informatics, we have to provide components of infrastructure that can be used by others across the region, whether those others are affiliated with us or compete with us. They have to be able to incorporate our components into their internal systems. As our relationships change, we need to dynamically, on demand, link or not link the information so that it can look integrated or not integrated. Fortunately, our architecture has allowed us to create reusable components, which we should be able to be transfer externally. Planning for that type of inter-organizational interaction is more complex than what we had to do within Vanderbilt.

I ask the three panelists to consider the perspectives of IAIMS that they are representing and to tell us how they would start with planning, architecture, or organization to establish a regional or national inter-organizational IAIMS. What would be the first step from each of those perspectives?

Mark Frisse—I think IAIMS is local. It is opportunistic. It requires good luck, and there is no substitute for having at least one person spearheading it who is supported by the institutional leadership. If that is not possible, having someone who is identified as a clearinghouse is a key first step. Understanding your limitations is important as is knowing where you can make a difference early into the process. Given the fragmented nature of our institution, our approach has been one of opportunism. We have succeeded in putting people in hybrid positions within the organization. Progress occurs, but not in the way that the classic Matheson and Cooper article would have articulated. This strategy should also work at the regional level.

Joyce Mitchell—An interorganizational effort must be spearheaded. To get people from different schools, different hospitals, different integrated delivery systems to cooperate requires that they sit down together and get to know each other. In order to define a common direction, individuals have to understand what other individuals are presently dealing with and their points of view. Individuals have to communicate either electronically or physically. It is difficult to dictate anything within the academic environment; it is easier within the hospital environment because the hospital is traditionally more organized.

Mark Frisse—Somewhere in the middle of those two settings lies the answer. In a rapidly changing environment, some organizational chaos can allow small mistakes that show what is working and what is not. An evolutionary approach may be preferable to where some health care systems are headed. They are going to make well-orchestrated, well-financed, highly effective, catastrophic errors. They are like giant cannons pointing in one direction; they are going to shoot whether it is the right direction or not. A little bit of chaos might be helpful.

George Hripcsak—If you have a good architecture, you are on the road to success. If you don't get the architecture right, you're doomed. Without the right underlying architecture, a CIO can have the most proactive rhetoric you have ever heard, but be inherently, 100% of the time, reacting. Without the basic architecture, CIOs are totally trapped in legacy systems. They can never get out. They can never do anything other than just react to yesterday's problem.

Ed Hammond—It seems that each of you expects the medical schools to be the instigators of regionalization. That is not going to work. There will have to be an identified neutral authority to provide the platform where people can come together and work. The academic side, the medical school, is too far removed from the nonacademic environment in terms of the art-of-the-possible and in terms of what they believe needs to be done.

Mark Frisse—I agree that it is generally the hospitals and health care systems that are the drivers of change. The medical schools, in most instances, are totally reactive and have very little money and very little organization. The neutral-person model may not work either. A more viable alternative may be one person who reports to two masters or a group of people who get along well together.

Peter Tarezy-Hornoch, University of Washington—How do we help physicians who have grown up in a legacy system environment to understand the opportunity of an environment in which they can redesign processes and work differently? Given the fact that everyone has started with a legacy architecture, how do we proactively transition to a new architecture?

George Hripcsak—There are two ways to move to a new architecture. Some people have the luxury of starting from scratch—that is obviously one answer. The other way is one step at a time. As each new step is reached, the institution moves forward a little without being aware that it is moving. Much of the architecture is conceptual; therefore, not all systems need to change. Sometimes minor adaptations can make the old systems fit into a better architecture.

Joyce Mitchell—Incremental work is also possible in terms of organization. If an employee leaves, and there is a plan toward which your organization needs to move, change can be achieved as that employee is replaced. I am notified every time a position with an IT title is vacated. I initiate a conversation with the hiring department to determine whether we can do something cooperatively rather than having them hire a person autonomously. Sometimes it works and sometimes it doesn't, but we usually move in the right direction just by having that conversation. When you get external money, there are opportunities to do things faster. Because of our IAIMS planning process, we were ready to move when the University of Missouri said they had money to provide campus-wide support for end-user computing. I can use that support to split-fund positions without having to extract the positions back to the individual departments. The departments don't see any net loss.

George Hripcsak—The planner would now say to a medical school, "Consolidate all of your billing systems if you haven't already done so." "If you have not established your master patient identifier, do it now." "Establish a clinical data repository program that is fed by your legacy systems." "Don't spend a lot of time with the computer-human interface without getting the back end right."

Joyce Mitchell—There are some other things that need to be mentioned. You need to pull together all of your transcriptionists now so that you can eliminate FTEs as the role goes away. People have secretaries who do secretarial work, answer the phone, and transcribe at the same time. Separate those roles and figure out which roles are going to disappear in the long run as you squeeze costs out of your system.

Tom Rindfleisch, Stanford University—How can the planning model accommodate the rapid change of technology?

Mark Frisse—If you are referring to a centralized computing facility, it is destined to fail when economics get tight. You either provide marginal service at marginal costs and eventually run into capacity problems, or you try to allocate the fixed costs. The inability to see ahead can be dealt with by a process that allows small mistakes in a supportive environment, where you can pick people up and learn from the mistakes. A highly monolithic plan is much more likely to result in large catastrophic failures.

Joyce Mitchell—We should avoid becoming fixated on any one piece of technology—it is going to become obsolete. However, a bigger failure is to not do anything because you are paralyzed by the fear of everything changing underneath you. What we hope for is to have some successes along the way, and that enough people recognize the value of those successes, so that we are not crucified for our failures.

Bill Stead, Vanderbilt University—Putting in systems that become obsolete is not a failure. We are replacing shared workstations in the hospital and clinic on a three-year cycle. We budget for depreciation with that expectation. We do the same thing with network technology. Most of our electronics are now four years old, and we are replacing about a third of them this year. We knew that we would have to do that—it was part of the plan. The architecture gives us that flexibility to evolve because we can do the replacements in pieces.

Ed Hammond—What do we expect the vendors to do? It almost sounds like a hopeless situation from their perspective.

George Hripcsak—The vendors are producing good modules that can be plugged into other systems. No vendor currently can provide an architecture across a medical center. The consultants are the ones who should be doing that, not the vendors of individual software. The consultants who are trying to fulfill that role are not successful. They are looking for technology problems that require technology solutions when it is planning, resources, and leadership that are needed.

Mark Frisse—I have been impressed by the extent to which IBM has adopted open systems in terms of HL7, databases, and HTML front-ends. There are better things to buy all the time, although I confess I still don't know how to make the little ambulatory care systems talk to the other systems. It seems that a lot of vendors will fail, and some of us will fail with them.

Joyce Mitchell—The vendors don't know nearly as much as those of us here about the direction for the future. Yet, to decide that you are going to build everything yourself is digging a hole so deep you could never get out of it. You have to find the right vendor who is willing to work with you. We are in the process of doing that right now. Our approach is to look at the functionality of current systems, but to put greater emphasis on the long-term vision of the corporation and its leaders in terms of where they think health care is going, where they think technology is going, and how they are planning for the future. We want to know what they think they will be doing five or ten years from now. It is almost like buying futures in the vision of the company. You have to pick a company that either is going to be around or is going to be acquired because they have the right vision. We don't yet know whether our approach will work because we haven't actually gotten to the step where we choose a company.

Bill Stead, Vanderbilt University—You need to catergorize vendors by the types of products they sell. The health care software vendors have not built a strategy around open systems. They are buying a set of niche products so that they can claim to have a complete solution. This is the wrong answer, because the products do not work well together. The real question is whether Vendor A's product accepts a plug-in module from Vendor B. The health care software vendors do not buy into this concept. There is another set of vendors who are information-technology-based. The health care industry has not taken advantage of these vendors. To the degree that people are building technology solutions that plug and play nicely, they give an institution the ability to plug the pieces together in the way they want their architecture to look without having to build very much at the institutional level. This is the model that will likely emerge. I believe that the current health care software vendors will be replaced by a mixture of consultants and information technology companies.

The Computer as a Focus of Organizational Change in the Hospital

Coralie Farlee

Administrators and other organization heads often decide to adopt Hospital Information Systems (HIS) in order to achieve greater control over the work of health professionals in the care delivery setting. Sometimes, such information systems are introduced in order to achieve organizational change. Whether introduced as a catalyst for change or for improved control over care delivery, the HIS produces changes rarely anticipated.

Reprinted by permission from Journal of Nursing Administration *(February 1978):2026 Copyright 1978 Nursing Resources. Coralie Farlee is senior staff associate with the Association of American Medical Colleges.*

Often, the healthcare administrator contracts for an automated system designed to support certain patient care functions. Rarely is the system assessed for its probable impact on the hospital as an organization (that is, its subunits and organizational structure).

This article is designed to help nursing administrators and others assess the potential impact of technological innovations introduced in healthcare organizations. The organizational changes often accompanying the introduction of hospital (or medical) information systems will be examined and discussed.

Hospital Information Systems: Functional Characteristics

The most sophisticated computer-based hospital information systems establish patient files in computer memory and make provisions for adding information into these files in an on-line, real-time basis, that is, as successive events occur. The most basic system sorts data entered and disseminates the information to departments throughout the hospital in the form needed and at designated time intervals. Lists, records, and reports can be assembled at scheduled times or on call. Some systems also possess other functions, such as patient billing (linked to the accounting department), or results reporting (linked to a laboratory system).

Input alternatives are of two major types, involving either (1) nursing personnel transcription or physicians' orders, or (2) direct physician input. The latter type usually requires input via the cathode ray tube on whose TV-like screen the physician or a person designated by the physician is presented with questions or choices for the sequence of decisions to be made in creating, extending, or canceling orders for patient care. Some hospital information systems propose to eliminate the patient's medical records file and other written records except for those documents that require patient signatures.

Whatever system is adopted, the major consequence of this technological change for the workers involved (physicians, nursing staff, pharmacists, dieticians, etc.) is to reduce the flexibility and options involved in decision making and to increase the standardization of the work.

The hospital (organizational and occupational) functions to be performed by the computer are specified in various ways. Typically, this sort of technological change is begun by documenting elements of information required or currency received by various units of the organization. Rules and procedures are derived to specify the elements of information and to structure the manner in which the information is to be entered into the computer terminal. Checks for missing data and for entries that exceed specified limits are programmed into the controls of the information system.

Cautions about certain combinations of information may be included (for example, drug incompatibilities, allergic reactions, or scheduling of meals versus lab tests). As the nursing staff or physician interacts with the terminal, it indicates deficiencies of information in the messages they are attempting to enter and, in such situations, will ask for re-entry or correction or confirmation of the input data.

Usually, rules are specified about who can enter information, who can have access to different levels of information, and what types of data elements should be entered at which points in time.

Among computerized hospital information systems, there is wide variation in the extent to which job functions will be formalized, or standardized. The extent of change depends largely on whether it is assumed that physicians will input directly to the computer terminal, or whether the nursing staff will continue to be responsible, as on a completely manual system, for transcription, interpretation, and, often, completion of physicians' orders. Increased job formalization (to be more fully described) is a byproduct of the procedural standardization required by a computerized system. A specific example of job formalization might be the requirement that medications be administered to all patients on all nursing stations within a half hour. Thus the computer system would expect all medications to be "confirmed" as "given" to patients by that time. If confirmations were not entered in the terminal by one half hour after the time of the ordered administration, reminder messages would be generated. This simplistic procedure allows for no difference in size of nursing units or in patient needs between geriatric, newborn, general medical, or surgical nursing units.

Other organizational changes generally accompany the increased standardization of job functions, rules, and procedures: new jobs or occupational specialties are often added. These jobs bring computer personnel into the organization, and may include new personnel located at nursing stations whose major function is to enter information, and not patient care or other medical or health-related work. During the process of change, the relative status of various departments and of occupational roles may be clarified—(by the priorities assigned and resources allocated)—even more precisely than many would have desired.

Theories of Organizational Change Relevant to Technological Change

A series of studies of technological change have reported a variety of outcomes relative to effects on the organization and the extent of workers' perceived control over work tasks.[1] While studies of automation in industry must be applied with caution to the clinical setting, Blauner's studies of the effect of technological change in various types of industries does set the tone for examining the functional change involved in technological change. [2] Changes of functions must be examined in order to assess more clearly the extent of change in worker control.

The most comprehensive yet comprehensible theoretical construct in which to view complex organizational change is that developed by Jerald Hage and Michael Aiken.[3] This paradigm details eight organizational variables, four of which describe the means (or processes) by which organizations operate and four of which describe the objectives (goals or outputs) that organizations expect to achieve. Following is a list of the eight organizational variables, each of which is defined.

Means

Formalization: The number of rules that define how a job is to be performed; the relative flexibility permitted within jobs.

Centralization: The organizational level at which decisions are made; the number of occupations allowed to participate in decision making.

Complexity, or Specialization: The number of occupational specialties or disciplines in an organization; the variety of levels of education or training among personnel.

Stratification: The differences in status among jobs as measured by differential power, income, or prestige; the rate of mobility between status levels in the organization (for example, the number of nurses who become nurse administrators, hospital administrators, or physicians).

Objectives

Productivity: The number of units produced per unit of time (such as patient days per year).

Efficiency: The average cost per unit of output (such as cost per patient day) and the manner in which resources are utilized.

Adaptability: The organization's rate of change and ability to change (often indicated by the number of new programs or new techniques introduced and accepted, or by the amount of time required to introduce change and bring about its acceptance).

Efficient and productive organizations are found to result from high-level decision making; extensive standardization of rules and procedures; rigid stratification; and low task specialization within jobs requiring only minimal skills, education, or training. This sort of static organization is also characterized by a low level of satisfaction among employees and consumers.

But hospitals, like educational institutions and other "people processing" systems, have generally been characterized by a concern with the quality of their output or service—concern that their patients are well cared for. They have also been noted for the diversity of medical and organizational specializations and their concern with innovation.

Recent financial pressures and demands for service are forcing hospitals to reconsider their priorities: efficiency (cost per unit of output) and productivity (effectiveness) are being defined as more relevant organizational goals than previously. Health care administrators hope these new objectives can be achieved without a deleterious effect on patient care and without reducing satisfaction among employees or consumers.

Hospital information systems have been promoted as one mechanism for improving efficiency and productivity. In the following section, we will discuss the four previously defined means of achieving organizational objectives in the context of the HIS.

Hospital Information Systems and Means of Achieving Organizational Objectives

The four means variables are presented in the order of the extent of change they would probably undergo as a result of the introduction of an HIS.

Formalization

The major effects of the introduction of an HIS are likely to be an increase in the number of rules and procedures, more formal or specific requirements for job incumbents, and more direct enforcement of these requirements through the automated system. Any change that increases formalization, or rule enforcement, tends to encounter opposition. The main characteristics of HIS—its provision of greater structure for codification of segments of jobs and its imposition of scheduling requirements on many roles—reduces the flexibility and autonomy characteristics of professions.

The essential task, then, is to examine the variation among hospital information systems' software in terms of specification of procedures. Procedural requirements contribute in various ways to increase formalization. These requirements include:

- Specification of the types of personnel able to enter or access information in particular locations. (Access to patient records is often controlled via coded badges or ID numbers.)

- Requirements that each order be complete, with all basic components uniquely identified, before the order can be entered and processed.
- Requirement that all orders be entered in advance (thereby decreasing flexibility to provide emergency medical care or procedures).
- Use of standardized formats for requests, order options, diagnoses, observations.
- Security requirement restricting modification of orders once entered (thereby limiting cancellations, refund options and billing updates).
- Use of schedules, lists, reminders.

Centralization

Decisions about change made at the highest organizational level—such as by boards of governors or federal agency administrators—are likely to be met with resistance by employees. Centralized, high-level decision making is often associated with an absence of channels of communication between organizational levels and limited access to decision-making channels. Consequently, when new ideas are suggested at the organization's lower levels, their approval (and implementation) may take a long time. In addition, if employees recognize that certain procedures and assumptions in packaged software systems are inappropriate for the specific organizational environment, their comments and suggestions will reach a limited audience of decision makers.

The decision to adopt an HIS should be made with the participation of nursing, medical, and administrative personnel. Following implementation of the system, their continued involvement in decision making can be ensured by designating a competent full-time staff member as HIS project director and by the formation of a users' committee to help make technical decisions on operational problems. (This delegation of decision making cannot be a substitute for commitment and support of the hospital management.) The users' committee should include representatives of nursing, medicine, pharmacy, laboratory, and other important hospital units.

Most suggestions to introduce HIS will not originate at the lowest levels. However, it is important to ensure that subordinates and users are free to participate in the selection of a system from the many available and, after its implementation, to suggest necessary modifications.

Specialization

Program change often introduces new occupations or skill clusters into the organization. If persons are recruited from outside, it is unlikely that they will be familiar with the organization's unique characteristics; consequently, existing staff may offer resistance to the program change—in part as a reaction to the introduction of the new roles and new personnel. If individuals from within the organization are selected for retraining, they may never become fully aware of the innovation's implications and potentials, for they may have a limited perspective and may remain oriented to the former status quo.

With the introduction of HIS, it is almost inevitable that increased specialization will occur. An organization may choose either or both of the above options for filling the new specialty positions. Vendor specialists may be introduced into the organization—in addition to or instead of recruiting matching specialties for the regular hospital staff. The hospital may have to integrate such new occupations as a data processing (DP) head and programming staff, DP nurses, DP clerical workers, HIS project officers, and others in liaison capacities to the medical staff, hospital departments, employees, and vendors.

Recruitment of competent in-house computer staff is not without its problems, of course. Programming for HIS requires sophisticated people who support efficient utilization of the computer technology through selection of appropriate trade-offs and alternatives in software procedures. If computer personnel are not added to the organization, the change in occupational specialization will be slight, but the decision not to add such personnel is based on the assumption that the HIS software and procedures are compatible with the organization's structure and goals, and that changes in the vendor's product and hospital procedures will be minimal.

Stratification: The Increased Structuring of Roles

The more that program change is accompanied by increased clarification of status differences in an organization, the greater the likelihood of dissatisfaction with the change, since high stratification tends to increase rigidity and reduce communication and interaction between levels of occupations and organizational units.

Hospitals are work settings where the occupational mix and the rights and obligations of occupations are governed by state and professional licensing agreements. The introduction of badges or regulations specifying which job occupants can perform which tasks results not only in the development of rules within jobs (formalization), but also in a clearer specification of which roles and which organizational units (e.g. nursing department, x-ray department) can have access to particular kinds of information or can perform certain tasks. This clarification of the hierarchy of access to information results in a more precise exposure of the differential rights, obligations, and distribution of rewards (status) among jobs and departments.

When the new occupations are introduced (specialization) with the HIS, the hospital has several options regarding departmental and hierarchical placement of the new personnel. The occupants of the new roles can be inserted into existing departments, or else new tasks can be added to old roles. In either case, the location of HIS-related tasks is generally clearly specified or easily assumed. This occurs, for example, when data processing is added to the finance and accounting department on the rationale that data processing serves the financial interests of the organization. Their status is also clear when DP personnel are introduced at a nursing station on the assumption that they work for the head nurse and do tasks similar to those of clerical workers.

On the other hand, if a new HIS department is created, at staff level, the status of HIS versus other departments may not be clearly defined. The HIS department can receive and consider requests from the finance and accounting department, from nursing, laboratory, dietary, and other departments, as well as from members of the administrative staff and physicians. This structure also permits a loose definition of the status of HIS staff or liaison personnel in other parts of the hospital; it may, for example, permit a colleague-type relationship to develop between the head nurse and the DP person taking on unit manager tasks.

Progress of Change

Low formalization, low centralization, high specialization, and low stratification are most conducive to employee acceptance of and accommodation to the sort of technological change introduced by the HIS.

It is also important that the time schedule of the system's introduction not deviate substantially from the expectations of those affected and that the change assume a steady though not necessarily rapid rate. Optimally, there should be a realistic implementation schedule agreed to by all major parties involved; this schedule along with the objectives for the HIS should be published, and the schedule adhered to as far as possible. If there is a deviation from the schedule or from announced objectives without the full participation and consent of those affected, interest will lag and confidence in the new system will wane. It is also important that users of the system know that the change has occurred, that is, when the parallel, or test, phase on particular segments is completed and that the information in the automated system is to be relied on.

Acceptance of Innovations: Socialization Models

A number of sociologists have developed models of the process by which new norms of behavior are internalized. These socialization models are presented here with a view to managing behavioral change in conjunction with technological change in organizations.

Talcott Parsons has outlined four major stages of socialization. [4]

Stage 1

In this, the "permissiveness" stage, crucial inputs from the socializing (or change) agent are information about the change and expected new behavior and opportunities to learn the new behavior. Lowered rewards for, and decreased satisfaction with, the prior behavior and achievements should provide some incentive to take on the desired new behavior.

Stage 2

In this, the "support" stage, the inputs from stage 1—information about the change and opportunities to learn new behavior—continue to be offered, but external rewards for the new behavior are given and confidence in performance of the new behavior is encouraged. The latter two elements should, theoretically, produce increased internal satisfaction with performance of new behavior. (The disorganization generated at the first stage will decrease as the sense of accomplishment increases with improved performance of the new behavior.

Stage 3

In this, the "denial of reciprocity" stage, the inputs from stage 1—information about the expected new behavior and opportunities for learning it—are still offered, but external rewards are decreased, while the new patterns of behavior are internalized. Rewards for the new behavior come from internal, rather than external, sources.

Stage 4

During the final stage, external rewards, gratification, self-rewards, and satisfaction for performance of the new task are all increased, while information about performance and opportunities for performing the behavior are maintained.

By the time stage 4 is reached, the target of change should have given up the old behavior because it is no longer rewarded (the costs of doing it are too high). It is assumed that the new behavior expected by the change agent has been adapted.

Bredemeier and Stephenson have summarized and elaborated upon Parson's scheme. [5] Their model indicates that to achieve the desired change, the change agent should reduce rewards for the prior behavior by reducing approval from the original reference group (that is, those whose opinions matter a lot); changing the definition of the original reference group so that their sanctions are no longer so important; increasing the interaction between change agents and change targets; providing opportunities for self-approval resulting from correct performance of the new behavior; and giving opportunities for pleasure for performance of the new behavior or for giving up the old behavior. Then change agents should increase rewards for the new behavior by providing a period of anticipatory socialization (where change targets are eagerly awaiting the change and its consequences); providing contingent rewards; deferring gratification for new behavior; and reducing feelings of relative deprivation. Further, the change target should be provided with a clear definition of his or her status and with consistent expectations from the change agents. Change agents should also allow for flexibility in learning, furnish adequate role models for the new behavior, and provide facilities for learning the new behavior.

The literature recommends that change agents in organizations gain the confidence of the change targets, for only when agents are trusted will their efforts at providing rewards for new behavior and negative sanctions for old be meaningful. [6] Often, change agents do not have a prior or stable base in the organization, and thus they must compete with existing reference groups in the resocialization effort. If this is, indeed, the case, efforts to reduce the importance of previous reference groups will be more difficult.

Relevance of Socialization Models for Hospital Information Systems

Most of the literature on behavioral change is derived from theories based on groups having little power, such as the young minorities or the handicapped. [7] However, in the case of HIS, the change targets hold a stable and powerful position in the organization, whereas the change agents are in a more tentative position. Nursing staff and physicians must learn new procedures that involve changes in task structures and in certain role expectations. Both groups are powerful and may resist change initiated by personnel whom they consider to be peripheral to circumstances surrounding the delivery of healthcare. Thus, in order to be effective, the change agents should be in occupational roles that traditionally have some leverage with the group whose behavior is affected. It is not realistic to expect that clerical workers or nurses can have a large impact on physicians. Nurses put in the role of change agents for the purposes of changing physicians' order writing practices are not likely to have the necessary leverage (they are not and will not become the important reference group needed) and they are likely to experience status inconsistency. Likewise, it is improbable that data processing staff will have an impact on the decision making and healthcare practice of either physicians or nursing staff. However, some software packages incorporate significant behavioral change and attempts at social control of the health professionals. It is thus extremely important that nursing administrators be actively involved in this technological change, for it is likely to have a major impact on the nursing staff.

It is important to examine the functional implications of any specific hospital information system being explored. If new occupations are to be introduced into the hospital, if older writing and other aspects of the practice of nursing and medicine are to be affected, hospital and nursing administrators should be aware of the probable restructuring of roles that will follow introduction of an HIS. If extensive formalization (reduction of flexibility) is to occur with respect to major job functions of health professionals, negative "unanticipated" consequences are likely.

When program change is attempted, it is followed by an effort to gain employee conformity, or compliance, with new procedures and behaviors required by the change. In this effort it is important to provide hospital personnel with accurate knowledge of the change; facilities and resources that will help them learn the new behaviors and procedures; rewards for conforming behavior; and negative sanctions for inappropriate behavior. Inappropriate behavior includes both irrelevant prior behavior and deviant or innovative behavior that may develop in response to the technology being introduced.

Change agents should be significant to others who are involved in communicating their expectations about the new behavior and should develop meaningful rewards for conformity and appropriate and negative sanctions for deviance.

Selecting Hospital Information Systems

Hospital information systems are said to produce increased formalization, centralization and stratification, all of which should result in increased efficiency and productivity. However, organization theory hypothesizes that these factors are inversely related to employee satisfaction and accommodation to change. Furthermore, sociological theory postulates that abrupt and extensive attempts to achieve increased efficiency, often effected via increased job structuring (formalization), will not necessarily result in improved productivity and effectiveness. This hypothesis is supported by the results of a study conducted by the author to observe the implementation in the hospital of HIS medications application. [8]

Administrators, including nursing administrators, must make a crucial decision when weighing the various approaches to HIS. In order to achieve the optimum effect on organizational and unit productivity and effectiveness, a moderate increase in organizational centralization, job formalization, and occupational stratification is recommended. The following guidelines should be helpful in this effort.

1. Permit only a moderate increase in job standardization. This can be achieved by ensuring that

   - health professionals have unrestricted access to patient data in order to carry out their functions of ordering, charting, and carrying out treatment plans.
   - orders can be entered and accessed in a manner as similar to the present (manual) procedures as is feasible. Some standardization between nursing units may still be felt necessary, since there can be wide variation in treatment plans and individual physician ordering patterns by type of patient diagnosis (and thus by type of nursing station).
   - there is flexibility in the technological system to accommodate organizational and health professionals' needs for lists, schedules, and ordering patterns.

2. Insist on sufficient participation in decision making by relevant sections of the organization. The increase in centralization can be moderated by ensuring

   - participation by health practitioners in decisions about applications, changes, vendor's role, etc.
   - participation by unit and department administrative staff in committees and decisions affected by the HIS.

3. Soften the effects of increased occupational stratification, which is often an unintended consequence of the introduction of an HIS, by

   - incorporating any change agent roles (e.g., DP nurse, HIS physician) within the organization or by selecting as change agents health professionals who are opinion leaders with a political base and constituency who support the change and will effectively communicate the need for new behaviors and routines.

- providing flexible options regarding access to patient record so that, for example, nurse aides, occupational therapists, are not prevented access to diagnostic and treatment information available to practically anyone looking through a manual, or paper, record.

In the initial phases, at least, the factors contributing most to successful implementation of the HIS are the organizational variables *formalization* and *centralization*. The author suggests that the HIS would be most likely to win acceptance in a hospital setting under the following conditions: (1) the HIS is not permitted to change the physician's role extensively or place excessive restrictions on the nurse or other health practitioners (formalization); (2) all occupations, departments, and users are allowed to participate in decision making about the system and its modifications (centralization); (3) excessive changes in hierarchical stratification of occupations are not introduced (stratification); and (4) the progress of change is definite, continuous, visible, and in conformity with the advance plans and schedule.

A Caveat

Frequently, reality does not turn out to be the way theories predict it will be. And schemes such as the one proposed above do not always encompass all the factors that bear upon decisions.

Vendors of HIS offer a variety of approaches to the same applications, and so a hospital's HIS committee may select the approach it favors. [9] Some hospital organization heads are fairly knowledgeable about the various alternatives, objectives, and probable effects of HIS. Members of the organization could, therefore, be more effectively involved in decision making about the HIS, even those with service or "turnkey" (software) arrangements.

In some instances, decision makers (with some assistance from federal or state governments and insurance companies) may determine that the HIS that does attempt to provide the most in standardization and control over particular roles and the one that has the most effect on restructuring the roles is the right system for their organization. [10] A hospital may select one particular HIS approach and philosophy precisely because it wishes to achieve more conformity to policies and procedures.

The above presentation should not be interpreted to mean that the system that attempts to achieve more administrative control over the documentation-related activities of all types of healthcare practitioners should not be attempted. Rather, the intent here is to point to the potential risks and outcomes involved in such an attempt and to outline possible unanticipated consequences for the organization.

When decision makers are aware of the risks and alternatives inherent in the various hospital information systems being promoted, they can make informed decisions regarding the selection, adoption, and implementation of one of them. It is hoped that knowledge of these factors can help make decision makers and implementors, including physicians and nursing administrators, aware of those areas in which reorientation and education programs are most necessary.

References and Notes

1. See, for example, the following studies: Karsh, B. and Siegman, J. Functions of ignorance in introducing automation. *Social Problems*, Vol. 12, No.2, 1964, pp. 141–150; Friedmann, G *The Anatomy of Work, Labor, Leisure and the Implications of Automation*. Translated by Wyatt Rawson. New York: The Fress Press of Glencoe, 1961, pp. xiv–xv; chapter VII and p. 50.

2. Blauner, R. *Alienation and Freedom: The Factory Worker and His Industry*. Chicago: The University of Chicago Press, Phoenix Edition, 1967, p 170.

3. Hage, J. An axiomatic theory of organizations. *Administrative Science Quarterly* Vol. 10 no. 3, 1965, pp. 289–320; Hage, J. and Aiken, M. *Social Change in Complex Organizations*. New York: Random House 1970.

4. Parsons T. and Bales, R. F. *Family Socialization and Interaction Process*. Glencoe, III.: Free Press, 1955, pp. 234–37; Parsons, T., et al. *Working Papers in the Theory of Action*. New York: Free Press 1953.

5. Bredemeier, H. C. and Stephenson, R. H. *The Analysis of Social Systems*. New York: Holt, Rinehart and Winston, 1962, chapter 4.

6. Bennis, W. G., et al. (eds). *The Planning of Change: Readings in the Applied Behavioral Sciences*. New York: Holt, Rinehart and Winston, 1961.

7. See, for example, Goslin, D. (ed.). *Handbook of Socialization Theory and Research*. Chicago: Rand McNally and Company, 1969, chapters 25–29.

8. Goldstein, B. and Farlee, C. a *Hospital Organization and Computer Technology: The Challenge of Change*. New Brunswick, N.J.: Health Care Systems Research 1972. Copies of the final report are available from the Social and Economic Analysis Division of the Health Resources Administration, NHCSR, DHEW and are on file with the Hospital Information Systems Sharing Group.

9. The Hospital information Systems Sharing Group is composed of several vendors with HIS software and various hospitals that are implementing different HIS packages with various structured assumptions and varied organizational consequences.

10. The TRI-service Medical information System (TRIMIS) is planned for introduction in "all" Department of Defense hospitals over the next five to ten years on the assumption that one standardized system can be implemented throughout all DOD hospitals and clinics.

MANAGING USER RESISTANCE

PERHAPS THE single most prevalent, yet underappreciated, negative phenomenon that accompanies information technology is user resistance. Both professionals and office staff have consistently tended to challenge the deployment of new information systems in their organizations. Because managers often have failed to deal with staff resistance, many technically sound information system applications have been inordinately troubled, or have failed altogether. Shoshona Zuboff (1988), a social psychologist at Harvard Business School, studied resistance to information technologies for a number of years. She reported that resistance is not isolated but, rather, is endemic and is " . . . an implied threat to the whole structure of authority." Pascale, Millemann, and Gioja's 1997 research supports this contention. They found that modern organizations have "a remarkable capacity to resist change." Let's check out St. Serena's experience in this regard.

CASE STUDY

Case Five: The Retarding Resisters

Andrew Able's day at St. Serena's nursing home facility had been hectic and stressful. After reflecting on the situation that had developed since the installation of the new integrated information system, he reluctantly decided to postpone his vacation planned for next week. As administrator of the nursing home facility, Andrew had been attending endless meetings recently with both professional and nonprofessional staff, trying to deal with mounting complaints about the new information system. Brenda, the facility's assistant administrator, called the situation "techno-stress" and was not optimistic about the future. "We have tried everything to convince them that their work will be easier with the new system but they don't seem to want to cooperate," Brenda quipped. "Heck, I'm not convinced myself that this new system is any better than what we had!"

Andrew thought about the transition efforts he developed with Stewart to help staff become accustomed to the new system. Andrew had held regular pre-implementation meetings, encouraged involvement, initiated training sessions, and spoke positively about the benefits of the change. Why were the staff still complaining? He was beginning to wonder whether coercion might be a better approach to the problem.

Brenda had kept a diary of occurrences as the new information system unfolded (see below). She gave a copy of it to Andrew for his record and review.

June 30: The user committee, convened by Stewart, met with the vendors and consultants and approved, with little argument, the hardware and software for the new information system.

July 1: The director of Nursing tells me at lunch that she thinks implementation of the new information system is being rushed. I suggested that she should speak with Stewart about her concerns.

July 7: Rumors are rampant. Some of our people are asking about layoffs; others are talking about other healthcare facilities that had problems with their system. Stewart is being described as an ogre who was brought in by Samantha to be a hatchet man.

July 15: We called a general staff meeting to address the concerns and unfounded rumors. The people there seemed to listen and calm down, but attendance was not good.

July 30: Stewart led a pre-implementation meeting with us and all department heads. Most attendees seemed bored or burdened by the session. About half the departments sent assistants to represent them.

August 12: Overheard Dietary staff in the elevator saying there was no way they would be able learn the new information system. It was too technical.

August 13: Spoke with Dan, the director of Dietary, about what I heard. He responded that the complaints were only idle gossip, but that the new system does seem a bit complicated.

August 21: A second pre-implementation meeting was convened by Stewart. Samantha was there, but left after 15 minutes for a board committee meeting. Mike, the chief of Medicine also left early but, before that, reported that a colleague at St. Ditmas Hospital in Denver tells him that they had mega problems with a similar system there. The representative for the vice president for administration, Ann Apple, asked Samantha about cutbacks in the clerical ranks. Samantha said there would be none.

August 30: Another meeting convened today apparently to allay lay-off fears. The younger representatives present seem to be more comfortable with the whole thing than are the more senior ones.

September 8: Sally from Social Services resigned today citing as one of her reasons St. Serena's disregard for patient privacy issues in the new information system.

September 22: The new hardware finally arrived today. Installation begins tomorrow.

September 23: Some of the new equipment disappeared overnight and some appears to have been damaged. Where the heck were our security people?

November 20: Training of staff on the new system has gone slower than expected. They complain that the new system is so different from the old one.

December 1: The director of Nursing sent a memo complaining of chronic staff shortages. She claims that all the time spent on the new information system has taken staff away from residents.

December 15: The new system went online today.

January 15: Stewart sent a memo stressing that the "bugs" in the new system are gradually being eliminated. He is asking for patience. Apparently Dan blew his top when the new system told him to send a hot fudge sundae to a diabetic resident. Fortunately, floor staff caught the mistake before the whipped cream was consumed.

February 30: Frank from Finance reported that last month's Medicaid billings were all returned because of coding errors. He is blaming Stewart's new system. What was Samantha thinking when she brought him aboard?

March 17: The Nursing staff called for a work slow-down to begin next week to protest the new system. They say that too many resident's charts have been erased inexplicably. Stewart has promised to get the software vendor on the problem pronto. Can this really be St. Patrick's Day?

Questions for Discussion

1. What forms of resistance are evident at the nursing home facility?
2. Can you explain why these problems have arisen at St. Serena's?

3. What do you recommend be done? Should Andrew go on his planned vacation?
4. Prepare a plan to deal with the problems at St. Serena's.

COMMENTARY

The phenomenon of resistance to information technology became a focus of research attention in the last decades. Charles Eberle, a noted information technology specialist, consistently found that with new technologies "resistance is enormous" (Zuboff 1988). A survey by Richard Walton of the Harvard Business School supports this contention. Of a large sample of organizations with serious commitments to information technologies, Walton found middle managers to be major barriers to change (*The New York Times* 1988). Demattia (1999) found physician resistance to be a major barrier to deployment of new electronic technology. Prompted by evidence of severe resistance to information technology at one hospital, researcher Alan Dowling surveyed a randomly selected sample of 40 public and private hospitals. He estimated that staff resistance to and interference with new information systems had occurred in nearly half the hospitals that have attempted to implement such systems. Furthermore, Dowling (1980) found that "interference can have significant consequences in terms of cost, lost earnings, organizational disruption, and poor quality of care." The magnitude of the problem is nationwide, and it can have an enormous effect on corporate America's drive to reengineer itself. Polls have shown that while 70 percent of large U.S. companies claim to be reengineering their information technology systems, nearly one quarter of these reengineering projects are failing. Experts attribute much of this failure to staff resistance (Cafasso 1993). Both the Dowling study and the 1993 polls revealed that the problem was much more widespread and serious than most managers, including Samantha and Stewart, realized. In fact, although Dowling reported that hospital managers generally thought resistance was rare or unique to their hospital, resistance to information management efforts appears to be the rule, rather than the exception, and it extends from front-line workers to clinicians, and even to top executives.

This resistance was illustrated by the multitude of articles, published in professional journals, that emphasize the drawbacks of information technology and express pervasive resentment by a wide range of health-care professionals, such as "Can a Computer Tell How Good a Doctor You Are?" (*Medical Economics* 1994), "Are Information Systems Your

Friend or Foe?" (*Chief Executive* 1986), "Nursing Views Computers as Both Friends and Foes" (*Hospitals* 1986), and "How Soon Will You Be at the Mercy of a Hospital Computer?" (*Medical Economics* 1987).

Based on his experience as a consultant in private business, Roger Hallock concludes, in his 1999 article in *Administrative Management*, that "many computer systems barely live up to half their potential" because of top management resistance. This conclusion is consistent with a *Fortune* magazine article that asserts "information technology cannot reshape an organization unless the organization finds some way to make workers comfortable with computers" (Kirkpatrick 1993).

These reports all indicate a need for healthcare professionals to deal with resistance effectively if "state of the art" information systems are to work at St. Serena's and elsewhere.

Recognizing Resistance

Recognition of the nature of resistance has frequently been impeded by its subtlety. Resistance consists of any number of acts, deliberate or subconscious, that interfere with the effective implementation or use of an information technology application. The range of such acts runs the gamut from clear, direct, active behavior—such as physical abuse of equipment which appears to have occurred at St. Serena's—to subtle, indirect, and passive forms, such as simple nonuse of a carefully designed system.

The first type of resistance is the physical sabotage of computer equipment, which has occurred with surprising frequency. Terminals smashed, paper clips inserted into scanners, and printer wires pulled are only some examples. The second kind of resistance is much more subtle and clever. Chief among these covert acts is absenteeism of some form including increased truancy, lateness, slowdowns, and nonavailability while at work.

"Badmouthing" the system is the third common expression of resistance. Comments like "This system stinks. I told you it wouldn't work!" "The terminals are always down. They're a danger to patient care" are at least occasionally heard during most information management efforts. Sometimes these complaints are based on totally fabricated woes, sometimes they blow up minor and anticipated problems, and sometimes they are based on intentionally faulty use of the system such as repeatedly hitting the wrong key on a terminal and then claiming that the system does not work or is too difficult to use.

Nonuse of an installed information system is the fourth, and frequently encountered, form of resistance. Unwilling to learn and depend on the expensive new information system, workers have been known to continue using old systems and supervisors have been known to influence unit workers to not use the new system. The result, as Hersher (1999) observes, can be expensive: "Spending money on new technology is useless if staff is either not using it or just working around the system by 'jerry rigging' old procedures."

Perhaps the most serious form of resistance is data tampering, which can consist of withholding data or inputting errors. For example, case workers incompletely fill out automated forms on clients or users intentionally input incorrect data or a wrong code to upset the system or arouse complaints. Could this be behind St. Serena's problem with Medicaid billings?

Who are the resisters? Resistance emerges at all levels of the organization (Dunbar and Yound 1992; Dostert 1993; Mutschler and Hoefer 1990). Dowling concluded that each form of resistance "can be used by almost any key staff member at any time during implementation." Indeed, the evidence suggests that professionals, whose tasks are more discretionary than routine, may be the more frequent and effective resisters (Gardner 1990). This resistance can be understood by examining possible causes.

Causes of Resistance

At least seven possible explanations for resistance to modern information systems exist. Despite evidence to the contrary, technology is associated with layoffs and unemployment (Applebaum 1990); therefore, the first and most basic reason may be an economic determinant. James Manuso, a specialist in reactions to technology, claims that economic factor is the key cause: "First, of course, is people's fear that they're going to lose their jobs, that some machine is going to come in and do the work instead" (Hodges 1980). This perception is evidently present at St. Serena's. Information technology is viewed as a timesaving and labor-saving device that decreases the need for labor and middle managers. However, research shows that automation does not usually cause job losses; instead, job displacement (e.g., transfer) is a frequent result. Zuboff notes that while executives typically try to justify new information systems by showing how they would enable efficiencies, including elimination of jobs, few managers face the fact that the jobs cut, or redefined, might be their own. Zuboff's (1988) work shows that organizations that have gone the furthest in using information technologies tend to have only about half the managerial layers as their rivals.

A second, and perhaps the most common, cause of resistance, however, is psychological. New information systems can easily be ego-threatening. Proud professionals who know very little about the technology may fear a loss of prestige and status in the organization if an unfamiliar system is introduced. Support staff members who control file cabinets may resist changes that would deprive them of the power to dispense information from the files. Supervisors might resist out of fear that a new information system would perform the scheduling function that previously was a source of power for them.

The third reason may be social. Plans to disperse various members of work groups to isolated terminals or PCs might encounter resistance. The prime satisfaction some workers derive from their job may well be the chance to talk, or interconnect, with coworkers; therefore, removing this social benefit can prompt strong dissatisfaction. Additionally, resistance could be caused by a socially acceptable attitude of enmity toward machines. Resisting information technology might simply be viewed as "the thing to do."

The fourth reason may be intellectual. Professionals, such as in healthcare and human services fields, who hold high human values may have ideological barriers to accepting anything that might produce less human contact or deprive them of some personal and professional freedom. We seem to see this at St. Serena's. As one commentator puts it: "Some feel that computers dehumanize the care of patients . . . computerization reflects an increase in technical quality at the expense of humanness (i.e., 'high tech' without 'high touch')" (McConnell, Summers, O'Shea, and Kirchoff 1989).

Historical reasons, such as a previous bad experience with an information technology effort, could be the fifth probable cause. This factor appeared at St. Serena's in the form of the medical chief's comment about another hospital's experience.

The sixth reason may be organizational. For example, new information systems might be resisted because some individuals see little connection between what the system does and what role they have in the organization. Just as it is unusual to enter any modern organization and find no PCs, it is equally unusual to enter the office of a chief executive and find a well worn PC. In her book, *Leadership and the Computer*, Mary E. Boone (1993) says that "the problem is that many executives don't know that computers are capable of extending their creative and leadership abilities." Similarly, many practitioners in human service organizations perceive that computers are irrelevant to the practice of their profession (Semice and Nurius 1991).

The seventh reason may be operational. "People love innovation, but hate change" according to an article in *Hospitals & Health Newtorks* (1993). If we subscribe to the notion that technology means ongoing operational adjustment, the increasing application of information technology in healthcare suggests an inevitable operational upset. This aversion to change may simply be that people are obliged to think, work, and interact differently, which are consequences often associated with information technology.

Other reasons for resistance undoubtedly exist. Determining why an individual, or a group, in an organization resists the introduction of a new information system is not easy; however, basic fears of job loss, failure, and change are common factors in general. The important point is that understandable, though subtle, human needs probably underlie the most overt, as well as the covert, expressions of resistance. With an understanding of how and why information technology might be resisted, managers can then develop approaches to dealing with the phenomenon.

Dealing with Resistance

The fundamental guideline for managing resistance is to focus on the user. Research has documented that modern information systems are more likely to be accepted if they are responsive to the needs of the users, and if users participate in the development and implementation of the system (Mutschler and Hoefer 1990). As Michael Ginzberg (1978) put it: "Being a change agent requires that management . . . really comes to understand the user; that he keeps the user involved through the entire project, making sure the user understands where the project is going and contributes substantially to setting this direction."

This tenet seems to be echoed by all analysts of resistance. For example, *Output* magazine published Hodges' recipe "for managers who want to introduce technology without fear" (1980):

- Consult your staff from the beginning when you're considering the feasibility of new systems.
- Make it clear from your actions that the interests and requirements of the users are being taken fully into account in the design of new systems.
- Explain as clearly and honestly as possible the consequences of these developments, and plan with the staff how problems can be overcome.

The importance of this user focus was supported by Gelderman's (1998) extensive study of organizations in Holland. He found that "user satisfaction" is the key to information system success. St. Serena's might well benefit from this kind of perspective.

Several specific steps can help professionals manage resistance. First, develop a strategy for minimizing resistance before it occurs, as well as for detecting and addressing it during implementation. Dowling's study is useful in such an effort. In the cases of resistance in hospitals, Dowling (1980) found that "appraisal of the presystem environment and *a priori* diagnosis of the system's effects on the staff would have alerted management to impending problems." Dowling recommended using feedback mechanisms for detecting staff reaction and identifying resistance-inducing factors as major elements of an effective strategy.

Second, focus on the causes of resistance. Education and training well ahead of implementation can alleviate threats to egos by equipping staff with the knowledge needed to maintain their status and power. Studies consistently show that a significant relationship exists between education and training and users' attitudes toward new technology (Dean and Shorter 1991).

Deliberate efforts to maintain existing social groups can help alleviate the social causes of resistance, and a policy of avoiding layoffs, even when new technology makes staff reductions possible, is needed to temper the economic fear of job loss. Studies indicate that a single layoff can abet this fear. Such alternatives as attrition or reassignment, though perhaps more expensive in the short term, have proven to be far less costly overall.

Third, take specific measures to sell the information management effort, much like a marketing professional sells a product. For this to be effective, the benefits of using the technology have to be identified, highlighted, and explained. Using orientation workshops well before installation, presenting examples of favorable results in similar organizations, and demonstrating strong top-management support are some good methods. Particularly important is clarification of the organizational and personal advantages of using the new information system.

Fourth, help and encourage users to get involved from the earliest stage of the information management effort to the design, implementation, and evaluation of the system. Although participation takes time and nontechnical users can frustrate technical designers, we have learned from our experience with information technology that technically sound systems are useless unless people use them. Past experience clearly dictates user involvement in system development. Pascale, Millemann, and Gioja (1997) second this assertion that rigorous "engagement" of staff in the whole process is essential to success.

Keeping organizational staff informed is part of that staff-involvement process. Few factors create more fear and resistance than mystery and surprise. Making an information management plan a closely guarded secret is a major mistake in information system efforts.

Fifth, consider time and timing. Rapidly introducing new information systems in healthcare organizations has nearly always failed or produced serious problems. A go-slowly approach in which employment of the technology evolves in stages as users become more comfortable with it is more time consuming, but also more cost effective and successful. Time and exposure do heal fears and antagonisms. In the same vein, timing the introduction of new systems with a perceived need for change and improvement can help. Automating a process or activity that already appears to work well can understandably inspire cynicism toward, if not outright rejection of, new information management plans.

In addition, a range of specific resistance-countering techniques should be undertaken. One such example is the use of "ergonomics." Ergonomics refers to the design of equipment and workspace that fits each employee, ensures comfort, reduces strain, and avoids injury. The designers of telephone technology, for example, went to great pains to develop a handset, dial tilt, and so forth that would be both easy and comfortable to use. Until recently, widespread efforts in developing ergonomic designs in the field of information technology had been rare. But research suggests that regular use of computer terminals causes eyestrain, migraine headaches, nausea, and back pain, which could also have caused resistance (Lesin 1994). Questions of safety have arisen because of persistent worries about monitors possibly posing a variety of health risks including cataracts, muscle strain, and miscarriages (King 1991). Many manufacturers now commonly take into consideration terminals and workstations with ergonomic features which, although more expensive, should be part of an overall user-focused strategy. Information system-related periodicals now customarily publish articles that deal specifically with user safety and comfort (Heller 1993).

Some organizations have sold employees on new technology by introducing the system with games on the terminals. They have found this friendly technique to be an effective means both for overcoming fear and for training users on terminal and system operations (Leo 1985). Winter, Chuboda, and Gutek's (1998) studies confirm the wisdom of this approach: "Improving workers' computer literacy enhances the relationship between attitudes and computer use."

Other organizations have employed error-detection devices, such as inaccurate inputting and data withholding, to monitor forms of resistance (Dowling 1980). Still, other organizations suggest the need to induce a feeling of naturalness in user interface design. Nonkeyboard interfaces such as pen-based computers and systems that recognize voice, handwriting, and gestures, which substitute for keystroke commands, are alleged to make information systems more transparent to users (Ryan 1992). In terms of receptivity, studies in nursing show that educational preparation, length of service in the nursing profession, and specialization make a demonstrable difference in nurses' attitudes toward information technology (Brodt and Strong 1986).

Of course, when all else fails, managers can order cooperation and use of the new system and threaten to fire resisters. Although most studies have found this approach to be counterproductive, some analyses suggest that it can work in certain cases (Schewe 1976). When employed, however, the approach is more likely to work in combination with other approaches. In one notable case, a state government mandated all its local hospitals to install a new information system that would monitor administration of prescription drugs. Hospitals were informed that failure to cooperate and install a successful system would result in reduced funding and staff and the transfer of clients to other facilities. The hospital administrators conveyed this order to doctors, nurses, and pharmacists. Intended to identify the extent of long-term drug use in the treatment of psychiatric patients, the system was resisted by doctors, nurses, and pharmacists. Doctors felt that it would be used to qualitatively judge the care they were providing, as well as place artificial constraints on their future ability to prescribe medication. Nurses expressed concern over the additional workload they would incur by having to fill out more and different medication forms. Pharmacists resisted because the new system would entail a major change in their processing, distribution, and dosage preparation procedures.

The system's managers met this resistance with fairly firm methods. Using a top-down approach, they first met with hospital administrators to explain the nature of the system. Then, they tried to reduce some of the user hostility by offering alternative solutions to various problems in the system. They agreed to intervene only if decisions were not made within certain time frames. Additionally, great emphasis was placed on adequate staff training to reduce the problems of learning to use the system.

Resistance from nurses was reduced by adapting the new system for use with the old drug-reporting forms, which eliminated increased work and training sessions. Doctors were presented with a benefit in the form of a drug-information database that would help them in prescribing drugs and dosages.

The greatest benefit was presented to the pharmacists. Computerization in the pharmacy often required a complete revision of departmental policy and procedures. The system managers made clear that the new system would increase the pharmacists' efficiency and control over inventories and distribution procedures. They also emphasized that the pharmacists' status would be greatly increased because the new system would expand their participation and impact in the process of developing therapeutic drug regimens.

The system has now been operating for a number of years, and system managers report that initial studies demonstrate that users are getting accurate and complete information from the system. The experience demonstrates the wisdom of Henry's (1997) contention that resistance is basically a healthy phenomenon which, if properly managed, helps bring information management efforts to fruition.

References

Applebaum, S. H. 1990. "Computerphobia: Training Managers to Reduce the Fears and Love the Machines." *Industrial and Commercial Training* 22 (6): 9–16.

Boone, M. E. 1993. *Leadership and the Computer.* Rockilin, CA: Prima Publishing.

Brodt, A., and J. Strong. 1986. "Nurses Attitudes Toward Computerization in a Midwestern Community Hospital." *Computers in Nursing* (March–April): 82–86.

Brown, S. 1987. "How Soon Will You Be at the Mercy of a Hospital Computer?" *Medical Economics* (2 March): 160–3.

Cafasso, R. 1993. "Rethinking Reengineering." *Computerworld* (15 March): 102–5.

"Can a Computer Tell How Good a Doctor You Are?" 1994. *Medical Economics* (24 January): 136.

Dean, R., and J. Shorter. 1991. "Preparing Your Networking Information Systems in Healthcare Organizations." *Health Care Supervisor* (September): 58–62.

Demattio, R. 1999. "It Pays to Be Connected." *Modern Physician* 3 (10): 60–3.

Dostert, M. 1993. "Candy from Strangers." *Computerworld* (29 March): 89–92.

Dowling, A. F. 1980. "Do Hospital Staff Interfere with Computer System Implementation?" *Health Care Management Review* (Fall): 23.

Dunbar, C., and J. Yound. 1992. "Expensive Iron Doesn't Equal High Technology." *Computers in Healthcare* (December): 16–20.

Friend, D. 1986. "Are Information Systems Your Friend or Foe?" *Chief Executive* (Summer): 26–7.

Gardner, E. 1990. "Physician Resistance Major Obstacle to Expert Systems." *Modern Healthcare* (12 February): 43.

Gelderman, M. 1998. "The Relation Between User Satisfaction, Usage of Information Systems and Performance." *Information & Management* 34 (1): 11–8.

Ginzberg, M. J. 1978. "Steps Toward More Effective Implementation of MS and MIS." *Interface* (May): 61–2.

Hallock, R. I. 1979. "With Computers, Administrative Attitude Is the Key to Success." *Administrative Management* (March): 80.

Heller, M. 1993. "Positioned for Success." *Windows Magazine* (November): 171–83.

Henry, P. 1997. "Overcoming Resistance to Organizational Change." *Journal of the American Dietetic Association* 97 (10): S2, S145–7.

Hersher, B. 1999. "Technology Transitions." *Healthcare Executive* 14 (5): 48.

Hodges, P. 1980. "Fear of Automation." *Output* (August): 34.

King, R. R. 1991. "Health Effects of Visual Display Terminals." *Nursing Management* (October): 61–4.

Kirkpatrick, D. 1993. "Making It All Worker-Friendly." *Fortune* 128 (7): 44–53.

Leo, J. 1980. "Coping with Computers." *Discover* (December): 97.

Lesin, B. E. 1994. "Safety Tips for PC Users." *Human Resources Professional* (January–February): 19–21.

McConnell, E. A., S. Summers O'Shea, and K. T. Kirchoff. 1989. "R.N. Attitudes Toward Computers." *Nursing Management* (July): 39.

Mutschler, E., and R. Hoefer. 1990. "Factors Affecting the Use of Computer Technology in Human Service Organizations." *Administration in Social Work* 14 (1): 87–101.

The New York Times. 1988. (7 February): B-1.

Packer, C. L. 1986. "Nursing Views Computers as Both Friends and Foes." *Hospitals* (November): 20.

Pascale, R., M. Millemann, and L. Gioja. 1997. "Changing the Way We Change." *Harvard Business Review* (November/December): 128.

Ryan, H. 1992. "The Human Metaphor." *Information Systems Management* (Winter): 72–5.

Schewe, C. B. 1976. "The Management Information System User: An Exploratory Behavioral Analysis." *Academy of Management Journal* (December): 577–90.

Semke, J. I., and P. S. Nurius. 1991. "Information Structure, Information Technology, and the Human Services Organizational Environment." *Social Work* (July): 354.

Winter, S., K. Chuboda, and B. Gutek. 1998. "Attitudes Toward Computers: When Do They Predict Computer Use?" *Information & Management* 34 (5): 275–84.

Zuboff, S. 1988. "Resisting Technology." *The New York Times* (7 February): B-1.

READINGS

The issue of resistance management is enlightened through the two articles below. William Umiker concisely sets forth the nature of the resistance phenomenon, emphasizing that user perception of information systems "is often more meaningful than reality," and that emotional reactions are central to the problem. He then provides concrete measures for preventing and attending to the phenomenon.

Kathryn Dansky et al. have produced one of the most managerially useful articles to date on information systems management with specific application to electronic medical records (EMR) systems. The authors brilliantly and concisely lay out the tremendous benefits of EMR, but then they soberly address the practical managerial challenges involved in reaping the potential. Before contemplating the introduction of EMR in your organization, the authors caution that managers "would be wise to assess the readiness of the principal end users—that is, the physicians." Right on! The article then proceeds to offer insightful results of the authors' empirical studies for helping managers practically deal with the challenge. St. Serena's would do well to have these articles discussed at the next steering committee meeting.

How to Prevent and Cope with Resistance to Change

William Umiker

Abstract

Resistance to workplace changes is always to be anticipated. It can be minimized by insightful planning, and overcome by competent leadership. This article provides practical advice for both planning and leadership tactics.

Resistance to change is not all bad. It can be a valuable protective device, sometimes keeping an Organization from making critical mistakes. For the most part, however, resistance is a roadblock that must be removed. The inability of employers and managers to cope with employee resistance can destroy organizations and careers.

Any significant workplace change alters established habits, responsibility roles, relationships, and operational procedures and causes some people to cling desperately to the past. Change always means giving up something; the greater the sacrifice, the more likely it is that people resist the innovation. Managers and specialists who worked hard to achieve their current status are likely to oppose, overtly or covertly, any threat to their hard-earned power or special niche in the organization. Most educational and health care institutions are divided into functional units like silos. When restructuring rocks the integrity of a unit, or when mergers, right-sizing, process reengineering, or crossfunctional teams require the integration of isolated functional units, the probability of resistance increases.

When employees do not accept change, it may be because they do not understand it, they think that it will be bad for them or for their organization, or they don't trust their leaders to make it work,

Reprinted with permission from William Umiker, "How to Prevent and Cope . . . ," Health Care Supervisor 15 (4), 35–41,
© 1997, Aspen Publishers, Inc. William Umiker is adjunct professor at the Pennsylvania State University Medical Center.

especially if they have witnessed failures in the past. Perception is often more meaningful than reality. A false perception or a negative mindset is frequently based on lack of information, misinterpretation, faulty assumptions, or irrational thinking. Employees are particularly prone to resistance when change occurs without proactive analysis, planning, or direction, or when they have supervisors who fail to say what they mean, or fail to mean what they say.

Emotional responses to change are portentous. The major emotion elicited by change, or even the threat of change, is fear. It may be fear of the unknown, fear of loss of job, fear of inability to measure up to new responsibilities, or fear of disruption of work relationships.

People with low self-esteem and a great need for security are more likely to become resisters based on fear. Altered relationships with former coworkers or the sudden appearance of new faces, new equipment, or new building contractors may be very upsetting. A major responsibility of leaders is to help their employees overcome these fears.

Getting Commitment

Successful change is not achieved until commitment is obtained from the people who must implement the change or who are affected by it. This commitment is best sought when a change first is contemplated. Competent leaders know that commitment will not be obtained if rational or emotional concerns are ignored. They understand why people resist change and persuade them to view change as normal—a journey, not a destination.

Knowing that preventing resistance is much better than trying to overcome it, change agents have designed practical techniques for confronting doubt, helplessness, and indifference. Employees then gain a clear understanding of what is to happen, why the change is necessary, and what the goal is. Even more important, the spoken or unspoken question "How does this affect me?" is answered.

These leaders are aware that people are most likely to commit to a major change when they perceive that the survival of their organization or their job is threatened without the change or that the change offers some kind of a payoff for them. Change specialists also know how to allay the fears of their employees and how to readjust employees' perspectives.

Change agents seek opportunities to involve people. Whenever possible they give them a voice in designing the change and determining them role in implementing it. Employees learn much and become more understanding when they find out the seriousness of the situation that must be changed. They also develop a greater appreciation of the difficulties involved. More specifically, proposals meet less resistance when employees note that there may be an opportunity to get their work done faster or with less interference, or when there may be pay increases or promotions in the offing. Resistance often diminishes or may even be replaced with enthusiasm when teams visit sites where similar changes have been introduced successfully. [1]

On the negative side, the more people involved, the more the process is slowed down. Group-think can dilute the quality of decisions, and a popular program may be poorly conceived. [2]

Exemplars of change are cognizant of the fact that changes stir up resistance somewhere and that by anticipating this one is better prepared to cope with it. They suggest that for major changes, opening moves be dramatic and convincing enough to overcome inertia. They claim that you do not need commitment from everybody before you move forward. For many people, buy-in will come later, after some favorable results are in.[2]

Principles of Preparing for a Major Change

The following principles should be followed whenever an organization is facing or plans any major change.

- Choose your opening moves carefully. Sometimes it's possible to make changes gradually and quietly so no opposition is aroused, but this is a big gamble.
- When cross-functional activities are planned, take special care to preserve the functional integrity of affected departments or units.
- Introduce initiatives by pilot projects, and use highly motivated teams to increase the likelihood that quick, favorable results are obtained.
- Provide comprehensive analyses, thorough planning, and proficient direction.
- Articulate a clear goal and identify an end point.
- Address concerns promptly. You can't expect people to be eager to change when they don't know how it's going to affect them, or when they feel threatened and vulnerable.
- Avoid stalling. Even when the change is not in people's best interests, getting closure helps to alleviate resistance.
- Avoid focusing only on the positives. Admit that things will get worse before they get better.
- Always remember that your job is to be a promoter and encouraged. Change requires lots of cheerleading.

The Importance of Communication

Extensive communication is essential. One must not rely on what filters down through the formal communication system or is transmitted via the "grapevine." Explain the need for change in pragmatic terms, and listen patiently to employees who elect to blow off steam. Employees feel a sense of relief when told that their concerns are normal and will pass. Answering all their questions satisfactorily and patiently is essential. By understanding the questions that people pose, and answering them conscientiously, you markedly improve the odds that innovations will succeed. Explain what is to change and why it is necessary. Consider the situation from the employees' perspective.

Communication is also crucial in keeping programs moving. People see and hear things that disturb them. They are often disappointed and frustrated by all the problems or bottlenecks that develop. When they complain, showcase the benefits or the progress that has been made. Make it easy and safe for them to express new concerns.

The Importance of Education and Training

Don't overlook the knowledge gap that change creates. There is usually a lot to be learned. Make certain that people have the necessary know-how. They must handle new kinds of equipment and face unfamiliar methods. There may be different supervisors, coworkers, or culture changes to accommodate.

What appears to be obstinance or lack of cooperation may be a simple lack of comprehension. Help them understand what must be done and to develop new skills. Instead of training everyone at the same time, and covering all material before they can utilize the training, provide the instruction as it is needed ("just-in-time" training), and provide it to those workers who are going to use it first. Make training manuals and other instructional materials readily available, and give the people enough time to get acquainted with them.

Exhibit Your Own Commitment

A lot of resistance dies out when people realize that the change is a done deal and that there is no turning back. If there is any indication that the initiative might be averted, resistance will increase. Your actions speak louder than your words in this regard, so "walk the talk." Be obvious and passionate in your determination to follow through. Don't try to reduce resistance by softening your position. It will only stiffen the resistance. Employees will fully commit only when they trust their superiors, and this trust must be earned.

Adjust Your Reward System to Support Change

Hanging on to old habits makes sense to employees when their old reward system stays in place. Therefore it is wise to restructure the way people are compensated. Rewards are more than promotions, awards, and bonuses. They include desirable assignments, praise, attention, and notes of appreciation.

Resistance should produce a more unpleasant set of results than change does. Pritchett [2] articulates this very forcefully: "Make an example of someone who resists. If this sounds ruthless, remember that it is their choice to resist. Something has to suffer, either them or the change effort."[2, p.21]

Monitor Progress and Measure Results

Major change efforts require constant monitoring. Things do go wrong. Unexpected situations develop. Some resistance is due to certain aspects of the plan that were wrong to begin with or that are carried out poorly. As people have to break their familiar routine, performance weakens, and there is more confusion, communication problems, and job stress. Some people conclude that the plan is not working. The grumbling grows louder unless the leaders have prepared people by making it clear that the change will not be trouble free.

Talk to people. Track results. Look for symptoms like slippage in timetables, productivity downturns, loss of customers, increased customer complaints, or signs of uncooperativeness, complaining, and criticizing of the people in charge. People may get confused, drift off course, or start regressing to the old way of doing things. If you're paying attention, you can address the problems before they get out of hand.

Monitoring performance and tracking results also enable you to identify the new heroes, the role models who are contributing the most to the change effort. You need to single these people out, honor them, and celebrate their achievements.

The Responses to Change

The very quickest way for my organization to pick up speed is for resisters to take their foot off the brakes . . . to stop their desperate attempts to preserve the status quo. [2 (preface)]

The happy campers

A minority of a work group embraces new marching orders enthusiastically. The better the preparation for change, the larger this percentage will be. Alert managers will make full use of these eager beavers. They will assign them to pilot programs and have them discuss successes during the early phases of a new initiative. They will give generous attention to the people who drive the change. Although these essential people deserve the best treatment, all too often they are taken for granted. [2]

Highly successful organizations employ only workers who are motivated, competent, and devoid of "me first" mentality. Selective hiring of new employees merits special attention. Most new supervisors inherit teams and must make do with the individuals who are already on board. But these managers can be more selective when screening new candidates, and they should be hesitant to hire people who have past histories of inflexibility, cynicism, or the inability to adjust to new situations.

The bystanders

Usually, the largest percentage of employees are fence-sitters who are neither obstinate nor uncooperative but who do fret over how a change may affect them and their work group. While not hostile to change, they are not enthusiastic about it either. Perhaps they have witnessed multiple rounds of workplace fashions that fizzled out. Bystanders withhold commitment. They want proof that the change will work. They want to know where it was tried and what the results were. They need time and support to make choices.

An easy out is tell them to lead, follow, or get out of the way. A better option is to prepare for the change carefully and thoroughly and then to ensure early success. Most of the members of this group will join in the endeavor when they see colleagues commit themselves, and the bystanders will then pitch in to help.

Get resistance out into the open. Make it safe and easy for people to express their feelings. Be patient enough to get beyond superficial answers so you can reach the true issues. Try to understand the various positions. Evaluate the legitimacy of their resistance. You might discover that some of their reluctance keeps you from doing something dumb. At the very least, they can educate you about why they are resisting and how you can elicit their support. [2]

When people say that things were better before the changes were installed, remind them of the problems that existed before the change and how we tend to forget the bad things of the past. For example, while people may have griped about a new computer system, few would elect to go back to the old one.

The resisters

Resistance can be overt or covert, active or passive, well intentioned or subversive. People fight change in ways that best fit their individual personalities, so expect a wide range of tactics at work when resistance emerges.

Among the resisters are a few firebrands who are loud and outspoken in their opposition to change. One or two highly vocal critics can infect an entire team, so it is hazardous to ignore them. You must get beyond the hostility and the high decibel level, because only then do you discover what is really causing all the fireworks. Sometimes you must turn your back on some of the racket; a lot of it is just pollution.

A larger group comprises the cynics. They are less brazen than the firebrands and often have some truth to support their pessimism. There may have been failures in the past, or upper management may have abandoned similar previous initiatives. More than likely, these prophets of doom believe their own propaganda. A favorite expression of these folks is some form of "We have been down that path before," and this statement can set the tone and carry the day.

Cynics lack faith in the leadership, and they express disbelief that management will do what it says it will do. They seek promises, reassurances, or certainty, knowing that these seldom can be guaranteed.

Cynics rely on a strategy of delay. Naturally, speed is the adversary they fear the most. Actually, they do not even want "slow," they want "not at all." They wag their heads and warn about the risks of rapid change. They condemn speed as reckless. They constantly want to sit down and talk things out, weigh the risks again, consider other options, and ruminate over what might go wrong. Careful deliberation is appropriate in the planning phase when trying to decide on the right course of action, but even there the resisters may bog things down—analysis-paralysis. Pritchett [2] warns that there are far more failures from going too slowly than from exceeding some imaginary speed limit.

Some resisters deliberately disguise their resistance to make it safer or more politically correct. People in this category are the most cunning. They operate under cover, resisting on the sly, fighting change carefully to minimize their chances of being caught. These are the saboteurs, the silent enemies of change.

Your job is to blow their cover. Look for signs of passive resistance, for example, foot dragging, quiet uncooperativeness, malicious compliance, etc. When you spot these people, corner them and get them talking.

Bureaucracy is the enemy of change. Its primary virtue lies in its ability to stabilize things. It provides structure, role clarity, and predictability. However, it causes work patterns to stiffen and to become inflexible routines. It lets once-serviceable guidelines deteriorate into procedural ruts. Its emphasis on petty rules and proper forms stifles innovation, interferes with progress, and legitimizes resistance.

Bureaucrats like saboteurs, rely heavily on covert tactics. Passive resistance is their forte—not taking a clear position or rationalizing the need to go slow to avoid mistakes. They wage their private turf battles by means of red tape and standard operating procedures. They circulate behind the scenes to spread doubt and sabotage the change game plan.

Expect the bureaucrats to wrap themselves in the corporate flag and warn that the change is ill conceived. Even if you give them the benefit of the doubt as to their motivation, you must dismiss their rhetoric. And you must override their argument for preserving the status quo. Frankly, you won't have much luck selling change to these people, so proceed in spite of them. Make it happen.[2]

Responses to Resistance

The instinctive response of leaders to employee resistance is to argue, to persuade the doubters that this particular change is special, that it is different from the previous ones that failed. However, cynicism may be so potent that rational argument and a cogent vision are not enough to overcome that skepticism. [3]

Rational arguments such as pointing out that a new initiative is unlike previous ones that failed may not have the desired effect. These damage-control efforts are worthwhile, however, because while they may not convert the cynics, these efforts limit the influence of the skeptics on other members of the team. In other words, we don't need every scoffer to join our effort, but we do want to contain the influence they have over the others—to neutralize their power.

Occasionally, the critics can be converted simply by giving them more of the action or involving them more in the decision process. For example, a person with a negative attitude toward a change that involves a new piece of equipment may change that attitude after being sent to a training unit to learn how to use that equipment.

It's hard to ignore resisters, but this group gives you the least return on your efforts and giving them your attention reinforces their problem behavior. Be willing to let squeaky wheels squeak. Save your grease for the quieter wheels that are carrying the load. Lombardi [4] notes that the change dynamic provides an excellent opportunity to appraise substandard performance and to provide the genesis for terminating a nonplayer for inferior performance.

Block [3] recommends replacing persuasion and coercion with an invitation to the cynics to choose to have faith in the experience. No attempt is made to disagree with their version of history. Block even supports them in their doubts. He would say something like 'I understand what you say. The doubts and perhaps bitterness you express I share to some degree. However, I have decided to have faith that this time we can do something here that will matter, and I'm going to give this my best shot. I hope that you will make the same choice and join in the effort.'

Resistance to change can be minimized when supervisors select new hires carefully, weed out the hard-core resisters, keep people informed, solicit and respond to concerns of their reports, and engage them in the planning activities. You must also provide the training needed to get the job done. Employees who cooperate and commit must be rewarded. Earning employees' trust and demonstrating empathy are also critical to success.

References

1. Carr, C. "7 keys to successful change." *Training* 31 (February 1994): 55–60.
2. Pritchett, P. *Resistance: Moving Beyond the Barriers to Change.* Dallas, Tex.: Pritchett 1996.
3. Block, P. *Stewardship: Choosing Service over Self Interest.* San Francisco, Calif. Berrett-Koehler 1993.
4. Lombardi, D. N. "The Healthcare Manager's Guide to Managing Change in Challenging Times." *Clinical Laboratory Management Review* 10 (January/February 1996): 18–24.

Electronic Medical Records: Are Physicians Ready?

Kathryn H. Dansky, Larry D. Gamm, Joseph J. Vasey, and Camille K. Barsukiewicz

Executive Summary

The use of electronic medical records (EMR) in healthcare organizations will require substantial changes in the way physicians and their staff

Reprinted with permission from the Journal of Healthcare Management 44 (6): 440–455. (Chicago: Health Administration Press, 1999). Dansky, Gamm, and Vasey are on the faculty of Pennsylvania State University. Camille Barsukiewicz is assistant professor at University of Memphis, TN.

provide patient care. This study is the first part of a larger study assessing factors that influence successful implementation of EMR in ambulatory care settings. The purposes of this study were to identify specific attitudes or factors that should be targeted before implementing an EMR project, and demonstrate empirical support for a model of perceived usefulness of EMR. We found that computer experience, computer anxiety, and perceptions of organizational support predict the degree to which physicians and mid-level practitioners view the EMR effort positively.

Strategies for the successful management of EMR implementation include engaging the physicians and practitioners in computer activities prior to implementation and providing strong organizational support before and during the redesign effort. Acceptance of EMR by physicians and their support staff is essential if computerization is to be successful, yet anecdotal reports of resistance and negative attitudes are frequently reported. Empirical studies indicate that physicians have not yet embraced this technology. As part of strategic planning and deployment of a computerized patient record, attitudes of end-users must be assessed. Using an integrative framework from the job design literature and management information sciences, we propose that multiple factors influence attitudes toward EMR, offer a conceptual model of end-user acceptance, and present findings from an empirical test of our model.

Computers in Healthcare

Computerization in ambulatory healthcare is generally classified into four types of applications: (1) electronic medical records (EMR); (2) office or practice management; (3) medical literature integration; and (4) telecommunications. Although any of these can be used as stand-alone products, computerization in healthcare organizations is most effective when all applications are integrated, with the EMR forming the "hub" of the system in which all clinical, administrative, and financial data move electronically among users. The focus of this study is EMR.

With EMR, all elements of the patient's record exist in a computer file. In most contemporary software packages, different elements of the chart are accessible through graphic user interface methods that allow the user to move easily from one part of the record to another. In addition to having the ability to enter text, the user may navigate through the record by pointing to icons on the screen to generate progress notes and flowsheets, complete insurance forms, prescribe medications, or perform countless other clinical and administrative tasks.

An extension of EMR is the decision support system, which assists physicians in medical decision making. Computerized systems are designed to perform case analysis in the traditional sense by producing a differential diagnosis given a rich set of inputs and generating a therapeutic course of action (Middleton, Detmer, and Musen 1995). Diagnostic decision support systems integrate clinical findings (e.g., signs, symptoms, and test results) with disease profiles to produce probability-based pairings of findings and diseases, while therapeutic decision support permits the physician to generate a patient-specific, disease-specific treatment plan, including medication prescriptions, patient education, and diet therapy.

The Push Toward Electronic Medical Records

The increasing use of computers in healthcare has largely been the result of two forces: cost containment and quality improvement. Cost-containment efforts by employers and managed care organizations have led to increased productivity requirements. At the same time, physicians are being asked to improve the quality of their work, document their results, and benchmark against their peers. Measurement of patient satisfaction, compliance with health maintenance practices, and physician practice profiles are examples of current documentation requirements (Edelson 1995).

The EMR is viewed by many as a panacea for contemporary management problems. Although research on electronic records in ambulatory settings is limited, empirical studies of pharmaceutical practices have found that the EMR is effective at identifying drug interactions (Haumschild et al. 1987), generating physician pharmaceutical reminders (Rind et al. 1991), and monitoring the use of antibiotics in hospitals (Evans and Pestotnik 1994). EMR studies have also evaluated the use of electronic records to enhance preventive care. In a study of 49 physicians, EMR-generated reminders improved preventive services such as cholesterol measurement, mammography, and immunizations (Ornstein et al. 1991). A study that compared computer-based health maintenance tracking with a manual flowchart-based tracking system found that the former resulted in significantly higher provider compliance for 8 of 11 procedures (Frame et al. 1994).

In the current environment of integrated delivery systems, the connectivity attribute of the EMR enhances its value further. Marshall and Chin (1998) conducted a study of 497 clinicians in a large northwest HMO to investigate perceived benefits of the EMR. They reported that 82 percent of the respondents felt that the EMR improved their ability to care for patients with other providers.

In sum, a properly configured EMR system enables the routine generation and collection of data, provides decision support, and facilitates workflow. Productivity is gained from increased quality of work and fewer information handling errors, with numerous studies indicating cost savings as a result of the EMR (Hamdy et al. 1995; Tierney et al. 1993). Despite its apparent benefits, however, acceptance of the EMR is far from universal.

End-User Acceptance

Little doubt exists that EMR will change the way physicians and other clinicians work. Before beginning such a significant job redesign, managers of EMR projects would be wise to assess the readiness of the principal end-users—that is, the physicians.

The job design literature suggests that characteristics of the job (Hackman and Oldham 1976) as well as cues in the work environment (Salancik and Pfeffer 1978) influence an individual's responses to the job redesign effort. Oldham and Hackman (1980) argue that technical, personnel, and control systems can all constrain the implementation of job redesign and propose that job satisfaction is a function of personal characteristics, job characteristics, and organizational practices.

In the management information sciences (MIS) literature, perceived usefulness is considered to drive behavioral responses to computer use in the workplace. Davis (1989) defined perceived usefulness as the tendency to use or not use an application to the extent that a person believes it will help improve job performance. Davis developed a scale to measure this construct and found that perceived usefulness was significantly correlated with both current usage and self-predicted future usage. Adams, Nelson, and Todd (1992) replicated Davis's study and found strong support for perceived usefulness as a predictor of subsequent use.

Integrating the MIS concept of perceived usefulness with job design principles provides a meaningful framework for understanding predictors of end-user acceptance. Forsythe (1993) argues that end-user acceptance should increase when system-builders understand both the needs of potential users and the context in which a system will be used. Thus EMR implementation efforts must consider individual and contextual factors that drive physician responses.

Predictors of Perceived Usefulness

Individual characteristics. The effect of individual characteristics on user attitudes toward computer use has been investigated extensively with mixed results. Several studies report that older individuals tend to have unfavorable attitudes toward computer use (Dyck and Smither 1994; Laguna and Babcock 1997), but Clayton, Pulver, and Hill (1994) found that age was not a predictive factor of computer acceptance and use.

The effects of individual characteristics may be indirect, however. For example, age is positively correlated with computer anxiety (Igbarria and Parasuraman 1989) and negatively correlated with computer experience (Dyck and Smither 1994). Both computer anxiety and computer experience are negatively related to end-user acceptance (Laguna and Babcock 1997).

Although early studies on gender and computer use found that women were more likely than men to report computer anxiety (Gilroy and Desai 1986), this does not appear to be true today. More recent studies have found that gender is not a predictor of computer attitudes (Aydin, Rosen, and Felitti 1994; Brown and Coney 1994).

Patient care values. The work involved in patient care reflects high skill variety, task identity, task significance, autonomy, and feedback—requisite features of the job characteristics model (Hackman and Oldham 1976). The tendency for a physician to feel that the EMR will change these characteristics adversely may be influenced by her or his values regarding patient care. A value is an enduring belief that a specific mode of conduct is preferable to a converse mode of conduct (Rokeach 1973). Thus, the extent to which EMR characteristics support underlying values about patient care is expected to have an effect on end-user acceptance of EMR implementation.

Medicine has been described as both an art and a science. Computers make medical care more scientific by improving data accuracy and by enhancing the precision of decision making. Thus, a physician who values a scientific approach to medical care may be more receptive to computer applications in healthcare. Conversely, physicians who value patient care as an art rather than a science may rely more on personal insights and intuition. These physicians may view computers as ineffective and intrusive. PROMIS, an EMR developed in the late 1970s, failed to gain acceptance because it attempted to make medicine more scientific by reorganizing the medical record and using logic to guide patient care decisions (Teach and Shortliffe 1981).

Another important value is the physician's view of the doctor-patient relationship. Aydin (1994) reported that many physicians, fearing a depersonalized examination room, are concerned about the effect of computers on the patient relationship. Physicians who value a highly subjective and personal relationship with their patients may view the computer as cold and technical. Although a few studies have evaluated the effect of compute usage on physician-patient relationships (Warshawsky et al. 1994; Pringle, Robins, and Brown 1985), the target has been the patient rather than the physician. Lacking are studies that address computer use from the physician's perspective and how values related to patient care influence these attitudes.

Office/clinic conditions. Maintenance of the patient record is a core function of a medical practice, with literally hundreds of administrative tasks performed as part of healthcare delivery. Inefficient management of these tasks may be one incentive to implement EMR. Physicians and their staff communicate directly and indirectly about clinical and information tasks that are the most problematic in their office or clinic. From a job design perspective, the perception of current office conditions can be viewed as a cue in the work environment. The premise of Salancik and Pfeffer's (1978) job design model is that cues are identified and interpreted in a social context. Thus, how physicians and staff view these conditions should influence their regard for computerization as a solution to office management problems.

Organizational support. Forsythe and Buchanan (1992) note that consideration of the social context is often lacking in systems evaluation: "Developers tend to think of systems as isolated technical objects . . . they do not necessarily consider who will work with the system . . . how that work will be accomplished . . . [and] the organizational contexts in which they are to be fielded" (Forsythe and Buchanan 1992, 910). The culture of the organization, including its supportive elements, influences both implementation and persistence of the work innovation. Thus, it is critical to understand which organizational practices most strongly support or compromise work redesign efforts.

The term "organizational practices" can be interpreted broadly, such as the organization's culture, or more narrowly, as in traditional human resource management functions such as training. Igbarria, Parasuraman, and Pavri (1990) specify two categories of organizational support: (1) application development support, a specific domain that describes the infrastructure necessary for implementation; and (2) general support, which is more reflective of the organizational culture.

In summary, the healthcare literature is incomplete with regard to antecedents of perceived usefulness among physicians and other healthcare professionals. Furthermore, the few studies on end-user acceptance of computers in healthcare organizations have focused primarily on hospital staff. Our model, developed for physicians and clinical staff in ambulatory care settings, integrates principles of job design from the organizational literature with the concept of end-user acceptance from the MIS literature.

Conceptual Model

Although models of end-user acceptance have been tested empirically (Davis 1989; Adams, Nelson, and Todd 1992; Igbarria 1993), virtually all have studied perceived usefulness, end-user acceptance, and satisfaction simultaneously, without clearly defining the differences among these constructs. A methodological flaw in this approach is the potential for common method variance, which occurs when subjects are asked to respond to different but related measures in the same instrument.

An alternative approach is to articulate a two-stage model where perceived usefulness is analyzed as an antecedent to acceptance prior to job redesign and end-user satisfaction is studied as a separate measure after implementation. The rationale for this approach is based on Fishbein and Ajzen's (1975) theory of reasoned action, which states that attitudes precede behavioral intentions. In theory, perceived usefulness should precede behavioral intentions.

The model developed for this study includes predictors of perceived usefulness prior to implementation of an EMR project. We propose that perceived usefulness is influenced by individual characteristics as well as by contextual factors (see Figure 1).

In keeping with the MIS literature, we propose that age and computer experience predict the level of individual anxiety. These relationships are hypothesized as:

- **Hypothesis 1**: Age and lack of experience with computers will be positively correlated with computer anxiety; and
- **Hypothesis 2**: The greater the level of anxiety about computers, the more negative the attitudes toward computers, reflected as a lower score in perceived usefulness of the EMR effort.

Drawing from the job design literature, we propose that contextual factors such as current office conditions and organizational support will influence perceived usefulness.

- **Hypothesis 3**: Dissatisfaction with current office conditions will result in more positive attitudes toward computers, reflected as a higher score in perceived usefulness; and
- **Hypothesis 4:** Beliefs about the organization's ability to effectively support EMR use will result in more positive attitudes towards computers, reflected as a higher score in perceived usefulness of the EMR effort.

To summarize, the purposes of this study were to (1) identify specific attitudes or factors that should be targeted for successful EMR

Figure 1 Predictors of Perceived Usefulness

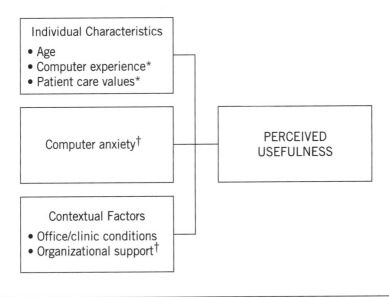

* Statistically significant: $p = .05$.   † Statistically significant: $p < .001$.

implementation, and (2) demonstrate empirical support for the predictors of perceived usefulness model.

Methodology

This study is the first part of a larger assessment of factors that promote successful EMR implementation in ambulatory care settings. The sample was pooled from five private medical practices, nine group medical practices that are part of a staff-plan HMO, and a university-based health center. All sites are located in Pennsylvania and all are healthcare organizations where electronic medical records were not in use at the time of the study.

Surveys were distributed during the fall of 1996 and winter of 1997. Respondents were asked to return the survey directly to the investigators. A stamped envelope was attached to the survey. Response rates ranged from 53 percent from the private practices to 85 percent from the HMO sites.

This convenience sample consisted of 67 physicians and 18 mid-level clinicians (nurse practitioners and physician assistants). Respondents ranged in age from 25 to 65, with a mean age of 40.12 for physicians and 36.22 for mid-level clinicians. The sample consisted of 57 percent males and 43 percent females, although most of the physicians are male and most of the mid-level clinicians are female. Table 1 illustrates a profile of the sample.

Measures

Perceived usefulness. Perceived usefulness, the dependent variable, was defined as the degree to which an individual believes that the EMR system will improve healthcare delivery. We used nine items that measured the individual's overall assessment of perceived usefulness of electronic records. The items were adapted from Davis (1989) and used response categories anchored on a five-point Likert-type scale. The reliability of the scale, using Cronbach's alpha, was .92. A description of the items is found in the Appendix.

Individual characteristics. Respondents were asked to indicate their age and gender. Years of work-related and personal computer use and the extent and source of computer training were measured. Seven items that measured years of computer use, computer ownership, and use of different types of computer application were recoded and summed to compute a new measure, "computer intensity."

The scale developed by Raub (1981) and validated by Igbarria and Parasuraman (1989) was used to measure computer anxiety. Ten items asked individuals to indicate agreement or disagreement with statements reflecting apprehension, confusion, hesitation, and so forth in using computers. Response categories ranged from strongly disagree (1) to strongly agree (5), with high scores reflecting high levels of anxiety. Two items were dropped from the original scale because they were not appropriate for the current setting. Reliability for the eight items was calculated at .82.

Patient care values. To measure individual values about patient care, six items were constructed expressly for this study. Response categories used a semantic differential format with five response categories. The respondent was asked to indicate whether her or his view was closer to one word or its opposite. "I view medicine as: art. . . . . . science" is an example of an item with word pairs. Scores were coded from 1 to 5, with 5 being closest to a scientific orientation.

Office/clinic practice conditions. Twenty-four items were developed by the investigators to measure satisfaction with specific medical practice conditions. The items reflected a range of conditions specific to a medical office or clinic, such as "number of incomplete medical records" and "turnaround time for tests." The response categories ranged from very

Table 1   Profile of Respondents

	HMO Sites	University Health Center	Private Practices	Group Total
Physicians				
Number	57	5	5	67
Age (y)	40.1	46.2	43.2	42.7
Mid-levels				
Number	9	9	0	18
Age (y)	36.2	40.8		38.5

Total participants = 85.

unsatisfactory (1) to very satisfactory (5). After pilot testing, twenty items were selected for use. These items were summed and averaged to obtain a scale score labeled "satisfaction." This scale score had a reliability of .88.

Organizational support. We defined organizational support as those practices under the purview of senior management that support or impede the effective use of an EMR. Four items, adapted from Igbarria, Parasuraman, and Pavri (1990), were used to measure the respondent's belief that the organization was able to provide adequate time and resources for EMR implementation. These items were summed and averaged to obtain a scale score labeled "organizational support." The reliability for this scale was .85.

Analysis

Descriptive statistics—frequencies, means, and standard deviations— were calculated for all variables. Correlations between major variables (scale scores and demographic data) were calculated. Regression equations, using ordinary least squares, were used to test the hypotheses. A hierarchical procedure (i.e., entering blocks of variables in separate steps) was used to test the unique contribution of each variable, or set of variables.

Results

The mean for perceived usefulness, the major variable of interest, was 3.47, reflecting a neutral-to-slightly positive attitude overall about the perceived benefits of the EMR. Means and standard deviations for major variables are shown in Table 2.

Several individual characteristics were significantly correlated with computer anxiety. Results showed that female gender, not owning a

Table 2   Descriptive Statistics

	Mean	Range	Standard Deviation
Perceived usefulness	3.472	1–5	.594
Age	39.85	25–65	7.44
Computer intensity	3.154	1–5	2.05
Computer anxiety*	2.316	1–5	.756
Satisfaction	3.259	1–5	.473
Organizational support	1.179	1–5	.386

*High scores reflect computer anxiety.

computer, and few or no years of computer use were positively and significantly correlated with computer anxiety, but that age was not significantly correlated with computer anxiety. Correlations between patient care values and perceived usefulness were calculated. Results showed that only one value, "maintaining distance vs. a close patient relationship" had a statistically significant correlation with perceived usefulness.

Regression equations were then constructed to test the hypotheses. In the first equation, age, gender, computer experience, and the significant patient care value were entered in the first block of variables as individual characteristics. Computer anxiety was entered in the second block. Satisfaction with office conditions and organizational support were entered as the contextual variables in the third block. Results showed that computer experience and organizational support were positive predictors of perceived usefulness, and computer anxiety and valuing a close patient relationship were negative predictors. The demographic factors (age and gender) were not statistically significant predictors of perceived usefulness.

Discussion

This project assessed end-user attitudes toward computerization prior to implementation of an EMR project. Using a model of individual and organizational factors to predict end-user attitudes, we found that perceived usefulness is influenced by both categories, suggesting that EMR use is a complex job redesign intervention.

Consistent with both the job design and MIS literature, individual characteristics were found to be predictors of perceived usefulness. Age and gender did not have main effects, but computer anxiety, after controlling for age, gender, and computer experience, was significant and underscored the effect of psychological phenomena in job re-design. The importance of experience with computers is noteworthy. Computer intensity, a scale that captures the breadth and depth of computer experience, was a statistically significant predictor of perceived usefulness. Other individual factors, such as cognitive style, may have an effect on user attitudes (Alavi and Joachimsthaler 1992) and should be investigated.

Dissatisfaction with current work conditions that might be influenced by an EMR system was not a predictor of perceived usefulness; thus, hypothesis 3 was not supported. This finding may be a result of the salience of office conditions—physicians and other practitioners who are not routinely exposed to office inefficiencies may not be aware of computerization benefits. The "perceived usefulness" scale, although validated as a global measure, may actually capture two distinct sets of expectations among physicians, that is, contribution to improved patient care versus contribution to improved office productivity. Further analysis may help to clarify this distinction.

Organizational support had a positive relationship with perceived usefulness, supporting hypothesis 4. As a contextual factor, this finding is consistent with the social approaches to job redesign and helps to explain the degree to which senior managers' expectations and attitudes about the computer system influence staff responses. By providing strong support for the redesign effort, management can communicate its commitment to the EMR investment. A useful next step would be to study managers' and employees' attitudes during the actual redesign process to determine how issues of control, participation, and feedback can be resolved.

Finally we found that physicians who value a close patient relationship have less positive attitudes about the EMR. This is consistent with the Aydin (1994) study, which suggested that physicians may view computers as intrusive and depersonalizing. Because the doctor-patient relationship is often viewed as sacrosanct, this finding may be the most important. Again, we emphasize the importance of determining, from the physicians themselves, why the computer may be viewed as a barrier. Studies on patient satisfaction when the electronic record is actually used in the examination room would advance our understanding of this complex issue.

Implications for Managing an EMR Project

Practical strategies emerge from these findings. Previous research has identified older and female employees as having increased anxiety. We did not find age to be a significant factor, although gender was correlated with computer anxiety. Managers should, at a minimum, assess prior computer experience as one indicator of readiness. Since physicians may be uncomfortable with their keyboarding skills (Brown and Coney 1994), providing them opportunities to explore simple applications that use word-processing skills may increase their feelings of self-efficacy. Likewise, the use of e-mail may ease the transition to the next level. Hands-on training with a software demonstration program, or a simulated model, should occur early and often, and be tailored to the needs and work schedules of the physicians.

Given the current focus in many healthcare settings on cost containment and productivity, management and physicians must share their expectations regarding computerization. Prospective needs assessment is a starting point for system design and implementation (Strasberg et al. 1998); thus the preferences of physicians regarding functionality of the system should be assessed early in the planning stage and should be followed by feedback from management. Without common goals, expectations may be unrealistic and may result in negative attitudes and resistance.

Management of EMR implementation requires attention to multiple success factors that have been identified from research and experience (Tan 1995). User characteristics such as background, attitudes, and expectations, and organizational characteristics in the form of management support are among these factors. The research summarized here suggests that the ultimate success of computerization depends greatly on managers' use of this information.

Implications for Evaluating an EMR Project

Clearly, the importance of this topic suggests that a well-designed evaluation plan is necessary for understanding the dynamics that surround the implementation and use of an EMR. We offer several recommendations. First, the importance of a longitudinal design cannot be overstated. Valid conclusions regarding responses to the EMR can be made only after analyzing attitudes pre-implementation and post-implementation. Understanding the dynamics that lead to acceptance of EMR, and responding appropriately, requires a longitudinal design with data collection occurring before, during, and after implementation.

Second, the assumption of causal relationships in our analysis may not be appropriate for studying changes in the workplace. Rather than linear relationships between variables, organizational reality suggests multidirectional influences, thus we offer the caveat of using nonlinear analytic methods. Structural equation modeling or confirmatory factor analysis may be more appropriate methods for analyzing these data.

Finally, evaluation should include the use of qualitative data. Surveys that are coded with numerical values are efficient and relatively inexpensive to administer and analyze, but are limited in the scope and depth of questions that can be asked. They are necessary but not sufficient. Focus groups, structured interviews, and other means of obtaining feedback are important mechanisms for ensuring that physicians have ample opportunity to voice their concerns and provide input at each stage. Given the high stakes associated with EMR implementation, evaluation may be the most important component of the project.

APPENDIX

Items in Perceived Usefulness Scale
Computerization:

- Will contribute to work productivity
- Will be worth the investment
- Improves productivity
- Will save time
- Will assist in the delivery of patient care
- Will be a valuable aid in my clinical work
- Will improve the quality of patient care
- Would be rewarding
- Will enable people to set higher performance targets

References

Adams, D., R. Nelson, and P. Todd. 1992. "Perceived Usefulness, Ease of Use and Usage of Information Technology: A Replication." *MIS Quarterly* 16: 227–46.

Alavi, M., and E. Joachimsthaler. 1992. "Revisiting DSS Implementation Research: A Meta-Analysis of the Literature and Suggestions for Researchers." *MIS Quarterly* 16:95–116.

Aydin, C. 1994. "Survey Methods for Assessing Social Impacts of Computers in Health Care Organizations." In *Evaluating Health Care Information Systems*, edited by J. G. Anderson, C. E. Aydin, and S. J. Jay, 69–115. Thousand Oaks, CA: Sage Publications.

Aydin, C., P. Rosen, and V. Felitti. 1994. "Transforming Information Use in Preventive Medicine: Learning to Balance Technology with the Art of Caring." *Eighteenth Annual Symposium on Computer Applications in Medical Care*, 563–67. Philadelphia: Manley & Belfus.

BMI Medical Information. 1995. *BMI Medic Physicians Survey*. Arlington Heights, IL: BMI Medical information.

Brown, S., and R. Coney. 1994. "Changes in Physicians' Computer Anxiety and Attitudes Related to Clinical Information System Use." *Journal of the American Medical Informatics Association* 1 (5): 381–94.

Clayton, P., G. Pulver, and C. Hill. 1994. "Physician Use of Computers: Is Age or Value the Predominant Factor?" *Journal of the American Medical Informatics Association* 1 (5): 301–305.

Davis, F. 1989. "Perceived Usefulness, Perceived Ease of Use, and User Acceptance of Information Technology." *MIS Quarterly* 13 (Sept.): 319–40.

Dyck, J., and J. Smither 1994. "Age Differences in Computer Anxiety: The Role of Computer Experience, Gender and Education." *Journal of Educational Computing Research* 10 (3): 239–48.

Edelson, J. 1995. "A Physician Use of Information Technology in Ambulatory Medicine: An Overview." *Journal of Ambulatory Care Management* 18 (3): 9–19.

Evans, R., and S. Pestonik. 1994. "Application of Medical Informatics in Antibiotic Therapy." In *Antimicrobial Susceptibility Testing*, edited by J. Poupard, 87–96. New York: Plenum Press.

Fishbein, M., and I. Ajzen. 1975. *Beliefs, Attitude, Intervention and Behavior: An Introduction to Theory and Research*. Reading, MA: Addison-Wesley.

Forsythe, D. 1993. "Using Ethnography to Build a Working System: Rethinking Basic Design Assumptions." In *Proceedings of the 75th Annual Symposium on Computer Applications in Medical Care, American Medical Informatics Association*, 505–509. New York: McGraw-Hill.

Forsythe, D., and B. Buchanan. 1992. "Broadening Our Approach to Evaluating Medical Information Systems." In *Proceedings of the 15th Annual Symposium on Computer Applications in Medical Care, American Medical Informatics Association*, 8–12. New York: McGraw-Hill.

Frame, P., J. Zimmer, P. Werth, W. Hall, and S. Eberly. 1994. "Computer-Based vs. Manual Health Maintenance Tracking: A Controlled Trial." *Archives of Family Medicine* 3 (7): 581–88.

Gilroy, F., and H. Desai. 1986. "Computer Anxiety: Sex, Race and Age." *International Journal of Man-Machine Studies* 25 (6): 711–19.

Hackman, J., and G. Oldham. 1976. *Work Redesign*. Reading, MA: Addison-Wesley.

Hamdy, R., S. Moore, K. Whalen, J. Donnelly, R. Compton, F. Testerman, P. Haulsee, and J. Hughes. 1995. "Reducing Polypharmacy in Extended Care." *Southern Medical Journal* 88 (5): 534–38.

Haumschild, M. J., E. Ward, J. Bishop, and J.S. Haumschild. 1987. "Pharmacy-Based Computer System for Monitoring and Reporting Drug Interactions." *American Journal of Hospital Pharmacy* 44: 345–48.

Igbarria, M. 1993. "User Acceptance of Microcomputer Technology: An Empirical Test." *OMEGA International Journal of Management Science* 21 (1): 73–90.

Igbarria, M., and S. Parasuraman. 1989. "A Path Analytic Study of Individual Characteristics, Computer Anxiety and Attitudes Toward Microcomputers." *Journal of Management* 15 (3): 373–88.

Igbarria, M., S. Parasuraman, and F. Pavri. 1990. "A Path Analytic Study of the Determinants of Microcomputer Usage." *Journal of Management Systems* 2 (2): 1–14.

Institute of Medicine. 1991. *The Computer-Based Patient Record: An Essential Technology for Health Care.* Washington, D.C.: Institute of Medicine, National Academy Press.

Kralewski, J., E. Rich, T. Bernhardt, B. Dowd, R. Feldman, and C. Johnson. 1998. "The Organizational Structure of Medical Group Practices in a Managed Care Environment." *Health Care Management Review* 23 (2): 76–96.

Laguna, K., and R. Babcock. 1997. "Computer Anxiety in Young and Older Adults: Implications for Human-Computer Interactions in Older Populations." *Computers in Human Behavior* 13 (3): 317–26.

Lawler, F., J. R. Cacy, N. Viviani, R. M. Hamm, and S. W. Cobb. 1996. "Implementation and Termination of a Computerized Medical Information System." *Journal of Family Practice* 42: 233–36.

Marshall, P. D., and H. L. Chin. 1998. "The Effects of an Electronic Medical Record on Patient Care: Clinician Attitudes in a Large HMO." *Proceedings of the American Medical Informatics Association*, Annual Meeting, Lake Buena Vista, FL, November 7–11.

Middleton, B., W. Detmer, and M. Musen. 1995. "Diagnostic Decision Support." In *Computers in Clinical Practice*, edited by J. Asherof, 59–76. Philadelphia: American College of Physicians.

Murphy, G. F. 1996. "Computer-Based Patient Records—A Unifying Principle." In *Health Information: Management of a Strategic Resource*, edited by M. Abbelhak, 590. Philadelphia: W. B. Saunders.

Oldham, G. R., and J. R. Hackman. 1980. "Work Design in the Organizational Context." *Research in Organizational Behavior* 2: 247–78.

Ornstein, S., D. Garr, R. Jenkins, P. Rust, and A. Arnon. 1991. "Computer-Generated Physician and Patient Reminders." *The Journal of Family Practice* 32 (1): 82–90.

Pringle, M., S. Robins, and G. Brown. 1985. "Topic Analysis: An Objective Measure of the Consultation and Its Application to Computer Assisted Consultations." *British Medical Journal* 290 (6484): 1789–91.

Raub, A. 1981. "Correlates of Computer Anxiety in College Students." Unpublished dissertation, University of Pennsylvania, Philadelphia.

Rind, D., C. Safran, R. Phillips, W. Slack, D. Calkins, T. Delblanco, and H. Bleich. 1991. "The Effect of Computer-Based Reminders on the Management of Hospitalized Patients with Worsening Renal Function." In *Proceedings of the 15th Annual Symposium on Computer Applications in Medical Care*, edited by P. D. Clayton, 28–32. New York: McGraw-Hill.

Rokeach, M. 1973 *The Nature of Human Values.* New York: Free Press.

Salancik, G., and S. Pfeffer. 1978. "A Social Information Processing Approach to Job Attitudes and Job Design." *Administrative Science Quarterly* 23: 224–53.

Strasberg, H. R., F. Tudiver, A. M. Holbrook, C. Geiger, K. K. Keshavjee, and S. Troyan. 1998. "Moving Towards an Electronic Patient Record: A Survey to Assess the Needs of Community Family Physicians." *Proceedings of the American Medical Informatics Association*, Annual Meeting, Lake Buena Vista, FL, November 7–11.

Tan, J. 1995. *Health Management Information Systems: Theories, Methods and Applications.* Gaithersburg. MD: Aspen.

Teach, R. L., and E. H. Shortliffe. 1981. "An Analysis of Physician Attitudes Regarding Computer-Based Clinical Consultation Systems." *Computers and Biomedical Research* 14 (6): 542–58.

Tierney, W., M. Miller, J. Overage, and C. McDonald 1993. "Physician Inpatient Order Writing on Microcomputer Workstations." *Journal of the American Medical Association* 269 (3): 379–83.

Warshawsky, S., J. Pliskin, J. Urkin, N. Cohen, A. Sharon, M. Binztok, and C. Margolis 1994. "Physician Use of an Electronic Medical Record System During the Patient Encounter: A Descriptive Study." *Computer Methods and Programs in Biomedicine* 43: 269–73.

Practitioner Application

Larry Dansky, M.D., manager, General Medicine Department, University Health Services, Pennsylvania State University, University Park, Pennsylvania

Today, more than ever, the practice of medicine relies on the availability and use of highly sophisticated technology. Physicians as a group have generally been supportive of the use of technological advances to improve healthcare delivery. We have seen the advantages of technology when applied to diagnostic and therapeutic modalities that assist us in our work. Advances in laboratory techniques and equipment improve our abilities to diagnose and screen for disease processes. Diagnostic x-ray advances such as ultrasound, nuclear medicine, CAT scans, and MRIs are readily used and have become invaluable technological tools of our trade. Why then has there been such slow acceptance of the computer and the electronic medical record (EMR)? How can managers in healthcare delivery organizations assist physicians in valuing the use of computers in the office as well as for the organization?

As the authors discuss, computerization in ambulatory healthcare can be classified into four areas: office/practice management, electronic patient records, medical literature integration, and telecommunications. This article focuses on the EMR for good reasons, for I would venture to gamble that most physicians fully support the widespread use of computers for the other three areas. Like the lab and diagnostic x-ray advances cited above, computerization in practice management and use of the Internet can improve the quality of patient care without truly redesigning our work.

Analysis of physicians' attitudes about the use of the computer should look not only at comfort with computer use, but more importantly on how the computer changes what we do when we are with our patients in the exam room. In an era where physicians have already had to adjust to cost containment, productivity requirements, documentation issues, and practice profiles, changes that so dramatically affect the doctor/patient relationship will be viewed cautiously.

Healthcare organizations considering the implementation of EMR will face hard times without support from their physician staff and thus need to understand that physician acceptance will be influenced by factors that affect perceived usefulness. As outlined in the article, the factors that most dramatically affect perceived usefulness include computer anxiety and beliefs about organizational support. Enabling physicians to use computers for communications, work processing, and Internet searches long before instituting EMRs will allow for computer comfort and minimize anxiety.

The issue of organizational support is more complex. Physicians will have high expectations for implementation support, but issues such as financial resources and time management will need to be addressed. Most importantly, an organization embarking on such an important endeavor must assess its approach to "general support." How will it work with clinicians who are reticent to implement this new tool? Will physicians who see computerization as another intrusion on the doctor-patient relationship be supported in this transition, forced to accept its coming, or a combination of the two? By looking at issues such as where individual physicians stand relative to computer anxiety, doctor-patient values, and understanding of implementation support, management can identify potential problems and alleviate clinician fears. As the authors point out, focus groups are vital to ensure that physicians have ample opportunity to voice their concerns.

I am not surprised that office/clinic conditions did not predict acceptance of EMRS. As stated earlier, the effect of computerization in office management does not strike home in the exam room. In that respect, the computer, like the chemistry analyzer and the CAT scanner, is a tool others use to assist us in our work. Alert managers in healthcare organizations will help physicians to look at computerization in healthcare delivery as a tool like the stethoscope, not the telephone.

MAINTAINING SECURITY

A FEW years ago, mystery author Louis Charbonneau wrote a novel, *Intruder*, about a character who electronically penetrates the computer system of a municipality in the northeast United States. The book's plot centers around the intruder's threat to "crash" the computer system and put government services into chaos unless a $5 million dollar ransom is paid. Fiction, right? Wrong! Remember the eighth graders at New York's Dalton School who penetrated the computer system of major corporations in Canada? These school children disrupted the operation of one system and actually seized control of another, destroying some data in the process all from a small terminal in their Upper Eastside school. More recently, students at the Russian Academy of Science penetrated the Pentagon's information systems, which contain highly classified sensitive defense data (Vistica 1999). Most recently, the "love bug" invaded thousands of computers around the world, causing millions of dollars in disruptions (Kaisey and McCann 2000).

The growth of PC use has dramatically increased the number of people who are familiar with and, worse, can manipulate information systems. Additionally, new communication technology allows access to private systems with relative ease. For example, one company found that some of its employees had set up a computer and, with sophisticated software, connected to their PCs at home. The set up required no password and allowed the employees to read, delete, or change data or software on the company's entire computer network (Charles 1991).

Most technology experts agree that breaking into the computer systems of nearly all government and healthcare organizations, as well as corporations, is both technically feasible and much less complicated than most of us realize. Take, for example, the case of two young "hackers" who were charged by the government with using a home computer to break into data systems at a federal court and at the Boeing company. According to the U.S. Attorney who was prosecuting the case, the motive appeared to be simply "the challenge of breaking into the computers. . . . Hackers have a name for it called 'network navigating' " (*The New York Times* 1992).

Acknowledging that the nation's computers are not secure, the National Academy of Sciences reported that the government's critical computer systems are extremely vulnerable to abuse and that "there is reason to believe our luck will soon run out" (*The New York Times* 1990). The Russian students seem to have proven the point! At a congressional hearing on this subject, one representative blasted those responsible for maintaining information systems safety by asserting: "Our economy, our traffic control system, the IRS and the entire Social Security program depend upon computer systems that are at risk because federal agencies have failed to put simple computer security controls in place" (Newlin 1990).

Studies by the Inspector General of the U.S. Department of Health and Human Services acknowledge the rapid growth and profitability of computer abuse. According to a 1989 article, theft and abuse by computer appears to be more lucrative, much safer, and carry less punishment than many other criminal activities (Knotts and Richards). To compound the seriousness of the situation, the same article predicted that computer crime will increase more rapidly than the controls that detect and thwart those crimes. With the increase in computer literacy, this trend has the potential to create serious management issues for all healthcare organizations.

Legions of horror stories about computer security breakdowns have been chronicled. Virtually every week another computer scandal comes to light. Almost everyone has experienced virus alerts like the "Cornell Worm," a rogue program that went out of control and stalled thousands of computers connected to the Internet. Another example is the trial of the "Legion of Doom" hackers, who were accused of stealing secrets from BellSouth Corporation (Newlin 1990). These stories are by no means limited to the United States. A pair of British computer hackers, who boasted they could "tap into anything," even America's defense network, challenged British authorities and the FBI to catch them. The hackers proved their claims by tapping into Fort Knox, Fort

Leavenworth, and the Pentagon. Especially disconcerting to the British authorities was the hackers insistence that they had Queen Elizabeth's unlisted phone number! (Levy 1980).

Yet, despite the apparent extent and severity of the problem, little seems to have been done about it. In 1992, *Newsday* reported that most computer system users do not have safeguards and, of those who do, many do not bother to use them. In healthcare, this sentiment is substantiated by Dennis Van Auken, vice president of Source Data Systems, who in 1994 said that "Until recently, many healthcare institutions simply have not paid attention to security" (*The New York Times*). In reflecting upon this problem, Jeff Schiller, who looks after a network of computers called Project Athena at the Massachusetts Institute of Technology, comments that computer vulnerability is common because "people who use computers generally don't worry about security" (Charles 1991).

The result is that those traditionally in charge of protecting and maintaining the resources of an organization often have very little understanding of the degree of exposure and vulnerability they have. One commentator goes so far as to say that if managers really understood the liability and risks to the assets of an organization, and to their professional reputations, they might shut down all networks and data centers (Weis 1990). The highly respected Research Foundation of the Financial Executive Institute defined the increasing reliance on poorly understood and managed computer information systems as the "Achilles's heel" of modern organizations (*The New York Times* 1980). According to the institute, healthcare managers who are cognizant of the security problem are "in an endless arms race pitting new systems of security against new weapons of intrusion." The situation at St. Serena's can help understand the challenge better.

CASE STUDY

Case Six: Phil's Pills

The litany of security problems seemed endless for Phil Palmer, director of pharmacy at St. Serena's. His assistant had prepared a report that lists the security breaches that have occurred since installation of the new information system. Phil had worked at two other hospital pharmacies in his 15-year career and had seen that the majority of pharmacists' time was spent writing orders, pricing medication, or doing clerical work. To increase productivity, when he arrived at St. Serena's he had supervised the installation of a stand-alone pharmacy information system that virtually eliminated most of the time-consuming paperwork in his pharmacy. He estimated that annually $50,000 was saved through processing efficiencies, which included more accurate Medicaid-automated documentation, better inventory controls, and nursing workload reduction through automatic writing of stop-order reports and compilation of administrative medication records.

When St. Serena's converted to the new integrated information system, Phil was assured that a similar pharmacy program would be part of it. But now, the security problems that have developed with the new system appeared to be threatening to wipe out all cost savings and, in fact, produce increased costs. Rex Rufus, his assistant, summarized the recent round of problems as follows:

> First of all, one of the new printers was stolen last week. Unfortunately it was the new laser printer that we use most. Additionally, we have lost about 300 of our outpatient files and it's not clear whether there's a way to get them back. The supervisor of Nursing came in yesterday while you were at a meeting and complained that the automated stop-order reports and medication records for 12 ICU patients were not consistent with their manual backup system records. Aside from these hassles, it looks like someone has tampered with the inventory files. The physical inventory amount of valium is different from the inventory records that appear in the information system. Beyond that, it seems that our MBA intern is using our system to write his research reports. When I confronted him, he responded that he assumed it was okay since 'everyone uses the system for personal purposes'.

Phil was dumbfounded as well as irate. He called Stewart's office demanding explanations and assistance with a fix.

Questions for Discussion

1. What specific security problems with the information system are evident at St. Serena's pharmacy?
2. What factors associated with the new integrated system are affecting the security situation in the pharmacy?
3. What operational considerations should Phil address in his dealings with Stewart and the techies?
4. What administrative and technical measures might be considered in trying to fix the security problems?

COMMENTARY

The problems at St. Serena's pharmacy may be the result of the rush to install a state-of-the-art system as well as an incomplete understanding of the nature of the security challenge in modern information systems.

The Nature of the Security Problem

Computer security is the very practical administrative and technical matter of protecting the organization's data and equipment. Breach in security is a critical issue given that billions of dollars are lost or stolen annually because of computer tampering, and most losses are never detected or reported. However, financial loss is only one aspect of the computer security breakdown problem. The problem has five major components: (1) equipment protection, (2) data loss, (3) data manipulation, (4) unauthorized access, and (5) system misuse.

Equipment Protection

This component involves the physical security of computer equipment. Some time ago, the computer system of a Vermont firm was destroyed by fire, a disaster which has also struck the computer systems of the Pentagon, some hospitals, and numerous other organizations (Williams 1980). Some systems have been physically sabotaged, others flooded, many vandalized and, as has occurred at St. Serena's pharmacy, stolen. As costly as these vulnerabilities can be, these risks are perhaps the easiest to guard against. Many sophisticated measures are available because the challenge of protecting the physical equipment is essentially the same as protecting any valuable equipment.

Data Loss

Loss of data is less easily protected by traditional security measures. A classic, "conscious-raising" case some years ago involved a firm in Chicago that lost its accounts receivable file stored on a computer tape. The firm's accounts receivable procedure was simple: every Monday the appropriate tape was taken from the tape library and used to process bills. One Monday morning, however, no bills were produced. Several hundred thousand of dollars in receivables were missing and the firm did not have duplicate records. What happened? The tape in question was stored on the bottom shelf in the new tape library and was accidentally erased by the magnetic coil in a new heavy-duty vacuum cleaner. The point of this example is clear: stored data can be lost, as St. Serena's pharmacy has discovered with its outpatient files.

Data Manipulation

A third component is data manipulation. Changing data stored on electronic information systems without leaving any trace of tampering is a fairly simple matter. At a New York college, for example, a "D" student received a Phi Beta Kappa key and was named to the Dean's list on the basis of an electronic transcript that showed all "As." The student had a friend in the college information system center who, for a small fee, was willing to raise "Ds" to "As." Three years after the student graduated, the ploy was accidentally discovered by a physics professor who noticed a discrepancy between his handwritten grade sheet and the transcript printout.

Unauthorized Access

The following *Saturday Review* report illustrates the scope of the vulnerability of information systems to unauthorized access:

> At 19, Jerry Schneider was president of his own thriving electronic equipment business, Creative Systems Enterprises. The "creative" aspect of the business was that the equipment he sold belonged to the Pacific Bell Telephone Company. Posing as a magazine reporter, Schneider toured Pacific Bell's computer installation; he asked a lot of questions and pocketed a handful of discarded punch cards. Armed with this information, a basic high school knowledge of computers, and a touch-tone telephone, the teenager keyed into Pacific Bell's inventory and supply computer and robbed the company blind (DeWeese 1995).

Another example of unauthorized access that can and has halted the flow of information is the lethal presence of "computer viruses" (Sanford 1993), which have become so threatening and common that, like hurricanes, they are sometimes given human names such as "Melissa." Viruses are snippets of computer codes that are deliberately introduced into an information system by way of a software program "downloaded"—received and captured electronically—from another system. Some viruses have even turned up in commercial software packages. The most common destructive virus infects a disk and scrambles or erases files. Other viruses are used to open "trap doors" in an information system, allowing an individual to gain information or exploit the system. Common terms associated with viruses are "trojan horse" and "logic bomb." A trojan horse is an unauthorized set of hidden instructions in a computer program that directs the system to perform certain functions. A logic bomb is an unauthorized computer program designed to be executed at a designated time or when certain conditions occur. Put in place by a trojan horse, the unauthorized program will cause the "bomb" to detonate, and any number of malicious acts might occur (e.g., removal of a terminated employee's name from a personnel file, erasure of a payroll file, or issuance of a big check to the perpetrator).

The prevalence of these viruses has changed the way we think about electronic information systems. Technical defenses known as "firewalls" have become essential but, as discussed below, broader technical "architecture" is now viewed as necessary (Gerberick, Huber, and Rudloff 1999).

System Misuse

Misuse of both equipment and data by authorized and unauthorized users is also a big problem. Incidents include using the organization's computers to do personal business, as is happening at St. Serena's pharmacy. In one notorious case, two employees established their own company on $2 million of time on a large government information system in San Jose, California (*The New York Times* 1992). A more serious example is the misuse of sensitive data. Examples include the use of sensitive personal information by criminal justice or healthcare workers to embarrass, bribe, or otherwise harm individuals (*The New York Times* 1992).

These security problems are so widespread that most organizations have probably been affected by them at one point or another. Security breaches affect the availability, integrity, or confidentiality of information systems. A major cause of the problem is technology users' ignorance of the particular security vulnerabilities that come with information technology.

How Information Technology Affects Security

Protecting modern information systems is far different and more difficult a challenge than protecting a file cabinet with diamonds, gold, and organizational secrets. While criminal acts—fraud, theft, larceny, embezzlement, extortion, sabotage, espionage—have remained the same, electronic information systems have created a new, unique environment in which crime can be committed. Access codes, passwords, and encryption all help, but none is by any means a foolproof defense. Kleinschrod (1987) notes that "crooks constantly 'think security' because security is their business. Business people only rarely think security because 'thinking business' is their business." Practical understanding of some fairly unique conditions, listed below, that technology introduces into the information environment is crucial to understanding the genesis of security breaches.

Invisibility

First, whereas traditional security procedures deal with visible, physical items, information security involves protecting invisible property. Once data are stored electronically, they are imperceptible to the human eye. We cannot see whether the data have been removed nor can we directly notice whether changes have been made because no jimmied locks on file drawers, no missing folders, no erasure marks on the paper would alert us to a break-in. Moreover, an intruder can instruct a computer to erase any invisible electronic evidence of an invasion.

Remote Access

Second, the remote access capability of electronic information systems means that intruders can invade an organization's system from the privacy of their own home or from another organization's computer, or even from a phone booth, with the aid of a laptop. Dead bolt locks on doors provide little, or no, protection from a system intrusion.

Strange Forms

Third, computers involve strange forms and codes so that even a visible indication of data manipulation, such as an unauthorized change in software, might go undetected. Nontechnical users can look at the screen or printout of their own application program and not notice a change.

Techies

Fourth, perhaps the most significant security factor is technical personnel—the information experts who are, as Kleinschrod (1987) observes, "in almost total situations of trust." Many of them, he insists, "know how to do anything to a computer without being detected."

Integration

Fifth, the sheer scope of electronic information systems affects security. Technology enables the collection and storing of more information than was ever possible in manual systems. Moreover, much of this information is integrated or networked, as at St. Serena's pharmacy, so that a violator can obtain a variety of data at once. As a consequence, unauthorized manipulation of electronic data can affect hundreds of users. As Muldoon and Sardinas (1999) put it: "The interconnection of subsystems through data communication networks and data bases promotes quick access to relevant information. It does, however, have drawbacks. One undetected error (intentional or unintentional) can have a serious impact by rippling throughout the system and causing many other errors to occur."

Social/Psychological Realities

Social, legal, and psychological realities are associated with the technology. The psychological challenge to "beat the machine" makes breaking into electronic systems a socially acceptable mindset. Take, for example, the aforementioned young hackers who used a home computer to break into data systems simply to meet the challenge of breaking into sophisticated computer systems. Or, consider the second-generation hackers known as "cyberpunks" who roam the electronic pathways of cyberspace and break into systems for the sheer joy of damaging, destroying, or capitalizing on the data they find (Caniglia 1993). This kind of mindset raises the information security bar.

Our legal system has lagged behind technological realities so that prosecuting security violators is difficult. Legal sanctions are ineffective because prosecutors have been unable to document theft given that the stolen data are invisible and physically breaking and entering have become unnecessary. The 1987 Computer Security Act—the legislation intended to proscribe using government information systems in an unauthorized manner—has had limited results. A congressional study found that a number of government agencies have simply failed to implement procedures mandated by this legislation (Newlin 1990). While progress is being made in this regard, our legal system still struggles to stay apace with the technology.

Some organizations lie about the status of information security in their organizations. One of the most common rationales for denying security problems is the "principle of secure image," which holds that if an organization is perceived as vulnerable, it invites attack and exploitation. Operating on this principle, many organizations choose not to disclose that they have been victimized by breaches of security for fear that disclosure would invite similar breaches, loss of confidence, and investigations into the adequacy of supervision (Wood 1992). Will St. Serena's pharmacy be tempted to do this in view of its forthcoming JCAHO inspection? Organizationally, the efficiency and speed of computers can prompt users to avoid efficiency limiting procedures, such as security measures, which can seem to impede operations. End users of the technology want user friendliness and do not always understand the nature of security threats, potential methods of abuse, or the value of some of the information resources they are using; and, often, users resist anything that they perceive as delaying their work (Weiss 1990). A typical pattern involves the security measure of access codes for terminals. To save time from forgetfulness, users will often write the access code on a strip of paper and tape it to their machine, which undermines security efforts. Other common behaviors include the indiscriminate sharing of passwords, unattended, but logged on, terminals, and improper disposal of printed reports. This "efficiency syndrome" is all the more evident in technicians who in the view of some "are adverse to the establishment of controls" because of the technical inefficiencies that accompany security measures (Muldoon and Sardinas 1996).

In sum, securing electronic information systems is a different task from securing the organization's visible valuables. For this reason, managing the security of information systems like that at St. Serena's pharmacy requires some creative action.

What Healthcare Professionals Can Do

Managing the security of electronic information systems is a technical and administrative task that requires creative user–manager action (Radding 1987). It cannot be left to the technician alone. Managers must be guided in this effort by a sober awareness that a completely secure system is not available today and that more security means more cost and less efficiency, as Phil is realizing at St. Serena's pharmacy. Therefore, the first issue is to decide how much security is needed. Several areas for action can be examined.

Organize and Classify Data

Probably the most effective action that managers can take is to better organize the information they collect and maintain because poorly organized information systems are easier to breach. Organizing information for security is a three-step process of (1) reviewing data needs; (2) eliminating unneeded data; and (3) classifying needed data into security-related categories such as routine, sensitive, and critical.

Many organizations maintain sensitive data that are not needed; eliminating them immediately reduces the problem. Because an estimated 10 percent of most organizations' required information is highly sensitive or critical, and because security measures are expensive and sometimes cumbersome, classifying information can be important. For example, once sensitive information has been identified and classified, it can be stored on a small, dedicated, highly secure system for security purposes, while less sensitive information is secured in less-expensive and cumbersome ways.

Assess Risks

Managers can also assess vulnerabilities and risks to determine how much security is needed. Consider asking the following questions:

- How attractive and valuable is the data?
- Who can be hurt and how badly?
- What is the probability of an intrusion?
- How vulnerable is the system and what are its major vulnerabilities?
- What could be the legal or replacement costs of a security breakdown?

Focus on Personnel

Nearly all studies have shown that the greatest vulnerability is the insider—the technician who has access and knows the system and its security measures. Therefore, a third measure for managers is to devise a careful personnel strategy to counter a dishonest, disgruntled, or careless employee. This strategy may entail special recruitment procedures, such as more extensive background checks; organizational separation of duties, such as not allowing programmers to operate terminals; special attention to technician morale; and continual security training for users and technicians as part of a "security consciousness" effort.

Employ Technical Measures

Managers can install a range of technical measures such as fire safety devices to protect the physical hardware, access codes, programming instructions that shut the computer down when anything unusual happens, and encryption of data. The technology can indeed be used to protect itself. Many organizations program their terminals to automatically record the user and the information input and to specify which terminal was used in the transaction. Still, other organizations restrict access to certain files and processes. The use of so-called firewalls—a dedicated computer that examines and restricts incoming and outgoing communications as a means of protecting networks—has become common in major healthcare systems (McKenzie 1997). In effect, through creative programming, an electronic information system can be instructed to be its own watchdog, which immediately alerts a manager when anything unusual or suspicious occurs. Rapidly developing technical measures that will soon be available include retinal identification, fingerprint, and voice recognition software.

Use Administrative Measures

Similarly, managers can take a range of administrative measures including restricting physical access to the computer facility, using burn bags for discarded papers, and checking identities of all visitors. These measures encompass traditional management functions such as the establishment of plans, screening, selection and training of personnel, development of performance standards, and insistence on documentation (Muldoon and Sardinas 1999). Ideas on possible administrative and technical procedures are catalogued in various manuals, such as Leibholz and Wilson's *The Users Guide to Computer Fraud* (1994) and John M. Carroll's *Computer Security* (1998).

Conduct Security Audits

Finally, nothing can better disclose the effectiveness of security measures than trying to break into the system. The practice of "hiring a hacker" has become organizationally acceptable because of today's security challenges. Some organizations actually hire former computer criminals to intrude into their systems, while others use legitimate "computer busters," such as the System Development Corporation in California, whose business is to break into computer systems to disclose their weaknesses. A recent *Newsweek* article (2000) reveals how broadly this kind of enterprise is developing:

> Last week a scraggly band of hackers known as "Lopht Heavy Industries" joined with some straitlaced tech execs to form @Stake, an internet-security consulting firm. The group of wily programmers, who have broken into security systems and testified before Congress that they could shut down the Internet "in 30 minutes," go only by their Net "nicks," which include Mudge and Space Rogue. They also insist they've never broken the law. Venture capitalists have already thrown $10 million at the start-up.

In any case, all healthcare organizations are well advised to conduct a periodic audit of their information system security.

In short, information security requires a package of measures. The challenge is considerable, and its resolution depends on the understanding and action of user–managers as well as technicians. In healthcare, in particular, because of the sensitivity of personal information, concentrated attention to this reality is critical. Stewart, Phil, and Samantha need to talk.

References

Caniglia, J. 1993. "Cyberpunks Hate You." *Utne Reader* (July–August): 88–96.

Charles, D. 1991. "Can We Stop the Databank Robbers?" *New Scientist* (26 January): 24.

DeWeese, J. 1975. "The Trojan Horse Caper." *Saturday Review* (15 November): 10.

Gerberick, D., D. Huber, and R. Rudloff. 1999. "Defining a Technical Architecture For Healthcare Security." *Information Systems Security* 8 (2): 37–50.

Hard, R. 1992. "Keeping Data Secure Within Hospitals." *Hospitals* (20 October): 50.

Kaiser, R., and T. McCann. 2000. "New E-Mail Bug Wreaks Havoc." *Chicago Tribune* (5 May): 1, 22.

Kleinschrod, W. 1987. "Thinking Like a Crook." *Administrative Management* (January): 62.

Knotts, R., and T. Richards. 1989. "Computer Security: Who's Minding the Store?" *Academy of Management Executive* 3 (1): 63–6.

Levy, L. 1980. "The Crime of the Future Has Arrived." *Newsday* (18 February): 7.

"Making Homes into Prisons." 1992. *New York Times* (15 November): 5.

Markoff, J. 1992. "Science Academy Urges More Computer Security." *New York Times* (6 December): D2.

McKenzie, D. 1997. "Legal Review: Protecting the Confidentiality and Integrity of Patient Records." *Topics in Health Information Management* 17 (4): 65.

Muldoon, J., and J. Sardinas. 1996. "Confidentiality, Privacy, and Restrictions for Computer-Based Patient Records." *Hospital Topics* 74 (3): 33.

Newlin, E. 1990. "A Better Way Is Needed to Keep Computer Systems Under Lock and Key." *The Business Journal of New Jersey* (September): 17.

New York Daily News. 1994. (7 February): 4.

"Tech Notes." 2000. *Newsweek* (17 January): 57.

"Pivotal Role of Data Processors Stressed." 1980. *New York Times* (10 June): D-13.

Radding, A. 1987. "Plans for a Safer System—Strategic System Security." *Computer Decision* (6 April): 38–41.

Sanford, C. 1993. "Computer Viruses: Symptoms, Remedies, and Preventive Measures." *Journal of Computer Information Systems* (Spring): 67.

Vistica, G. 1999. "We're in the Middle of a Cyberwar." *Newsweek* (20 September): 52.

Weiss, K. 1990. "One Time Passwords: The Key to Secure Systems." *Datacenter Manager* (September/October): 42.

Williams, D. 1980. "When the Computer Goes Up in Smoke." *Output* (August): 27–33.

Wood, C. 1992. "Lying About Information Security." *Computer World* (10 February): 2.

READING

Discussions that focus on the line manager's role in information security are rare. The following article, inspired by information policy developments in Great Britain, is among the most comprehensive and managerially enlightening reports in print. Fleur Fischer and Bruce Madge analyze seven specific managerial responsibilities in the realm of information security, which are responsibilities that Stewart would do well to heed.

Data Security and Patient Confidentiality: The Manager's Role

Fleur Fisher and Bruce Madge

Abstract

The maintenance of patient confidentiality is of utmost importance in the doctor patient relationship. With the advent of networks such as the National Health Service Wide Area Network in the UK, the potential to transmit identifiable clinical data will become greater. Links between general practitioners (GPs) and hospitals will allow the rapid transmission of data which if intercepted could be potentially embarrassing to the patient concerned. In 1994 the British Medical Association launched a draft bill on privacy and confidentiality and in association with this bill it is pushing for encryption of all clinical data across electronic networks. The manager's role within an acute hospital, community units and general practice, is to ensure that all employees are aware of the principles of data protection, security of hospital computer systems and that no obvious breaches of security can occur at publicly accessible terminals.

Managers must be kept up to date with the latest developments in computer security such as digital signatures and be prepared to instigate these developments where practically possible. Managers must also take responsibility for the monitoring of access to terminals and be prepared to deal severely with staff who breach the code of confidentiality. Each manager must be kept informed of employees' status with regard to their 'need to know' clearance level and also to promote confidentiality of patient details throughout the hospital. All of the management team must be prepared to train new staff in the principles of data security as they join the organization and recognise their accountability if the programme fails. Data security and patient confidentiality is a broad responsibility in any healthcare organization, with the Chief Executive accountable. In family practice, the partners are responsible and accountable. The British Medical Association believes as a matter of policy, that allowing access to personal health data without the patient's consent, except in a legally allowable situation, should be a statutory offence.

Reprinted from the International Journal of Bio-Medical Computing *43 (1–2)*, Fisher and Madge, "Data Security . . ." 1996, with permission from Elsevier Science. Fleur Fisher and Bruce Madge are staff members with the British Medical Association, London, UK.

Introduction

Although many papers have been written on data security and patient confidentiality [1–3], few [4,5], have looked at the role of the manager in ensuring privacy and confidentiality.

The confidentiality of patient information must be of first importance to all healthcare staff and must be implemented throughout the health care organisation and owned by all staff[5]. The protection of patient information must be ensured through policies implemented and audited by managers and the senior manager is accountable for ensuring that the technological solutions adopted enable the requisite level of security to be enforced. If technologically adequate policies are not enforced, the organisation could leave itself open to major litigation. Amongst many examples there is, for instance, the recent case of a patient's AIDS diagnosis being revealed, without authorization, to a friend. The patient successfully sued for damages of $4.5 million, claiming deprivation of seclusion, emotional distress, worry, anxiety, fear and humiliation [6].

The increasing use of networks in healthcare and the potential for the electronic patient record has led to increasing threats to the security of confidential patient information, a precondition of implementation of an electronic network must be the implementation of a viable security policy.

Much has been said about patients' right to confidentiality but little about staff's need for integrity. Most healthcare professionals are bound by a code of ethics which needs to be extended to encompass all healthcare personnel. The General Medical Council which licenses and disciplines doctors in the UK in its recent publication on guidelines for confidentiality says:

- when you are responsible for confidential information you must make sure that the information is effectively protected against improper disclosure when it is disposed of, stored, transmitted or received;
- you must make sure that, when patients give consent to disclosure of information, they understand what will be disclosed, the reasons for disclosure and the likely consequences;
- you must make sure that patients are informed whenever information about them is likely to be disclosed to others involved in their health care, and that they have the opportunity to withhold permission.

Recent work by the British Medical Association has highlighted the shortcomings in the UK's National Health Service Wide Area Network.

The concerns have been echoed by the whole medical establishment and the other professional health care bodies. This has led to a rethink of the whole question of security and confidentiality within health service networks.

The main problem with electronic networks is one of 'granularity'. With paper records a person wishing to obtain private data could possibly put on a white coat, walk into a ward and take a handful of records from a trolley. Nowadays, with electronic networks, someone with a password can potentially gain access to the complete set of records for a whole country! The main threat to electronic networks is not the expert 'hacker' but the employee of the health service who can provide patient information for monetary gain through blackmail or through selling a story to the newspapers.

Data security within an organisation is therefore a prime concern of the Chief Executive and IT Manager. Of equal importance is the integrity of the data kept within the secure environment, i.e. what is the quality of the data and how up-to-date is it? This is a major concern for the patient.

Who Is a Manager?

The manager's role in purchasing organisations—whether government or insurance funded, e.g. the USA or the UK, whether a regional health purchaser or a family practitioner—is to specify standards of security and confidentiality in handling identifiable health data in the provider organization and the arrangements for independent audit. Audit and audit trails could be considered as quality measures.

The role of managers in provider organisations is perhaps more obvious. These organisations range in the UK from government funded hospitals, clinics and outpatients services to general practice, community services and private institutions providing services contracted out by the NHS, e.g. private mental hospitals for the management of patients with psychiatric illness or mental handicap or severe behavioural problems. Community nursing, physiotherapy and dental services, etc would be included. In the UK, nursing care in the community is contracted by local authority social service departments in mainly private nursing and residential homes. Both purchasers and providers must have a role, purchasing and specifying technologically effective and well managed information systems that can protect the confidentiality of identifiable health data by using both effective audit trails to monitor unauthorised data access, and, independent audit of the system.

This is a major quality issue. It is also an issue of human rights and the individual's right to personal privacy. Security of identifiable personal health information is equally important in any setting where healthcare is delivered, e.g. in prison and in the armed forces. Whilst officers may need to be aware that the prisoner or soldier is ill or unfit for certain duties, there is no need for the medical diagnosis or details to pass outside the perimeter of the healthcare professionals involved with the patient.

Protecting the privacy of patients' records in epidemiological research, i.e. allowing access to the total record without patient consent has exercised the British medical profession.

The Role of the Manager

The role of the manager within healthcare must be to ensure that the strictest possible rules apply to data security. A culture that is 'privacy aware' and the continuous education and updating of staff is also a major task, so that everyone in the organisation knows their responsibilities under the data protection acts. To ensure full implementation of adequate security measures in a healthcare environment, managers must accept ownership of, and involvement in, the problem. Of equal importance is the question does a healthcare manager need identifiable access to confidential data or should he only have access via a clinician and with patient's consent. The BMA believes the latter.

To achieve adequate security the following measures could be implemented.

1. *Employment of a security manager*

The employment of a specific person to deal with all aspects of security within an organization is generally the rule in business. With the market approach to healthcare a security manager, preferably with a clinical/technical background, to oversee all aspects of data security and adherence to data protection standards is essential. The Chief Executive or Healthcare Manager should support this post fully and it must command a high rank and adequate respect within the health care organisation. This person should also be involved in setting up the independent security audit and training in all aspects of security procedures including the use of digital signatures and encryption where necessary [3].

2. *A punishable code of connection*

A code of connection for each member of healthcare personnel which is signed would highlight the area of security and would allow disciplinary procedures against those who transgress the code of connection. Current data protection legislation is usually powerless to deal severely with breaches of confidentiality which may have far reaching effects on the life of the patient. For instance, recent work by the British Medical Association with its publication of a draft bill to protect patient confidentiality calls for legislation to enable suitable punishment to be accorded to healthcare personnel who break confidentiality, together with a culture that makes revelation of personal health information without the patient's consent a dismissing offence.

3. *A policy of encryption of data of a sensitive nature*

Data of a sensitive nature must be protected by some form of encryption especially in transit between two different locations. The use of public key encryption would be recommended for maximum security as it is cheap and easy to implement. A central trusted body would be required to hold public keys. However the whole question of encryption is one that is enmeshed with government policy on freedom of information and in some countries health care institutions can and have run up against security agencies.

4. *Audit of security by an independent security advisor*

All secure systems should be regularly audited by an independent expert. This would ensure that the particular healthcare institution adhered to regulations. This would also support the proposal by Hayam that a Security Audit Centre is essential in health care informatics [7] and one that is preferably administered by a clinician.

5. *An information security policy*

An essential requirement in any healthcare setting would be an Information Security Policy [1,8]. The management of the healthcare institution would then ensure that this code was strictly adhered to. The first step to an effective security policy is the creation of a comprehensive 'threats and vulnerabilities' document to list all of the potential attacks upon a system. In addition a policy for data protection including all relevant laws should be included in the security policy which includes a description and explanation of all relevant legislation. This can then lead to the formulation of an effective policy to counter the threats from these sources.

6. *Implementation of audit trails*

The use of audit trails in hospital information systems appears to date to be the exception rather than the rule. There is no mandatory requirement for this procedure but a 'security aware' Chief Executive should be ensuring that the requirement for an audit trail is mandatory in any tendering procedure.

7. Finance

No good security system is free although promotion of the idea of security to employees should be mandatory and be able to be implemented at little cost. In the UK the purchaser/provider split could provide a method for imposing security standards on hospitals through contracting mechanisms, i.e. if the hospital has a poor record of security then that hospital will not get the contract with the local purchasing agency. In general practice and on the purchasing side however, it would require a different method for imposing controls and this would have to be implemented at ministerial level through some sort of penalty system. What every Chief Executive must realise, however, is that good security will cost money and should be built into the budget.

Conclusions

It is essential that the healthcare manager and the clinician work together to promote patient confidentiality. Patient associations need to keep a sharp awareness of the issue, with competent technological advice. If patient confidentiality is not maintained, especially in an electronic environment, then litigation against healthcare organizations will increase rapidly as patients become increasingly empowered to question procedures in medicine. Valuable work on the subject of security has been done by the AIM SEISMED project [9].

Security can be achieved through good modelling procedures for threats and vulnerabilities and an ensuing security policy can then be implemented. A member of staff or a team must be then put in place to ensure the security policy is implemented and adhered to using spot checks on staff as necessary. Encryption of sensitive patient data in transit is essential as is a high level security policy such as C2/B1 of the Orange Book or its counterpart in ITSEC [10,11]. End user access must be controlled through passwords, digital signatures and other access controls which must be future proofed to ensure that advances in security technology, such as hand and retina scanning, are implemented when sufficiently stable.

Managers in agencies both purchasing and providing healthcare, in all settings, must provide clear leadership and accept accountability for data security—and personal health information confidentiality.

There must be no ambiguity about disciplinary procedures being implemented and enforced.

National legislation to protect the privacy of identifiable health information should be put in place immediately.

References

[1] Lawrence LM: Safeguarding the Confidentiality of Automated Medical information. *Joint Commission Journal of Quality Improvement*, 20(11) (1994) 639–646.

[2] Marr P: Maintaining patient confidentiality in an electronic world, *Int J Biomed Comput*, 35(suppl 1) (1994) 213–217.

[3] Barber B and Douglas, S: An initial approach to the security techniques required by the electronic patient record, *Int J Biomed Comput*, 35(suppl 1) (1994) 33–38.

[4] Iversen KR: Security requirements for electronic patients records: the Norwegian view, *Int J Biomed Comput*, 35(Suppl 1) (1994) 51–56.

[5] Peterson HE: Management and staff issues in data protection. In *Data Protection and Confidentiality in Health Informatics*, edited by the Commission of the European Communities DGX111/F AIM, IOS Press, Amsterdam, 1991, 9-051-99052-9.

[6] John Doe vs Shady Grove Adventist Hospital et al., *MD App Lexis* 221. Court of Special Appeals of Maryland. 1991.

[7] Hayam A: Security Audit Centre: a suggested model for effective audit strategies in health care informatics. *Int J Biomed Comput*, 35(suppl 1) (1994) 115–127.

[8] Katsikas SK and Gritzalis DA: The need for a security policy in healthcare institutions. *Intr J Biomed Comput*, 35(suppl 1) (1994) 73–80.

[9] Van Dorp HD and Dubbeldam JD: The AIM SEISMED guidelines for system development and design, *Int J Biomed Comput* 35(suppl 1) (1994) 179–186.

[10] Department of Defense: *Trusted Computer Systems Evaluation Criteria*, DoD 5200.28-STD, Department of Defence, USA. December 1985.

[11] Information Technology Security Evaluation (ITSEC): *Harmonisation criteria of France, Germany, The Netherlands, The United Kingdom: Version 1.2.* ISBN 92826 3004 8: CEC. Luxembourg. June 1991.

MAINTAINING INFORMATION PRIVACY

J UST AS the computer security issue has inspired many books, so too has information privacy. Jeffrey Rothfeder's *Privacy For Sale*, for example, is based on the notion that information technology has made everyone's private life an open secret, a contention widely supported by investigatory reports (McGrath 1999). Rothfeder (1992) describes the random carnage sometimes caused by the carelessness and false assumptions of powerful institutions, and portrays the computer sharks who have learned to invade theoretically secure information systems for private gain. Suggesting that the misuse of personal information in the United States is on the increase because of the growing use of information technology for medical, financial, and other sensitive records, he warns that millions of Americans are violated or otherwise abused by privacy invaders. This chapter focuses on what healthcare professionals can do to skillfully manage the realities of information privacy.

CASE STUDY

Case Seven: Protecting Private Parts

St. Serena's Lance Larue returned from a stimulating healthcare management conference only to find two distressing reports, among many other matters, awaiting his attention. As the executive vice president of St. Serena's, Lance was known in the field as a leader in strategic planning and marketing for healthcare. Upon his return to work, the following correspondence were waiting to challenge his managerial skills.

MEMO

From: Feona Furie, M.D.

To: Lance Larue, M.B.A., FACHE

Probably in a misguided effort to maintain the "privacy" of our patients, the hospital has put some patients in danger of not getting proper care. Yesterday, a woman came to the emergency room with an acute infection. Before she collapsed, she mentioned that she had been a patient here some time ago and that she had been an intravenous drug user. Access to her past medical history was essential for evaluating her present condition so I immediately consulted the new "information system." But, not knowing her physician, I was unable to access her record from the system without a long delay. "Access may be allowed" repeatedly appeared on the screen as a response to my inquiry, then it informed me that this patient's file was "private information." I was required to acknowledge that the access desired was deliberate and then I had to provide a lengthy explanation. After finally getting the information subsequent to a considerable waiting period, I finally accessed the needed information. I was then informed that the appropriateness of access would have to be reviewed by another party. Had I not been able to ultimately access the record, the patient might have died. On the other hand, I later discovered that some of the information in her record had not been updated and that some was even erroneous. Is St. Serena's now having machines rather than physicians mediate care?

Lance saw the makings of a major problem. Although he had instructed Stewart and his techies to work with the legal staff to ensure that St. Serena's system was compliant with JCAHO privacy standards, this locked, unwieldy system was not what he expected from the effort. Privacy was essential, but Dr. Furie's experience was disturbing. Trying to follow the system's commands obviously had been frustrating for her while trying to treat the patient, but efforts to safeguard privacy do come with a price. But, was the difficulty she experienced necessary in today's healthcare environment or had Stewart gone too far? Then, Lance read the second document—a letter from a former patient forwarded to him by Samantha.

Ms. Samantha Savage

President

St. Serena's Hospital

Dear Ms. Savage:

As a former patient at your hospital and a resident of this community I feel it is necessary to bring a problem to your attention. Are you aware that personal information about your hospital's patients is apparently made available to almost anyone?

I recently entered your hospital to deliver my first child. As a single mother I chose, for personal reasons, to minimize the publicity that might be associated with this event. My hospital stay was wonderful and I returned home with a beautiful child. Soon afterward, however, several disturbing things happened that led me to believe that your hospital is violating my rights. First, a representative from Single Mothers of America called asking me to join her organization. Although it is undoubtedly a fine organization, I was irate that they knew my name, address, phone number, and situation. I had never contacted them nor had any of my family and friends. They told me that they received my name from St. Serena's and that I was now on their mailing list. They also knew my religion and listed me as a mother of five children!

Are medical records at St. Serena's so accessible that this kind of thing can happen? In speaking with some of your staff, I learned that most of my record is created by a variety of caregivers and that it is now electronically accessed. I find it shocking that such sensitive information is not held in strict confidentiality and that this kind of intrusion can happen. And by the way, at least get my record straight: I have only this one child!

Sincerely,

Tammy Smith

Attached to the letter was a note from Samantha telling Lance to get on the matter fast.

Apparently, Stewart and his techies had not overdone privacy protection from Ms. Smith's vantage point. How could the emergency room physicians have such difficulties, while outsiders could easily get patient information, like they did on Ms. Smith?! Lance called Stewart for answers.

Questions for Discussion

1. Assess the privacy problem as it appears at St. Serena's.
2. What should Lance ask Stewart about the issue and what should he have Stewart and his techies do?
3. Develop a set of principles for Lance to convey to Stewart.

COMMENTARY

First, clarifying the relationship of confidentiality, privacy, and security is helpful. Are the incidents reported to Lance matters of security or privacy? and what, if anything, is the difference between the two? Although the terms are sometimes used interchangeably, security, confidentiality, and privacy are not synonymous. Confidentiality refers to the notion of secrecy, whereas privacy refers to the broader notion of safeguarding, the former being only part of the latter (see Figure 7.1). Privacy and confidentiality are policy, social, and ethical issues. What personal information should be kept secret or restricted only to certain "need-to-know" standards? Should some personal information specifically not be restricted? What kinds of safeguards or managerial measures should be applied to personal information about patients and staff?

As discussed in the previous chapter, security is a technical and administrative matter on which there is general agreement about the nature of the problem and its solution. Privacy, on the other hand, is a social and political issue that involves considerably less certainty and consensus. Security questions include: What measures are available to implement the decisions made on the confidentiality and privacy questions? Are they in place? Are they working? The privacy issue concerns what *should* be done to control personal information, while the security issue deals more with what *can* be done to protect information.

That information privacy is a serious matter is suggested by a report of the United States Privacy Protection Commission (1990). This concern for privacy is discussed at length in healthcare conferences, healthcare literature, and the general press. The following examples illustrate an increasing consciousness of the importance of information privacy (Miller 1993):

- The Director of the U.S. Office of Information Systems and Development Agency for Health Care Policy and Research (now known as Agency for Healthcare Research and Quality) listed privacy as one of four primary issues being addressed in federal healthcare reform.
- The American Civil Liberties Union is mounting a campaign to tighten the laws protecting the confidentiality of medical information.
- JCAHO revised the Manual for Accreditation to include an information management chapter, which addresses a number of security requirements that guard against abuses of privacy.
- Court decisions on lawsuits such as *Behringer vs. Princeton Medical Center* have confirmed the patient's right to privacy, and have held healthcare organizations and their managers liable for preserving that privacy.

The privacy matter becomes complex because the right to privacy is not explicitly defined. Most people would probably agree with Supreme Court Justice Louis Brandeis who once identified "the right to be left

Figure 7.1 Conceptual Distinctions

Confidentiality	Privacy	Security
↓	↓	↓
Information Secrecy Policy	Information Safety Policy	Implementation Mechanisms

alone" as a prerequisite for a tolerable life. Nonetheless, as Lawrence H. Tribe, a professor of constitutional law at Harvard University notes: "The debate over the outer boundaries of a right to privacy will continue for some time" (Labaton 1988). Let's try to bring some clarity to the concept.

The Nature of the Information Privacy Problem

A major misconception, occasionally presented in the popular press,[1] holds that privacy is a small matter chiefly concerned with keeping information secret. Consider the following representative anecdotes that illustrate privacy as a multifaceted issue with serious implications for healthcare organizations like St. Serena's:

- "Do you have any skeletons in your closet?" Millstone was asked by his insurance broker. "No," he answered with a surprised laugh. "Why do you want to know?" "Some problem with your car insurance. The company wants to cancel it." So began a four year, $4,000 ordeal for James Millstone, assistant managing editor of the St. Louis *Post-Dispatch*. He asked the company for specifics and they directed him to a consumer credit investigating firm. It said that Millstone had been much disliked by his neighbors when he was in Washington, D.C., that he was a hippie with a beard and long hair, and was strongly suspected of being a drug user. He was accused of lacking judgment, failing to discipline his children, and driving peace demonstrators to and from demonstrations. Millstone was outraged. Not only did he dispute every piece of adverse material, he wanted to know where the damning allegations came from. He sued the investigating firm (Linowes 1978).

- On a blustery day in late November, a woman was filling out papers at an automobile dealership in suburban Vienna, Virginia, on a new car she and her husband were buying. She needed her husband's social security number but couldn't remember it, so she asked to use a phone to call him. "Oh, don't bother him," a clerk said. "I'll get the social security number for you." He turned to a computer console at his desk typed in a code number and her husband's name, and within 30 seconds the computer was printing out the couple's life history: where each worked and their salaries; where they lived, the cost of their home and size of their mortgage; the fact that the husband had been married before; the credit cards each held, and a credit rating for each card, and details of the husband's recent prostate surgery (Heller 1978).

• Dateline Miami (AP)—A 35-year-old North Miami man, released after spending five months in jail for two robberies he didn't commit, was rearrested because someone failed to clear his name from a police computer. Charges from the first arrest were dropped, with apologies from the prosecutors, on January 6, about a week after Matthews had been released on bond. On Wednesday, Matthews was walking down a northwest Miami street when a police cruiser pulled up behind him. Two officers stopped him, got his name and ran a computer check. It showed two outstanding robbery warrants (*Times Union* 1980).

These, and other, experiences with personal information suggest that information privacy, in connoting "safeguarding," means not only designating certain information as secret or restricted—that is, safeguarding access—but also:

1. Determining what personal information can or cannot be collected in the first place;
2. Ensuring that the information collected is accurate, complete and up to date;
3. Deciding whether and when certain personal information should be purged from the system; and
4. Limiting the purposes for which the information collected can be used.

Six major aspects of the privacy issue, thus, need to be clarified. They involve information collection, use, updating, purging, accuracy, and secrecy.

Information Collection

The information-collection issue concerns limitations on the kinds of information that healthcare and other organizations collect and maintain. For example, should healthcare organizations be restricted to collecting only what is demonstrably needed, and prohibited from collecting certain kinds of information? A *Time*/CNN (1991) poll has confirmed the public's concern about this issue. The poll found that 76 percent of the respondents are "very concerned" about the amount of computerized information collected about them. In response, federal and state policy development initiatives show a clear tendency toward limiting collection of personal information to that which the collecting agency can demonstrate is necessary to provide its service. At St. Serena's, for example, is collection of the marital status of Ms. Smith demonstrably needed to provide the healthcare she seeks, or is the collection just a "habit?" Lance might want Stewart and department heads to analyze and reduce the personal information they enter on the information system.

Information Use

Once collected and maintained, should information collected by healthcare organizations be limited in its use? The strong trend in privacy legislation is to limit information use solely to the purpose for which it was collected and given. For example, information obtained by a health clinic to treat a drinking problem could not be provided to an insurance company or to an employer. In this regard, the Clinton administration has recently proposed legislation that would prohibit healthcare organizations from releasing patient information for purposes unrelated to treatment and payment without the written consent of the patient (*Newsweek* 1999). Furthermore, the proposal restricts information disclosure for treatment and payment only to what is minimally necessary. For example, when paying for medical services, no treatment information would be provided to banks or credit card companies. If St. Serena's had such a policy in place, might Ms. Smith have been spared her ordeal?

Information Updating

Should requirements be in place to update information collected and maintained; that is, to keep it current? In the case vignettes above, for example, the Miami man was subjected to a police investigation simply because computerized information had not been updated to show that the charges against him had been dropped. Many people have been denied credit because a computerized data bank said they had unpaid debts, even after the debts had been paid. And the emergency room incident reported to Lance appears to involve outdated information on the patient. Given the danger of using outdated information in the provision of healthcare, we might wonder whether Lance's new information system includes rigorous updating procedures and checks.

Information Purging

Should personal information be automatically purged after a reasonable period of time? For example, should a person's medical record always include the fact that he/she contracted venereal disease as a teenager, or should that fact be dropped from his/her record after, say, 10 years? Should teenagers convicted of burglary, who never again stray, have the conviction on their record into middle age, or should records be cleared after a reasonable time period without an offense? Should notation of a delinquent bill at St. Serena's still be on a patient's record after the bill is paid? Should Lance and Stewart be considering some policies and procedures in this regard?

Information Accuracy

Perhaps the most serious aspect of the privacy issue concerns information accuracy and verification (Harris 1987). Should healthcare organizations be required to ensure the accuracy and completeness of the data they maintain, and should there be penalties for using erroneous or incomplete information? Should individuals have the right to inspect and verify personal information? Should patients have a right to verify their medical files? The new Clinton proposal gives a resounding affirmative answer. A Computer Science professor offered the following foundation for such a policy (Early 1978):

> Most errors in computer files remain undetected. They are the simple keypunch errors, simple in execution but devastating to the person whom they affect; programming errors which remain undetected long enough to cause untold anguish to many; errors of omission and commission which cannot be rectified except by the action of the party whose reputation is besmirched.

Aggravating this inaccurate-information situation is the victim's own ignorance of the cause of the problem, either because he or she has not seen the file or is unaware of its existence and use. Lance could well ask Stewart about accuracy and verification aspects of the new information system. Surely, Ms. Smith would appreciate the chance to correct the number of children assigned to her.

Information Secrecy

Finally, information secrecy is a significant part of the privacy issue (Dewitt 1987). Should organizations be prohibited from holding information about people without their knowledge? Should organizations be required to notify any person on whom they maintain a file? Should there be a ban on secret information files? Relatedly, should patients be informed of the release of information in their file to, say, a single mothers group, or should they be left in the dark?

Other Information Privacy Complications

All of the above questions concerning information collection, use, updating, purging, accuracy, and secrecy are complicated by legal, political, fiscal, operational, and inferential factors.

Legal Factors

The legal dimension of the privacy issue comprises laws, court decisions, and accreditation standards. The United States now has federal, state, and local laws that place legal requirements on the organizational use of information. At the federal level, for example, the Privacy Act of 1974 protects the confidentiality of medical information in the patient records system maintained by federal agencies. While these laws currently apply only to governmental data banks, legislators and healthcare organizations continue to push for a federal law that specifically protects the privacy, confidentiality, and security of information for everyone. The 1999 Clinton administration proposal is an example of the movement. As efforts to get specific legislation continue, many healthcare organizations are taking a wait-and-see approach (Bergman 1994).

One particular problem relevant to healthcare organizations today is the disconcerting fact that providers and payers that operate in more than one state must comply with a multitude of often "inconsistent" laws and regulations (*Hospitals & Health Networks* 1993). For example, as Pendrak and Ericson (1998) observe, "protecting patients' privacy is problematic because state laws regarding confidentiality of patient information vary, and federal requirements are unclear." Organizations, information users, and managers who do not know the applicable privacy laws are in considerable jeopardy. These privacy laws, however, are further complicated by freedom of information or "sunshine" laws that provide no clear legal solution to the dilemma between disclosing data or maintaining confidentiality (O'Brien 1979). Ms. Smith's episode with St. Serena's may well stem from the ambiguity involved.

While a considerable ambiguity still exists, courts are beginning to recognize personal information as private property, and misuse could result in profound privacy implications. For example, personal harm from a violation of privacy is currently judged under the law of torts, which means that it is a civil matter involving financial penalties. If the law of property is applied, the violation of privacy becomes a criminal matter involving possible jail sentences. Recent litigation in the courts supports the contention that personal information raises serious privacy considerations (Hard 1992); consider the following examples.

- A physician who worked for a medical center was diagnosed as having AIDS, but the information was not kept confidential. The physician filed suit against the hospital and some of its employees, claiming breach of confidentiality and violation of the state's anti-discrimination law.
- An individual sued a hospital for unauthorized release of patient records. The individual, an employee of the U.S. Postal Service, was judged unfit for the job by a psychologist who reviewed the employee's inpatient records without the individual's permission.
- A patient sued a regional health center. The patient charged that employees of the hospital shared test results with individuals who were not associated with the hospital.

A pseudo-legal dimension of accreditation is also a factor. For example, the accreditation standards of JCAHO (1994) require that medical records be "confidential, secure, current, authenticated, legible and complete." A healthcare organization that fails to meet this requirement can lose its accreditation. Samantha is certain to be concerned about this.

Political Factors

Politically, the atmosphere is charged as a result of studies and policies in other countries. In Great Britain, for example, lawmakers were trying to protect information in computers with a statute that makes unauthorized prying into a computer a crime punishable by up to six months in jail (*The Economist* 1991). Sweden has enacted strong privacy policies that are being used as a model by grass-roots interest groups in the United States. Under several acts of parliament, Sweden (1) requires that all data banks be licensed before being implemented; (2) prohibits any information gathering unless authorized; (3) recognizes a new felony crime, "data trespass," for unauthorized collection or use of personal data or for maintaining inaccurate, incomplete, or outdated information; and (4) applies these to all data banks in the country, whether private or public.[2]

In light of increased use of electronic patient records, the U.S. Congress continues to examine proposals for new federal medical records confidentiality laws that would preempt state laws and require protection that goes beyond current responsibilities of individual institutions (Bergman 1994). These proposals include (1) requiring hospitals to permit patients to inspect and correct their records; (2) making it a crime to obtain medical records under false pretenses; and (3) authorizing suits for breaches of confidentiality or other mismanagement of personal data.

Some states have general statutes governing the confidentiality of patient records and patient information. For example, both Montana and Washington have adopted the Uniform Health Care Information Act. California has also adopted a statute governing release of individually identifiable patient information by providers (Waller and Fulton 1993).

Fiscal Factors

The fiscal dimension of the privacy issue is simply that privacy protection can be expensive. After the first year of the federal Privacy Act, the Department of Defense complained that the new policy "put a heavy administrative burden on the Department and had proved very costly to implement" (Gerow 1976). Double checking for accuracy, providing for inspection, periodically purging, and other monitoring procedures are expensive. How much privacy protection can organizations afford?

Operational Factors

Operationally, the key problem is the dilemma—central to the St. Serena's case—between the information needs of healthcare organizations and the harm that can result from the collection and use of personal information. As Lee (1999) has expressed in a recent *Newsweek* article: "Confidentiality is a vital component of the trust between patients and physicians, and protecting it is worth some inconvenience. But information is the lifeblood of good healthcare." Lee was reacting to stories similar to Dr. Furie's experience, and concluded that "privacy can be hazardous to your health."

Restrictions on data activities imposed for the sake of privacy can make it difficult for an organization to function efficiently. What are realistic limits? For example, in Texas, an employee of a mental hospital who raped a patient was later found to have previously been convicted of rape. But a state law had denied the hospital the right to screen his arrest record before employment. And what can be done when the medical record of an unconscious patient is needed for treatment but cannot be released because it was collected for other treatment? As a CBS reporter once complained, privacy can be carried too far (Graham 1978).

Inferential Factors

The inferential aspect of the privacy issue should concern even those of us with "nothing to hide." Currently, credit card and phone call records are two easily accessed sources of information about the range of personal interests and activities. What people read, where they travel, who they call, what they wear, what organizations they support are the sort of information that can easily lead to false inferences.

For example, consider the kinds of records that are kept on individuals. Could someone infer from your large credit card purchase at a liquor store that you have a drinking problem, not knowing that your job entails heavy entertaining? Could someone infer from your record of frequent blood tests that you are concerned about venereal disease, not knowing that you are monitoring your cholesterol level? Could an employer who sees a psychiatrist's report of your treatment infer that you are unsuited for a high-pressure job? Might someone infer that St. Serena's patient, Ms. Smith, is irresponsible or even promiscuous? The power of information, even accurate and complete information, to generate unwarranted impressions is considerable, and is a legitimate concern in the matter of information privacy (Bologna 1987; Rothfeder 1992).

How Technology Affects the Issue

Clearly, information privacy is a concern even without modern information technology. So why do many believe that, " . . . by far, the most important high-tech threat to privacy is not an exotic surveillance device but a familiar storage system: the computer" (*Time* 1992).

One reason is that computers remove information from a guarded medical environment to a technical one in which patient contact may be lost and intuitive concern for privacy may be preempted by billing and data-storage needs. The tendency of information technology to depersonalize can aggravate the problem.

Another reason is that the integration capability of information technology poses an additional threat to privacy. With computers, scattered pieces of data can easily be compiled into a profile, which was never before possible. With computers, an erroneous piece of data that previously would remain isolated in a manual file cabinet can now be integrated with other data and widely disseminated. The computer also facilitates wide access to data, as Ms. Smith can testify; it enables personal information to be "passed on and on at lightning speed from one user to another all over the world" (Linowes 1978), as Jergesen and Schrier (1979), medical lawyers, point out:

> In the past, hospitals could restrict access to confidential information about patients simply by preventing unauthorized persons from entering the medical record area. However, with medical information potentially available to anyone with a connected terminal, there is a danger of multiple breaches of confidentiality without the knowledge of the hospital.

Also, the storage capabilities of information technology make keeping personal information easy. In fact, computers often make storing data less expensive than destroying them, which can, in turn, result in a failure to purge outdated or erroneous data and encourage more data collection. As a consequence, more personal data are now collected and maintained. The more complicated and sophisticated the technology becomes, the more challenging its management. "There are two broad dangers," said Gary Marx, a sociologist at MIT. "One is that the technologies work and the other is that they don't work" (Markoff 1998).

In addition, technical and psychological factors involved with information technology aggravate the privacy problem. Many people are inclined to regard computer-generated data as infallible. In fact, a University of Missouri research team found that even the brightest people "tend to take the word of a machine over their own good sense" (Tomnick 1982). Whereas a handwritten notation on a person might be questioned, a computer-generated item might appear so "official" looking as to dispel any inclination to question.

Finally, did you ever try to correct an erroneous computerized bill? Doing so takes a while. Correcting an electronic record is a technical task that involves more than erasing or lining out a sheet of paper. The use of information technology does magnify the privacy problem, as St. Serena's is learning.

Managerial Implications

Dealing with the privacy issue in information management is a serious responsibility that requires wise use of the perception and sensitivity of the user–manager. What can a manager do? What can Lance do? Blithely leaving the management of privacy to the technicians while using the technology is ill-advised, as well as irresponsible.

A first step in managing privacy is to reduce the amount of personal data collected and maintained to that which is actually needed. The storage capability of computers often prompts a tendency to collect and store whatever data might be useful. As long as the client is available and has to fill out a form, why not collect all the data possible? Clearly, the more personal data maintained, the greater the privacy problem for the organization.

Second, user–managers should know the privacy laws and regulations that apply to their work. Many managers unwittingly break privacy laws and rules simply because they have not kept abreast of legal and regulatory developments on privacy. An ongoing monitoring mechanism is advisable.

Third, managers attuned to the problem can establish in-house information handling policies that exceed legal obligations to clients who entrust the organization with personal data. These policies should outline what data can be collected, how they can be used, who must verify their accuracy, when they will be updated, and so forth.

Fourth, managers and users can provide training on the nature of the problem and on policies to develop an organization-wide "privacy consciousness." Most privacy breaches occur because information handlers are unaware of the power of the data they collect and hold. Training can develop this awareness.

Fifth, protecting privacy is largely a matter of properly managing information—that is, establishing verification procedures and updating, purging, and protecting data collected and scored. To collect and use an inaccurate piece of personal data is mismanagement of the first order. Weak or nonexistent information management procedures breed the kind of carelessness that makes privacy breaches simple, likely, and serious, as Lee (1999) illuminates: "These safeguards cost money and time, and doctors will grumble about the extra keystrokes. But with a little creativity and common sense, we'll find a way to protect privacy while ensuring that doctors have the information they need to take good care of people."

Sixth, managers must institute technical and administrative security measures as were discussed in Chapter 6. Electronic personal data that are otherwise well managed can be easily accessed and altered unless solid security measures are employed.

Seventh, managers should periodically audit privacy protection measures. The business of some firms is to attempt to obtain sensitive data from an organization, test verification and updating procedures, and measure staff alertness to potential privacy problems. Employing a firm to conduct periodic privacy audits can disclose weak areas and produce better privacy safeguards.

Finally, managers could opt not to computerize certain particularly sensitive personal data. Automation does aggravate the privacy problem; therefore, a deliberate decision not to computerize certain data can sometimes be a wise policy.

Notes

1. For example, see D. Singleton, "Privacy Study: Another Peek." *New York Daily News* (6 May 1979); and J. Caper, "The Privacy Scam." *Newsweek* (18 June 1979): 3.
2. For an overview of privacy policies in other countries, see Gabriel Rach, "Data Privacy." *Telecommunications* (May 1980): 43–8.

References

"A Question of Privacy." 1999. *Newsweek* (8 November): 67.

Bergman, R. 1994. "Laws Sought to Guard Health Data from Falling into the Wrong Hands." *Hospitals & Health Networks* (20 January): 62.

Bologna, G. J. 1987. "The Ethics of Managing Information." *Journal of Systems Management* (August): 28.

Dewitt, P. 1987. "Can a System Keep a Secret?" *Time* (6 April): 68–70.

Early, E. 1978. "Letter to the Editor." *New York Times* (12 December): 29.

The Economist. 1991. (4 May): 21.

Gerow, A. 1976. "DOD Officials Wage 'Hell' to Curtail Privacy Act." *Navy Times* (February): 4.

Graham, F. 1978. "Carrying Privacy Too Far." *The Washington Post* (12 September): 18.

Hard, R. 1992. "Keeping Patient Data Secure within Hospitals." *Hospitals* (20 October): 50.

Harris, D. 1987. "A Matter of Privacy: Managing Personal Data in Company Computers." *Personnel* (February): 34.

Heller, J. 1978. "Not-so-Private Lives at a Finger's Touch." *Newsday* (29 May): 4.

"Innocent Man Cleared Again." 1998. *Times Union* (15 June).

Jergesen, A. D., and S. V. Schnier. 1979. "Medical Legal Forum." *Hospital Forum* (September–October): 24.

Joint Commission on Accreditation of Healthcare Organizations. 1994. *Accreditation Manual* MR3. Oakbrook Terrace, IL: JCAHO.

Labaton, S. 1988. "Privacy." *The New York Times* (5 June): E-32.

Lee, T. 1978. "Too Much Privacy Is a Health Hazard." *Newsweek* (16 August): 71.

Linowes, D. F. 1978. "The Privacy Crisis." *Newsweek* (26 June): 19.

Markoff, J. 1988. "A New Breed of Snoopier Computers." *New York Times* (5 June): E-2.

McGrath, P. 1999. "Knowing You All Too Well." *Newsweek* (29 March): 49–50.

Miller, D. 1993. "Preserving the Privacy of Computerized Patient Records." *Healthcare Informatics* (October): 72–4.

"Nowhere to Hide." 1991. *Time* (11 November): 36.

O'Brien, D. 1979. "Freedom of Information, Privacy, and Information Control." *Public Administration Review* (July–August): 323–8.

Pendrak, R., and R. Ericson. 1998. "Information Technologies Need to Protect Patient Confidentiality." *Healthcare Financial Management* 52 (10): 66.

Personal Privacy in an Information Society, no.052-003-00339-3. 1990. Washington, D.C.: U.S. Government Printing Office.

Rothfeder, J. 1992. *Privacy for Sale*. New York: Simon & Schuster.

Time. 1992. (11 November): 34.

Tomnick, L. 1982. "Electronic Bullies." *Psychology Today* (February): 10.

Waller, A., and D. Fulton. 1993. "The Electronic Chart: Keeping It Confidential." *Journal of Health and Hospital Law* (April): 105.

"Washington Outlook." 1993. *Hospitals & Health Networks* (20 November): 14.

READING

Currently, numerous initiatives regarding information privacy are evolving toward standards that healthcare managers will face in the near future. The following article is as comprehensive and up to date a discussion as is available that would help healthcare professionals prepare for this future of compliance with mandated information privacy standards. The authors do a terrific job at bringing conciseness and focus to an otherwise complicated reality. St. Serena's is sure to latch on to this article as part of its effort to get to the forefront of information management.

Driving Toward Guiding Principles: A Goal for Privacy, Confidentiality, and Security of Health Information

Suzy A. Buckovich, Helga E. Rippen, and Michael J. Rozen

Abstract

As health care moves from paper to electronic data collection, providing easier access and dissemination of health information, the development of guiding privacy, confidentiality, and security principles is necessary to help balance the protection of patients' privacy interests against appropriate information access. A comparative review and analysis was done, based on a compilation of privacy, confidentiality, and security principles from many sources. Principles derived from ten identified sources were compared with each of the compiled principles to assess support level, uniformity, and inconsistencies. Of 28 compiled principles, 23 were supported by at least 50 percent of the sources. Technology could address at least 12 of the principles. Notable consistencies among the principles could provide a basis for consensus for further legislative and organizational work. It is imperative that all participants in our health care system work actively toward a viable resolution of this information privacy debate.

Responding to the information needs in our health care system and a heightened public awareness of health information privacy, many organizations are struggling to develop principles addressing the privacy, confidentiality, and security of health information. Some of the many

Reprinted with permission from the Journal of American Medical Informatics Association *6 (2) March/April 1999: 122–133. The authors are analysts with the Health Information Technology Institute at Mitretek Systems, McClean, VA.*

factors contributing to public awareness are the growth of managed care and integrated delivery systems, the increase in the number of entities and persons accessing health information for various reasons, and legislative developments such as the Health Insurance Portability and Accountability Act of 1996 (HIPAA).[1] HIPAA mandates the development of a national privacy law, security standards, and electronic transactions standards and provides penalties for standards violations and wrongful disclosures of health information. In addition, the Department of Health and Human Services' proposed rule on security and electronic signature standards (HCFA 0049-P) is also dependent on privacy policy decision making.[2]

Other contributing factors to this heightened awareness include the 1995 European Union's enactment of the Data Privacy Directive, which requires that all 15 European Union member states establish national privacy laws by October 1998. There is concern that this directive could limit data exchange between countries that do not have strong privacy protections in place, including the United States.[3,4] Awareness of privacy issues has grown, too, with the increased use of technology in health care (e.g., electronic medical records), advancements in genetic testing, and news reports on the misuse of information, such as the sale by CVS and Giant of consumers' prescription information to a marketing company.[5,6] In addition, the public is becoming aware of an inadequate legal environment, since no comprehensive federal law and only a patchwork of inconsistent state laws protect health information.[7] This inadequacy can serve as an obstacle to health care providers and organizations when they transmit data electronically across state borders. Legal uncertainty also makes it difficult for consumers to be aware of and understand their privacy and confidentiality rights. However, a number of congressional[8,9] and administrative [10,11] initiatives may improve this environment.

The authors compiled a set of 28 independent draft principles on privacy, confidentiality, and security, which was primarily a consolidation of principles from numerous sources, as discussed below. These draft principles are summarized in Table 1. The purpose of this paper is to provide a comparative analysis of the draft principles with those from ten identified sources, to serve as a guide in moving the discussion and development of a uniform set of principles forward. This paper also identifies those principles that technology can address and suggests ways technology can be utilized to help protect health information. It is the authors' purpose not to endorse the principles or detail potential conflicts among them, but rather to provide them as a means of generating further ideas and giving discussants parameters for decision making. We recommend that these principles be thoughtfully and thoroughly discussed in legislative, executive, and organizational settings and that exceptions as well as potential implications be determined. Any discussion of these principles must also take into account their potential interactions with other laws (such as ERISA) and local and state requirements, which are outside the scope of the paper. Last, discussions must also address the balance of sometimes competing needs-to protect privacy while ensuring access to information by those with a need to know.

Definitions

For this paper, the authors adopted the following definitions of privacy, confidentiality, and security:

- *Privacy*: "The right of individuals to be left alone and to be protected against physical or psychological invasion or the misuse of their property. It includes freedom from intrusion or observation into one's private affairs, the right to maintain control over certain personal information, and the freedom to act without outside interference."[12]

- *Confidential*: The "status accorded to data or information indicating that it is sensitive for some reason, and therefore it needs to be protected against theft, disclosure, or improper use, or both, and must be disseminated only to authorized individuals or organizations with a need to know."[12]

- *Data Security*: "The result of effective data protection measures; the sum of measures that safeguard data and computer programs from undesired occurrences and exposure to accidental or intentional access or disclosure to unauthorized persons, or a combination thereof; accidental or malicious alteration; unauthorized copying; or loss by theft or destruction by hardware failures, software deficiencies, operating mistakes; physical damage by fire, water, smoke, excessive temperature, electrical failure or sabotage; or a combination thereof. Data security exists when data are protected from accidental or intentional disclosure to unauthorized persons and from unauthorized or accidental alteration."[12]

- *System Security*: "The totality of safeguards including hardware, software, personnel policies, information practice policies, disaster preparedness, and oversight of these components. Security protects both the system and the information contained within from unauthorized access from without and from misuse from within. Security enables the entity or system to protect the confidential information it stores from unauthorized access, disclosure, or misuse, thereby protecting the privacy of the individuals who are the subjects of the stored information." [12]

Methodology

As members of the IEEE-USA Medical Technology Policy Committee, the authors began to consolidate these draft principles in September 1997 and drew on established principles from the following five sources: the Administration, Secretary of the Department of Health and Human Services (DHHS) Donna E. Shalala,[10,11] the Koop Foundation (Koop),[13] the National Research Council (NRC),[7] the Center for Democracy and Technology (Center),[14] and the Association of American Medical Colleges (AAMC).[15] In March 1998, the authors revised the draft principles to incorporate language and principles from five additional sources: the Computer-based Patient Record Institute (CPRI),[16] the American Society for Testing and Materials (ASTM),[12] the draft Model Privacy Law of the National Association of Insurance Commissioners (NAIC), [17] the Medical Privacy and Security Protection Act, introduced by Senators Patrick Leahy (D, Vt.) and Edward Kennedy (D, Mass.) (S.1368),[9] and the discussion draft of the Medical Information Protection Act of 1998 (Bennett-Jeffords), written by Senators Robert Bennett (R, Utah) and James Jeffords (R, Vt.)[8] Not all these sources had a set list of principles; therefore, the authors made interpretations based on the cited entities' materials.

These sources were obtained through a search that included personal contacts, congressional hearings, electronic files, and the Internet. . . . While reviewing the principles of the selected entities, it is important to take into account the specific purpose, charge, and perspective of each, to maintain objectivity. For example, the NAIC, S.1368, and draft Bennett-Jeffords legislation are focused on protecting consumers; the Center's purpose is to help designers of health information systems incorporate privacy and security mechanisms; recommendations of DHHS stem from governmental concerns; the CPRI and ASTM security guidelines are meant to help organizations that utilize computer-based patient records; Koop focuses on public health policy; AAMC has an academic research focus; and NRC, under charge by the National Library of Medicine, has a research focus to evaluate practices that can be used to better protect electronic health information. These perspectives may indicate why some sources do support or address specific draft principles and some do not.

Table 1   Draft Principles on Privacy, Confidentiality, and Security

1. Individuals have a right to the privacy and confidentiality of their health information.

2. Individuals have a right to access in a timely manner their health information.

3. Individuals have a right to copy in a timely manner their health information.

4. Individuals a right to amend and/or correct their health information.

5. Individuals have the right to withhold their health information from electronic format including being stored, managed or transmitted electronically.

6. Individuals have the right to segregate their health information from shared medical records.

7. Individuals have the right to the integrity of their health information. Entities and/or persons that create, maintain, use, transmit, collect or disseminate individual health information shall be responsible for ensuring this integrity.

8. Individuals have a right to control the access and disclosure of their health information and to specify limitations on period of time and purpose of use.

9. Outside the doctor-patient (other health care provider) relationship health information that makes a person identifiable shall not be disclosed without prior patient informed consent and/or authorization.

10. Informed consent and/or authorization for release of personal health information shall include identification of requester, declaration of purpose and boundaries, restriction of redisclosure, and explanation of potential harmful risks that could result from the release of this information.

11. Individuals harmed by the abuse or misuse of their health information shall be afforded individual redress through civil and criminal penalties.

12. Health care providers have the right to maintain private recordings of observations, opinions and impressions whose release they consider could be potentially harmful to the well-being of the patient. They shall not disclose this information without due reflection on the impact of such release.

13. The obligation of health care providers to maintain confidentiality and privacy of medical records shall not be undermined by outside organizations such as insurers, suppliers, employers or government agencies (i.e. forced disclosure without informed consent).

14. Personally identifiable information collected for one purpose shall not be used for another purpose without prior informed consent of the patient.

15. No secret databases shall exist.

16. No medical record demographics or other potential patient identifiers shall be sold, utilized for marketing purposes, or utilized for other commercial or financial gain without the prior informed consent of the individual.

17. Access to aggregate data shall be made available to support public health research and outcome studies as long as individuals are not and cannot be reasonably identified.

continued

18. Information gathered from available aggregate data shall not be used to the detriment of any individual in employment, access to care, rate setting or insurability.

19. Access to health information shall be limited to that information necessary for the entity's or individual's legitimate need and/or purpose.

20. Insurers have the right to access only that health information deemed necessary for claims administration and/or claims resolution.

21. Employers have a right to collect and maintain health information about employees allowable or otherwise deemed necessary to comply with state and federal statutes (e.g. ERISA, drug testing, worker's compensation). However, employers shall not use this information for job or other employee benefit discrimination.

22. A warrant requirement shall exist for law enforcement to obtain health information.

23. Health information and/or medical records that make a person identifiable shall be maintained and transmitted in a secure environment.

24. An audit trail shall exist for medical records and be available to patients on request.

25. All entities involved with health care information have a responsibility to educate themselves, their staff and consumers on issues related to these principles (e.g consumers' privacy rights).

26. All entities with exposure or access to individual health information shall have security/privacy/confidentiality policies procedures and regulations (including sanctions) in place that support adherence to these principles.

27. Current and new technologies should be continually incorporated in the design of information systems to support the implementation of these principles and compliance with them.

28. Support for these principles needs to be at the federal level.

Discussion and Analysis

We found no uniform set of principles across these entities that combines privacy, security, and confidentiality considerations. This lack may be due to the differences in purpose of these entities and the scope of coverage of their principles. . . . These differences add to the difficulty of comparison and contribute to the complexities of establishing uniform principles. For example, the NAIC model privacy draft law applies to all insurers. In contrast, the Bennett-Jeffords draft and S.1368 legislation apply to a wide range of entities, including health plans, hospitals, and health and life insurers. The CPRI security guidelines apply to organizations that utilize computer-based patient records. In addition, each entity delineates what type of information (and its format) is covered and protected. For comparison, the principles of the CPRI and NRC apply to protecting electronic information and electronic records, and Koop states that it protects "health information" (it does not provide a detailed definition). An important finding is that seven of ten sources utilize the same words to describe the information to be protected—information that makes individuals "identifiable" or "reasonably identifiable." This may indicate a possible consensus in the response to the public awareness for the need to safeguard health information from unauthorized disclosures and resultant discrimination.

We did find that many of the ten entities support specific draft principles, but they support them with exceptions. For example, eight entities support federal backing, but they differ on what type of pre-emption the law should have. If a federal law pre-empts state laws in such a way that no state may pass more protective laws, the term "floor-ceiling" pre-emption is used in the debate. A federal law that allows states to have more protective laws (such as protecting information about mental health and HIV diagnosis at a higher level than other health information), then the federal law is said to have a "floor" pre-emption. Bennett-Jeffords supports a floor-ceiling preemption, whereas DHHS, AAMC, NAIC, and S.1368 support the law as a floor. This is a notable and much debated distinction, as the NAIC reported concerns that health information regulations may be found in many places—insurance and probate codes, civil procedure, codes, and public health laws. Therefore, the NAIC points out that it will be difficult to determine which laws in which subject areas will be pre-empted.[17] Supporters of a floor-ceiling pre-emption argue for their approach because they view a floor pre-emption as leaving the door open for a continuing patchwork of state laws and thus not adequately addressing privacy concerns uniformly and completely. Advocates of floor pre-emption typically respond with support for allowing states to pass more protective laws in order to address and accommodate each state's unique needs.

Provisions regarding the ease with which law enforcement entities can access health information also differ. According to S.1368, Bennett-Jeffords, and Koop—but not DHHS—a warrant would be required. More specifically, Bennett-Jeffords supports the warrant requirement but also allows a less stringent legal proceeding for obtaining the warrant. The argument has been made that this could lead to law enforcement typically choosing the less stringent legal process.[18] In addition, we found that many entities support individuals' rights to access their own information. However, most create exceptions, such as when a health care provider determines that an individual may be harmed by access to mental health information. Similarly, there is broad support for the principle requiring informed consent or authorization by the patient before information disclosure but, again, some sources specify exceptions to this requirement, such as in emergency situations, for public health purposes, and for reports of child abuse or gunshot wounds. While exceptions may be warranted, it is important to recognize their potential impact. For example, there may be so many exceptions for a principle that they de facto "swallow up" the principle's primary intention, which is to protect privacy.

Principles That Entities Consistently Support

Although many of these entities represent different views in the analysis, we did find a "top ten" (plus one) list of consistent principles across them. Again, it is important to take note of the exceptions and their potential impact on the total support for the principles. The principles that obtained the most support and their specific exceptions are as follows:

- Individuals have a right to the privacy and confidentiality of their health information (Principle 1).
- Outside the doctor-patient relationship, health information that makes a person identifiable shall not be disclosed without prior patient informed consent and/or authorization (Principle 9). Nine entities have exceptions to this principle, for allowing disclosure without prior informed consent or authorization, including emergencies, current legal and public health requirements, law enforcement, and research.
- All entities with exposure or access to individual health information shall have security/privacy/confidentiality policies, procedures, and regulations (including sanctions) in place that support adherence to these principles (Principle 26).
- Individuals have a right to access in a timely manner their health information (Principle 2). Three entities have exceptions to the right to access, for specific state law requirements or for the protection of an individual.
- Individuals have a right to control the access and disclosure of their health information and to specify limitations on period of time and purpose of use (Principle 8).
- Employers have a right to collect and maintain health information about employees allowable or otherwise deemed necessary to comply with state and federal statutes (e.g., ERISA, drug testing, worker's compensation).

However, employers shall not use this information for job or other employee benefit discrimination (Principle 21).

- All entities involved with health care information have a responsibility to educate themselves, their staff, and consumers on issues related to these principles (e.g., consumers' privacy rights) (Principle 25).
- Individuals have a right to amend and/or correct their health information (Prmciple 4). One entity has an exception and refers to the exception as "under certain circumstances."
- Health information and/or medical records that make a person identifiable shall be maintained and transmitted in a secure environment (Principle 23).
- An audit trail shall exist for medical records and be available to patients on request (Principle 24). Five entities support an audit trail but do not specifically mention that patients shall have access to it.
- Support for these principles needs to be at the federal level (Principle 28). Five entities support this principle and then detail what that federal level should look like; four entities support a floor-level pre-emption, and one supports a floor-ceiling pre-emption.

Principles with Limited Support

Our analysis found that there are three draft principles that garnered limited support among the ten entities. We recommend that entities at least consider addressing and discussing the following principles and their potential implications:

- The obligation of health care providers to maintain confidentialitv and privacy of medical records shall not be undermined by outside organizations such as insurers, suppliers, employers, or government agencies (i.e., forced disclosure without informed consent) (Principle 13).
- No secret databases shall exist (Principle 15).
- Individuals have the right to withhold their health information from electronic format, including being stored, managed, or transmitted electronically (Principle 5).

Principles That Technology Can Address

Technology exists to facilitate the application of and adherence to at least 11 of these proposed principles. Technology provides a means to easily access, collect, manage, and distribute data and provides security mechanisms to protect health information through audit trails, encryption, strengthened authorizations, access controls, and such.[7] The principles and the subject areas that the technologic applications can address include the following:

- *Research.* Technology can make personal health data anonymous, removing identifying details[7] (Principle 17).

- *Access controls.* Technology can help ensure the granting and restriction of access to those users with legitimate needs, by means of passwords, access codes, and other identifying mechanisms [7,19] (Principles 1, 6, 8, 19, 20, 26, and 27).

- *Security in the maintenance and transmission of medical records.* Technology provides mechanisms for utilizing encryption, firewalls, digital signatures, system backups, and other requirements to secure data (Principles 1, 7, 19, 23, 24, and 27).

- *Maintenance and presence of audit trails.* Technology provides an electronic mechanism to track users, including details about information access, identity of the requester, the date and time of the request, the source and destination of the request, a descriptor of the information retrieved, and reason for access[7] (Principles 24 and 27).

- *Aid in developing and maintaining proper security and policy procedures in organizations.* Technology provides appropriate security mechanisms used for authentication such as passwords, digital signatures, biometrics, and access controls (Principles 19, 20, 26, and 27).

- *The need for new research and design of information systems to incorporate privacy, confidentiality, and security concerns.* Technology is utilized to develop and implement tools to address these issues (Principle 27).

Technology cannot be relied on solely to protect health information. Privacy, confidentiality, and security policies, regulations, sanctions, and organizational procedures must also be established and enforced.

Summary

While obtaining, analyzing, and discussing the draft principles, the authors discovered two concepts that were not specifically addressed by these sources and that could be considered in the principles framework. The first concept evolved from discussion of the ease of law enforcement access to health information and the differential status and treatment accorded the attorney-client and doctor-patient relationships. The second concept developed from discussions of the importance of ensuring that there is no obstruction, either deliberate or unintentional, to obtaining health information. The authors contribute these concepts for others to consider when discussing guiding principles and their implications.

- Privacy of communication in the doctor-patient relationship, including that documented in medical records, shall be afforded the same legal protection as attorney-client privilege.
- No entity or individual shall hinder timely access, when appropriately authorized to a patient's health information.

Others may be able to identify significant gaps as well. We encourage further discussion to generate more ideas and concepts, to ensure a comprehensive approach.

Based on our analysis, the following are summary statements and recommendations for working toward resolving privacy, confidentiality, and security issues:

- Health care providers should actively participate in the development of a uniform set of principles championing the rights of their patients and the doctor-patient relationship. Without establishing strong guidelines and enforcement mechanisms, health information may remain open to unauthorized access or disclosure that could have detrimental results.
- There appears to be general consensus in the support of the draft principles, in that 23 out of the 28 principles have garnered the support of more than 50 percent of these ten sources. There are consistently supported principles (ten plus one) that can serve as a baseline consensus and guidance for Congress, other entities, and individuals to discuss and a reference as they move forward to develop security standards and national privacy legislation.
- As important as the need to develop uniform privacy, confidentiality, and security principles is the need to establish clearly defined and uniform terms.
- There is also a need to clearly delineate exceptions and to study the impact of these on each principle, to determine whether the exceptions in fact erode the principle. For example, a principle may state that information disclosure requires previous consent by the patient but provide for many exceptions, such as in emergency situations or as required by law. In reality, if there are too many exceptions, then the individual may only have a very limited right. In

this comparative analysis, many of the entities' principles and guidelines were not explicit in their meanings, thus leaving much to interpretation. If consumer awareness and education of their privacy and confidentiality rights are a national priority, it is important that legislation, policies, and guidelines are clearly defined, understandable, and well researched.

- The current legislation in Congress could more adequately incorporate the exploration and use of technology to protect health information. However, the use of specific technologies need not be mandated, given the rapidly changing and improving technology industry. Public awareness of health information privacy concerns has increased, and the public should be apprised that technology can address some of these concerns. Existing technology can help protect health information through the use of tools to grant and deny access privileges, maintain and transmit data in a secure manner, provide audit trails, and such. Technology is not a barrier to protecting health information; rather, unresolved policy issues are the obstacles.

- It is important to note the differences and their potential implications of S.1368 and the draft Bennett-Jeffords legislation in Congress as compared to DHHS' because HIPAA mandates DHHS to promulgate national privacy legislation if Congress fails to enact legislation by August 1999.[20]

- "No secret database shall exist" is an important principle, especially in light of the rapidly growing uses and capabilities of information technology. Only the Center for Democracy and Technology addressed this principle by referencing the Code of Fair information Practices, which Includes this statement.

- Entities should consider including in their informed consent and authorization forms an explanation to the patient of the harmful risks that could result from the release of his or her information. Our research found that none of the ten entities explicitly incorporated this language into their consent and authorization forms. It would be helpful to research entities or states that have this language in their disclosure forms (e.g., Illinois) and find out about the impact of this inclusion.

- Privacy, confidentiality, and security requirements should be defined and implemented in future health information systems in a cost-effective manner.

- As important as utilizing the latest cost effective technology is the establishment of organizational policies, procedures, sanctions, and training that ensure privacy, confidentiality, and security

- It is important to continue the work and collaboration by many organizations and Congress toward consensus on privacy, confidentiality, and security issues. For example, committee members from number 2 Mar / Apr 1999 ASTM, CPRI, Health Level 7, and ASC X12N have already begun to coordinate data security standards for health care information.[20]

- Educating the public about their privacy and confidentiality health information rights should be a priority. Maintaining the public's confidence that their health information is protected is necessary to preserve the trust in the doctor-patient relationship. It is reassuring and important to note that all entities except the AAMC specifically emphasize educating consumers of their rights with regard to health information. The S.1368 and Bennett-Jeffords legislation even mandate that entities provide a "notice of information practices" to consumers.

Conclusion

The privacy, confidentiality, and security of personal health information have been long-standing needs and concerns in our society, especially to health care providers and the public. Also important to the public, health care providers, and organizations is the legitimate need to access information to deliver quality health care The increasing use of information technology in health care has heightened both of these needs as it has enabled easy access and exchange of vast amounts of information to more individuals and entities. In response to this changing health care environment, there is an urgent need to balance privacy and access and to proactively develop guiding principles, policies, and legislation to ensure that the information "near and dear" to the public—their sensitive and private health information—is protected now and in the future.

References

1. Department of Health and Human Services. Office of the Assistant Secretary for Planning and Evaluation . Administrative simplification. ASPE Web site. Available at: (http://aspe.os.hhs.gov/admnsimp). Accessed Feb 1995.

2. Federal Register, Aug 12, 1998;63(155):43241-80. Also, ASPE Web site. Available at: (http://aspe.os.hhs.gov/admmsimp/nprm/secnpm.txt). Accessed Oct 8, 1998.

3. Legislation relating to the confidentiality of medical information. Hearings before the Senate Labor and Human Resources Committee, Feb 26, 1998 (opening statement of James Jeffords, senator from Vermont).

4. Pasher VS: EU privacy law dangers cited. National Underwriter. Jan 12, 1998;102(2):1, 24.

5. Senate panel to study health privacy issue. Boston Globe. Feb 26, 1998: D2.

6. Pledger M. Patients worry about privacy, customers complain about telemarketing. The Plain Dealer. Feb 21, 1998: 1C.

7. Computer Science and Telecommunication Board. For the Record: Protecting Electronic Health information. Washington, D.C.: National Academy dressy 1997.

8. Discussion draft of the Medical Information Protection Act of 1998, introduced by Senators Robert Bennett and James Jeffords. Document O:/BAI/BAI 98.273. Obtained from the office of Senator Bennett in Washington, D C., Feb 1998.

9. The Medical Information Privacy and Security Act, S.1368, introduced by Senators Patrick J. Leahy and Edward M. Kennedy Available at: (http://thomas.loc.gov/cgi-bin/query/C?clO5:./temp/~clO5gQPqNe). Accessed Mar 18, 1998.

10. Remarks on privacy and health care by Donna E. Shalala, Secretary of Health and Human Services, at the National Press Club, Washington, D.C., Jul 31, 1997. Department of Health and Human Services Web site. Available at: (http://www.hhs.gov/news/speeches/pc.html). Accessed Mar 10, 1998.

11. Testimony of Donna E. Shalala, Secretary of Health and Human Services, before the Senate Committee on Labor and Human Resources Committee. Sep 11, 1997. Department of Health and Human Services Web site. Available at: (http://www.hhs.gov/progorg/asl/testify). Accessed Mar 10, 1998.

12. American Society for Testing and Materials Committee E31 on Healthcare Information, Subcommittee E31.17 on Privacy Confidentiality, and Access. Standard guide for confidentiality, privacy, access. and data security principles for health information including computer-based patient records. Philadelphia, Pa.: ASTM, 1997:2. Publication no. E1869-97.

13. Koop Foundation. Privacy principles. Draft dated Feb 25, 1997. (Written communication from Deborah Rudolph, Manager, Technology Policy Council, IEEE-USA.)

14. Goldman J, Mulligan D. Privacy and Health information Systems: A Guide to Protecting Patient Confidentiality. Washington, D.C.: The Center for Democracy and Technology, 1996.

15. Association of American Medical Colleges. Medical records and genetic privacy, health data security, patient privacy. and the use of archival patient materials in research. AAMC Web site. Available at: (http://aamcinfo.aamc.org/findinfo/privacy/start.htm). Accessed Jan 14, 1998.

16. Computer-based Patient Record Institute. Security guidelines for organizations with computer-based patient record systems. CPRI Web site. Available at: (http://www.cpri.org/docs/policy.html). Accessed Mar 18, 1998.

17. Legislation relating to the confidentiality of medical information. Hearings Before the Senate Labor and Human Resources Committee, Feb 26, 1998 (prepared testimony of Kathleen Sebelius, Commissioner of Insurance, National Association of Insurance Commissioners, Special Committee on Health Insurance).

18. Legislation relating to the confidentiality of medical information. Hearings Before the Senate Labor and Human Resources Committee. Feb 26. 1998 (prepared testimony of Janlori Goldman, Director, Health Privacy Project, Institute for Health Care Research and Policy, Georgetown University).

19. Morrissey J. Data security: as health care invests heavily in computer technology, confidentiality issues may be shortchanged. Modern Healthcare. Sep 30, 1996:35–6.

20. Blair J. Standards bearers: the standardization of healthcare information gains momentum. Healthcare Informatics. Feb 1998:113–4, 120.

UNDERSTANDING SOCIAL IMPACTS

I N HIS engaging book, *The Social Impact of Computers*, Richard S. Rosenberg (1992) asks the kind of questions that raises the subject of information management in healthcare beyond the merely practical level: "Will technology bring about Utopia, or 1984? Are we entering an age of unprecedented access to knowledge and power, or are we becoming a fragmented society of technology haves and have-nots?" While not proffering answers, he prods reflection on important questions for healthcare professionals. For example, is our use of information technology in healthcare organizations moving our caregiving more in the direction of "Utopia" or of "Planet of the Apes"?

Futurist Burt Nanus (1972), suggested an answer over a quarter of a century ago. He predicted that negative social impacts would inevitably appear if the implementation of computer systems were guided mostly by economic and technological considerations, with little managerial attention. According to some, his prediction has proven to be prescient (*Impact of Social Science on Society* 1987).

A case in point is the social effect of the effort of a "progressive" long-term care facility to automate its financial systems. During one weekend, the facility removed its manual systems and installed a computer. After the financial files, including the personal accounts of the residents, were restored on the electronic system, the old, hand-copied files were destroyed. On Monday, something happened that no one had anticipated: the elderly residents, to whom the computer age was a stranger and whose last vestige of independence was embodied by their small personal account in the facility's office, were bewildered and shaken when an imposing electronic printout was given to them in place of the familiar hand-written ledger. As a result, the happiness of these vulnerable people was disrupted. The managers and users of the technology had not thought of the "social" impact in planning and designing the new system.

Weighed against Kling's (1980) disturbing contention that "the social problems of information technology and strategies for alleviating them are relatively neglected and poorly understood," the seriousness of the social impact of information technology becomes apparent. What is the nature of the problem, and how can managers deal effectively with the responsibilities it entails? The following episode from St. Serena's might help our reflection.

CASE STUDY

Case Eight: Party or Produce, or Else . . .

Sonya Seemly, medical director of St. Serena's rehabilitation center, submitted her resignation yesterday. After 15 years at St. Serena's, Sonya was leaving for a position with a large pharmaceutical company. Her departure has taken Samantha by surprise.

"Things are just not the same as when I arrived here," Sonya told Samantha. "One of the things that attracted me to St. S. was the spirit of fun that always seemed to pervade our work. In those days we worked hard—we were very competent—and we partied hard. We enjoyed being with our colleagues and with our patients. Now, business seems to dominate everything. Forget about interpersonal relationships, just get patients through the clinical process as quickly as possible and don't waste time in idle conversation with them or with your staff. I hardly ever hear interesting conversations anymore in our facility. I feel like I answer to businessmen instead of doctors for what I do. So, I might as well be paid the big bucks the pharmaceutical is offering."

Samantha was taken aback. She asked Sonya what brought on this change in working environment. "It has been a gradual thing," Sonya reflected. "But it all seemed to take hold with the new and fancy information system you installed. I was so surprised when the new system came online without a hitch. It really has made my work easier. The time-consuming paperwork has been so much lessened by the electronic patient record system. And I love it when all I have to do is enter a name and my patient's entire record appears on the screen.

The diagnostic information system certainly helps with quality of care, but I miss the interaction with the clerks. My patients tell me that the staff now seems to be more interested in looking at the computer screens than looking at them. And many of the long-time staff seem unhappy. They used to be important here for the tasks they did, but now they seem to be intimidated by these new machines and programs that the new people relate to with ease. And, I worry that some of the doctors are not thinking as much anymore because the diagnostic system does it for them."

"But don't things run much more smoothly now?" Samantha asked. "Yes they do," responded Sonya. "But it just doesn't seem to be as rewarding." Samantha could not afford to lose more staff of Sonya's caliber. She wondered what she could do about the situation.

Questions for Discussion

1. What is happening at the rehabilitation unit?
2. Is there anything that management could have done to prevent the situation that Sonya describes?
3. What would you recommend to Samantha at this point?

COMMENTARY

The influence of information technology is apparent not only in health-care facilities like St. Serena's but in nearly every aspect of life today. Students are educated on terminals, and computers now even link parents to their children's schools so they can check attendance records, homework assignments, and lunch menus and have e-mail conversations with teachers. Clinicians use the technology to diagnose and monitor patients. Pharmacy information technology provides computerized dispensing units for medications. The technology of telemedicine enables caregivers to conduct two-way interactive video consultations. Elected officials use computerized mailing lists in campaigns and computerized opinion surveys in policymaking. The police use computerized fingerprints. The subway systems of San Francisco and Washington, D.C. are computer operated. Internet access services like those provided by Prodigy or America Online use the power of the computer to provide opportunities for social interaction as never before. New virtual communities are forming as a result of the Internet and other computer networks (*The New York Times* 1994). As Terrell Ward Bynum, founder of the Computing and Society Research Center at Southern Connecticut

State University, put it: "Computer technology and the information superhighway will change the world more than the inception of canals and roads . . . and by studying the effects of the computer revolution we can protect human values instead of damaging them" (*The New York Times* 1994). But what, specifically, are we talking about when we discuss this "social impact?"

The Nature and Meaning of Social Impact

Few people deny the social impact of information technology, but many question and debate its results. Is the impact positive or negative? Is the impact on the community of St. Serena's basically positive or negative? The dialogue, not unlike that between Sonya and Samantha, usually splits between those who focus on the objective, tangible impacts and those who see subjective, invisible, subtle effects (Danzinger 1985).

On the surface, the "social impact" of information technology in healthcare means better service delivery, faster response, greater efficiency, and more sophistication (Mandell 1986). Bringing telemedicine technology to rural areas, for example, could have considerable beneficial results on rural communities. But, significant impacts may also exist below the surface. The nursing home facility, mentioned in the example above, did indeed improve its financial management and increase revenues through its use of information technology; however, it also, in the process, produced anxiety in the very people for whose welfare the facility presumably exists. St. Serena's rehab unit seems to be running more efficiently but also less interestingly.

Similarly, *Time* (1993) magazine correctly predicted the dawning of a new age using information technology. The "electronic superhighway," a new world of video entertainment and interactive services combining the switching and routing capabilities of phones with the video and information offerings of the most advanced cable systems and data banks, will be in most of our homes in the near future. Instead of settling for whatever happens to be on at a particular time, subscribers will be able to select any item from an encyclopedic menu of offerings and have it routed directly to a television set or computer screen. Using relatively simple technological advances, such as translating audio and video communications into digital information, new methods of storing digitized information, and fiber optic wiring providing a virtually limitless transmission pipeline, users will have access to vast new video services. As *Newsweek* (1999) put it in its cover story: "There's no turning back. Once a novelty, the Internet is now transforming how Americans live, think, talk, and love; how we go to school, make money, see the doctor. . . ." Sound great?

"In the end," cautioned *Time*, "how the highway develops and what sort of traffic it bears will depend to a large extent on consumers. With economics driving the availability of services, a concern that this technology might endanger cultural diversity and pluralism may well be justified."

Most troubling to many skeptics is another kind of social impact. Neil Postman, a New York University professor and author of *Technopoly: The Surrender of Culture to Technology*, comments: "You already don't have to go out to the movies because you have your videos, T.V. and CDs. . . . With new technologies, you'd never have to go out and meet anyone. Is that great? It's a catastrophe" (*Newsweek* 1992).

Political Aspects

These kinds of subtle impacts can occur in several dimensions. Politically, the concern was that the efficient use of computers by elected officials could lead to manipulation of the electorate. In reporting on the wide use of computers by American congressmen, for example, the *Wall Street Journal* (1978) stated: "This causes concern both inside and out of Congress about whether the computer-using lawmakers can manipulate the voters back home in new and more sophisticated ways, thus making themselves even more invulnerable at the polls to opponents who have none of the perquisites the public purse supplies to incumbents." Could healthcare professionals similarly manipulate clients? An article in *Management Review* reported that survey results, from early 1990s, indicated that more than 70 percent of Americans were concerned with how medical information on national electronic databases will be used (Szwergold 1994). Should this be a concern at St. Serena's?

Psychological Aspects

Psychologically, information technology can cause feelings of alienation, fear, and depersonalization, which were conditions that Sonya appears to sense at St. Serena's (Dutton 1987). Consider this light-hearted illustration: A Los Angeles bank that uses computers to improve operating efficiency sends the following automated letter to customers who fall behind in loan payments: "This is a reminder from your friendly computer. You are $48.88 in arrears on your payments. Please remit. If you do not, next time you will have to deal with a human" (*Christian Science Monitor* 1978).

We might well ask, as some researchers have, whether information technology in healthcare could similarly depersonalize professional–client relationships and dehumanize medical care (McConnell 1989).

Intellectual Dimension

Considering the intellectual dimension of social impact, many commentators have expressed a concern about the proliferation of small, cheap electronic calculators among children who use them to count. Some writers go as far as warning that "today the question is no longer whether mental calculation is going to become less important but when it is going to disappear" (Nora and Minc 1980). Could healthcare information-technology applications, such as expert medical diagnosis programs, tend to program decision making and leave the thinking to the machines? Certainly, the recent technological advancements for medical applications of artificial intelligence and virtual reality tend to stimulate this kind of concern (Holusha 1993).

Sociological Dimensions

A sociological dimension is raised by many who, like Postman, view the encroachment of information technology in the home and workplace as a return to isolation in which people are removed from all, but basic, human intercourse. They see a society in which people never have to leave their homes because they can obtain what they need by ordering it on their home computers; they see workers isolated from other coworkers as they become "high-tech hermits" linked to coworkers only electronically; and they see a bipolarization of society into those who know the technology and those who do not (*The New York Times* 1994; *Time* 1993). For healthcare organizations, in which human service is the raison d'etre, such loss of personal interaction could be serious indeed, as Samantha is discovering.

The psychological and social commentator Bruno Bettelheim (1960) writes about "seduction" by technology in his book, *The Informed Heart*:

> The advantages we could enjoy from any new machine were always quite obvious; the bondage we entered by using it was much harder to assess, and more elusive. Often we were unaware of its negative effects until after long use. By then we had come to rely on it so much that small disadvantages that come with the use of any one contrivance seemed too trivial to warrant giving it up, or to change the pattern we had fallen into by using it. Nevertheless, when combined with the many other devices, it added up to a significant and undesirable change in the pattern of our life and work.

Bettelheim's words epitomize the concern of social-impact thinkers and the responsibility of professionals to address the social implications of using information technology. Healthcare organizations, specifically, can be viewed as micro societies in which these political, psychological, intellectual, and sociological impacts inevitably occur. Politically, for example, do and have power shifts occurred in healthcare organizations such that techies set the organizational tone more than caregivers do? Is this impact evident at St. Serena's? Intellectually, do caregivers tend to think less, as Sonya worries because the information technology is doing the thinking for them? If so, is this desirable? Sociologically, is organizational culture affected in ways like that described by Sonya to Samantha? Do people interact less, speak less, work more alone, etc.? Psychologically, are caregivers less happy and less satisfied in their work as a result of information technology? Sonya seems to think so.

Managerial Action

Jerome Wiesner, the former president of MIT and an eminent scientist and administrator, provides wisdom that is as relevant now as it was in 1971 when he talked about the impact of information technology:

> The great danger which must be recognized and counteracted is that such a depersonalizing state of affairs could occur without specific overt decisions, without high-level encouragement or support and totally independent of malicious intent. The great danger is that we could become "information bound" because each step in the development of an "information tyranny" appeared to be constructive and useful (Dresser).

Wiesner, and most writers, address the macro level; that is, society as a whole. We, as healthcare professionals, need to be concerned with the micro level; that is, the hospitals, clinics, nursing homes, etc., that we manage and work in. Deliberate managerial action at our micro-level organizations is required to prevent undesirable social impacts from occurring as a by-product of otherwise useful efforts at employing information technology (Gelman 1986). For example, in the case of the nursing home facility, its managers could have chosen to maintain hand-written personal accounts or they could have devised rituals to ease the residents into being comfortable with the change. With a little thought, they could have improved the human situation along with organizational efficiency. Similar efforts might have helped at St. Serena's. The point is that it takes skill and effort to maintain a managerial perspective; economics and technology can all too easily blind us to the obvious. Dealing with such a responsibility may be the biggest challenge that healthcare professionals face because anticipating such social impacts is as difficult as knowing how to counter them, and will inevitably take more time and money. Recognizing and managing social impact requires broad awareness and sensitivity and a conscious effort to adapt perceptions to a specific healthcare organization. Precise thought is essential. As

Bettleheim (1960) observed: "The most careful thinking and planning is needed to enjoy the good use of any technical contrivance without paying a price for it in human freedom."

Promoting social benefits and minimizing undesirable impacts require the institution of procedures and guidelines to safeguard such human values as individual respect and dignity, as well as interpersonal interaction. A need to focus on patients, clients, and workers in the design and use of information technology, instead of solely on organizational efficiency, must surely be a hallmark that makes using information technology a special challenge for healthcare professionals. As Sheridan (1980) has put eloquently: "We will have our computers, but our subjective sense of what is right, beautiful, and consistent with a just and sustainable society, and what contributes most to human fulfillment, ought to dictate our use of these exotic tools with their enormous potential. Productivity in human terms should prevail over productivity in machine terms."

In the past 40 years, computer scientists have tackled and overcome enormous scientific hurdles to produce today's powerful information technology. Now the challenge is managerial.

References

Bettelheim, B. 1960. *The Informed Heart.* Glencoe, IL: Free Press.

Christian Science Monitor. 1978. (1 June).

Danzinger, J. 1985. "Social Science and the Social Impacts of Computer Technology." *Social Science Quarterly* (March): 3–21.

Dresser, J. 1971. "The Information Revolution–And the Bill of Rights." *Computers and Automation* (May): 8.

Dutton, W., E. Rogers, and S. Jun. 1987. "Diffusion and Social Impacts of Personal Computers." *Communication Research* (April): 219–50.

"Electronic Superhighway." 1993. *Time* (12 April): 50–6.

Gelman, H. 1986. "Computers: The People Factor." *CMA: The Management Accounting Magazine* (March–April): 60.

Holusha, J. 1993. "Carving Out Real-Life Uses for Virtual Reality." *New York Times* (31 October): F–11.

Kling, R. 1980. "Computing People." *Society* (January–February): 14.

Mandell, P. 1986. "Computers that Humanize Health Care." *Ms. Magazine* (May): 103–5.

McConnell, E., S. Somers O'Shea, and K. Kirchoff. 1989. "R.N. Attitudes Toward Computers." *Nursing Management* (July): 39.

Nanus, B. 1972. "Managing the Fifth Information Revolution." *Business Horizons* (April): 7.

The New York Times. 1994. (27 March): 10.

The New York Times. 1994. (6 March): 10.

The New York Times. 1994. (13 February): Sec. 13LI 2.

The New York Times. 1994. (8 February): B–1.

Nora, S., and A. Minc. 1980. "Computerizing Society." *Transaction* (January–February): 30.

Perry, J. 1978. "Congressmen Discover Computer and Use It to Keep Voters in Tow." *Wall Street Journal* (15 March): 1.

Rosenberg, R. S. 1992. *The Social Impact of Computers.* San Diego, CA: Academic Press.

Sheridan, T. 1980. "Computer Control and Human Alienation." *Technology Review* (October): 72.

Szwergold, J. 1994. "Big Brother and Healthcare." *Management Review* (February): 5.

Symposium. 1987. "The Third industrial Revolution." *Impact of Social Science on Society* (146): 107–201.

"The Next Revolution." 1992. Newsweek. (6 April): 42–8.

Time. 1993. (12 April): 50–56.

READING

The social impacts of modern information systems are illuminated in the following article. Robert Brenning focuses on the environment of long-term care, but his analysis is equally relevant to most healthcare settings. He astutely articulates how the power of information can easily demean the people we are supposed to be serving unless we are alert and we institute protective measures. His reflection offers the kind of insight needed to keep our healthcare institutions ethical as we develop sophisticated information systems.

Ethics and Long-Term Care: Some Reflections on Information Management

Robert W. Brenning

Abstract

The ethical questions created by rapidly changing long-term care systems are demanding a much more intimate involvement of the information

Reprinted with permission from Robert Brenning, "Ethics and Long-Term Care . . . ," Topics in Health Information Management *18 (1), 59–67,* © *1997, Aspen Publishers, Inc. Robert Brenning is professor at The College of St. Scholastica, Duluth, MN.*

management professional. *No longer is confidentiality one of the prime considerations. The ethical principles of justice, autonomy, dignity of person, beneficence, truth telling, and utility are becoming a daily part of the information task in long-term care. The informal character of the long-term care facility requires a larger role for the information specialist. The result is that the information management role is being greatly expanded into the arena of ethical oversight of the information stream in long-term care facilities.*

Expansion of Ethical Issues

The ethical issues in long-term care are increasing with great rapidity as the structure of health care changes and the aging population begins a long-term explosion. Particularly relevant are those questions that pertain to information management and its linkages to the local and national system changes. In this article, merely a few of the basic implications will be highlighted, but they are fundamental to the way we understand the ethical dimensions of our work.

A couple of examples can serve to set the stage. With managed care creating economic and institutional shifts in where and how care is provided, the long-term care arena is facing major challenges.

For example, the move toward health campuses in which physicians, clinics, hospitals, and up to two-year long-term care facilities are located together, or where hospitals and clinics are purchasing long-term care facilities to augment their continuum of care, shows clear direction. The attempt is to capture as much of the health care dollar as possible. What is clear is that one consequence is to expand the information management function in new directions.

Another example of change is the awakening demand for more research on the aging population. Whether we are looking at Alzheimer's or acquired immunodeficiency syndrome (AIDS) research or at more basic studies in the risk factors of aging, the need for research and experimentation is already looking to the captive population in long-term care facilities.

Put this set of issues together with the increase in life–prolonging technology being placed in our facilities and questions about physician-assisted suicide, the nature of the ethical dilemmas presented not only to the health care staff but also to information management personnel is becoming increasingly complex. The perusal of a university's journal shelves will reveal the near explosion of journals associated with aging. A recent personal survey discovered 34, six of which had their inception in the last two years. This was not an exhaustive search. This article is based on the author's 22 years of experience working with hospital and long-term care facilities as an ethics consultant.

The Ethical Framework

The challenge to us is a multifaceted one because the personal and the professional sides of ourselves are intimately connected when we confront ethical questions. When we deal with issues of justice or dignity of the person or even confidentiality, our personal values are basic to how we think about ethical questions. To deny this connection is to play the dangerous game of hidden agendas in ourselves, which we call biases or prejudices. Our racism, ageism, classism, and sexism, as well as homophobia, are part of us if we have grown up in this culture. They sneak into our deliberations about ethical problems. To force them out into the open, to become conscious of how they work in us, is one of our first new tasks.

For example, if my prejudices about homosexuality are strong, how can I fairly and justly deal with the ethical questions arising from AIDS residents, who are becoming a larger part of our long-term care population? As I am forced to deal with their records, their experimental protocols, with the research information requirements, will I be able to be honest about my bias in order to offset its power in my work-related dealings? Are the confidentiality requirements as important for the AIDS resident as for the 80-year-old Alzheimer's patient who reminds me of my father or mother? What we call ethical slippages or fudging can lead to major ethical mistakes around personal dignity and justice, as well as confidentiality violations. A common violation found in all facilities is the loose talk at coffee and lunch, in which information is shared with those who have no right to it; we call it gossip. It is also easy to let persons having no right to records see them. Both actions occur daily in many long-term care facilities.

Another example highlights other ethical questions for information management. As we introduce more skilled care beds into long-term care facilities, and as hospitals use long-term facilities for longer term recovery and care, the more life-prolongation technologies will be introduced into our facilities. The result increasingly is that questions that usually resided only in hospitals are coming our way.[1] From more complicated cardiopulmonary resuscitation (CPR) and do not resuscitate (DNR) situations to residents requesting an end to their suffering, with residents being younger and with more complicated diagnoses (AIDS, etc.), the complexity of all types of information reception, information organization, and information referral becomes even more complicated.

Since ethics committees will be required to deal with the new kinds of questions, it is also becoming apparent that information management specialists need to be members. Not only are ethics committees dealing with individual consults with patients and families, but also increasingly, large issues of organizational ethics and policy are surfacing that involve information gathering and analysis. The long-term care facility has a different character from an acute-care setting. Usually the information specialist is one of a few who has the education and background in ethical reflection. The role is more broadly defined because the specialists' interactions cut across all aspects of the staff because of more informal structures.

Therefore, in order to understand this expanding world we need to remind ourselves of some basics having to do with ethical principles and their relation to our work.[2] When we examine ethical principles, we are looking toward finding sound reasons for our decision making. We look to principles to help us move beyond our subjectivity, our values and prejudices, to find a more objective basis for decisions for which we are accountable. While the context of each decision is certainly unique, we try to apply ethical norms in such a way that in other similar situations, we would make the same decision. In ethical terms this means that the reasons we use to support a decision have a more universal application beyond the specific case. Therefore, the consequence of consciously working with principles is to provide a consistency to our thinking.

There is one warning that must be given, however. A norm or principle does not lead us to a clear, definitive answer that applies to every situation. The actors, the diagnosis, the prognosis, the family history, the information requirements—all of these interact in unique ways in every context. Therefore, a single "answer" to a variety of situations is impossible.

The following principles are not meant to be an exhaustive list, but are the ones that appear most often in biomedical ethical decision making in all health care settings.

Autonomy

Autonomy has to do with the principle of the person being willing and able lo determine what is best for self—the person is never to be treated as a means but as an end. This principle also deals with the person being respected as autonomous. Different forms of residents' bills of rights should always reflect both perspectives. To be autonomous in one's actions is not to be constrained or controlled by anyone else. Persons have the moral right to have opinions and act upon them so long as there is no infringement on the rights of others and no ethical violation is involved. The issue of autonomy, of course, becomes complicated with diminished judgment or competence and the overriding of decisions that involve refusal of treatment, as in the cases of Christian Scientists, Jehovah's Witnesses, and those who come from one of the major Asian religious traditions. Governed by regulation as strictly as we are, these situations raise potential thorny information management problems.

Autonomy also presents a variety of subissues that relate to freedoms of residents. The following questions focus on this:

- How does the institutional policy structure and its practice at all levels give the freedom for residents to be free of dehumanizing hindrances to their desires and still have an effectively functioning institution? Are our biases, prejudices, and preconceived attitudes obstacles?
- Does institutional policy embrace, even guarantee, the freedom to know all the options regarding treatment, informed consent, right of refusal of treatment, freedom of speech, and the right to mix with other residents?[3,4]
- Do your policies at all levels, including information management, allow the freedom for residents not only to develop goals but also to achieve them, no matter how great or small these goals might be, and without infringing on the rights of others?
- Is the maximizing of the resident's freedom not only to take action but to be held accountable for those actions?
- Finally, does institutional policy and practice at all levels enhance the resident's chance to create new options or to give some sense of meaning to his or her existence no matter how demeaning, difficult, or limited his or her conditions may be?

The information specialist can in a variety of ways be a watchdog for these issues.

Beneficence

Simply stated, this principle means "above all, do the good." We are to act for the resident's benefit. Now, however, the issue becomes more complex. Who decides what is best for the resident? With what criteria? Does resident benefit mean physical health, or spiritual. or emotional, or even intellectual health? Or, holistically, are all of the aforementioned equally important? This principle needs usually to be balanced with a discussion of other related principles such as autonomy, utility, justice, and dignity. For example, is it justified by any one or combination of principles to use life-extending technology to keep a person alive at any cost with *cost* not being defined as primarily economic? Is it permissible for a resident to be allowed to die? With the prolongation technologies available in our facilities, this last question is no longer just for hospitals.

Some questions include:

- What happens when relief of suffering and preservation of life are not compatible? How do our policies and practices allow a death with as much dignity as possible?
- Since dying is not a scheduled phenomenon and your institution is a "schedule-based" operation, how can we free up our structures, policies, and staff availability (including at times, the information specialist) to humanize as much as possible the dying process?
- As a member of the utilization review process, is the information specialist watching for appropriate levels of skilled care, violations of patient autonomy, and ethical cost reimbursement?

Utility

In simplest terms, utility involves the consideration of consequences for the resident and for the wider community. Usually a second dimension is characterized as "acting for the common good." However, how is that defined and who defines it? Sometimes utility and beneficence conflict with each other. In looking at cost-effectiveness and the highest level of health for the most people, should we continue with use of some of our more sophisticated life-prolongation technologies in long-term care? For example, if only one respirator is available for two residents, one of whom will die soon anyway, how should we decide which resident receives treatment? Or do we let both die? We are dealing here with immediate consequences. Our decisions usually have immediate consequences, but are we perceiving the intermediate—and long-term consequences as well? Our immediate decisions may (and usually do) have consequences that can be precedent setting for the wider community in the future. How developed is our expertise at thinking consequentially beyond the immediate decisions with which we are faced?

How we use our staff and our technologies has many more implications. I mention only one. We are hopefully well aware of the grapevines that operate in large and small communities. How residents are cared for, how staff at all levels have resident and family interactions, requires of us a highly ethical posture and the ability to communicate effectively about all kinds of decisions both inside and outside our facilities.[5] Information management persons are a key element in this communication.

Dignity of human life

This principle is much misused and misunderstood in our culture today. Every human life has a sacred character or quality to it that must be inviolable. To violate this sanctity is to begin the larger process of dehumanizing the value of life for all of us. As caregivers, we would not choose intentionally to kill anyone. There may well be foreseen or even unforeseen consequences of our decisions that cause death; however, not every action we take that causes death, for example, is ethically wrong. We may give morphine to control pain, and the unintended effect might be to end respiration. The intent, however, is to relieve suffering and therefore our action is not morally wrong. Active euthanasia, however, is another story.

A further complication in applying this principle is to define what we mean by human. From fetus to severely handicapped to totally comatose presents a wide spectrum of possibility for defining human life. We need to be very clear what definitions are operating in the decision-making arena and from whom they stem, whether resident, family, physician, or Ethics Committee members, or even facility policy.

An example of the need for ethics review is the use of advance directions and their implementation. Retrospective review of cases is instrumental in avoiding abuses of advanced directives. In the context of the long-term care facility, the dignity issue is an everyday job. There are literally hundreds of ways we can deny residents and staff their dignity. Disrespect at any level to anyone is a denial of dignity. To treat one's own fellow staff from a power and control mode of thinking and acting is denial of respect. To "protect" information or to control it when it does not need controlling is disrespectful. With residents the violations are too numerous to mention.[6] The information specialist, however, must be an observer of the implementation of patients' rights with an eye toward the need for policy development when necessary.

Truth telling

This principle has often been much too simplistically defined in practice. From "always tell the truth" to "what is best for the resident to hear" allows a great deal of latitude. For instance, the resident may well give up the will to live if told the truth. Therefore, we will act paternalistically in the resident's best interest and lie or merely not give the resident all the information. In recent years this practice has come under severe questioning. Not giving the person all the information is a form of deception, but does that mean that what the person *is* told is true. Another trend is to argue that the resident will only be told as much or as little as he or she wishes to hear. This is a form of truth telling that respects his or her right to set the boundaries of honesty, which respects autonomy and dignity. Drawing the boundaries at their widest is to always tell the person the whole truth whether desired or not. Certainly, the telling of truth that respects autonomy seems normally to be the most "human."

This is an area in which information management may not have had much access. In the changing world of information, the monitoring of communication may well become a larger issue without developing a "big brother" mentality and practice. One important aspect to observe is to determine how much information a competent resident is getting versus what family members might be receiving. Often the star of the drama, namely, the resident, is left out of the communication loop when difficult information or decisions are involved. This is a simple human failing because we find it too challenging to face the resident. To allow this to continue is to violate not only the truth-telling principle, but also the dignity, autonomy, beneficence, and justice principles. A changing picture in long-term care has another consequence. Male residents will be coming to the facility for "recovery" care. That is one reason for increased life-prolongation technology. The DNR question then gets transferred to the facility, raising questions as to policy development and implementation. Is do not intubate (DNI) understood to *not* be an issue in DNR? How closely are DNR policies followed by health care staff? Is there misunderstanding between physician and nurse about this? Is the chart clear? Are you doing CPR when you should not be? The information specialist is an important person in this process.

Confidentiality

The literature in medical ethics terms this principle a form of contract. The issue here is that of a "need to know" contract. In long-term care facility practice, there is a great deal of looseness today. Too many persons who do not "need to know" have access to resident records, again a violation of privacy and autonomy. But there can be extreme circumstances in which confidentiality is not an absolute principle and must be violated for the good of the resident and/or the community. AIDS is a recent example of conflict in this area.

There is a good reason why this principle has been placed in the order it has. Among health information professionals, this is often the first, or the only, principle raised for ethical reflection. It is hoped that by intentionally deemphasizing confidentiality, the playing field for the variety of principles will be leveled in such a way that thy are all perceived as equally important in the information management sphere.

Hopefully, it is also clear that respecting the resident's ability to maintain privacy about medical care and other information requires protection in a regulatory and cultural climate, where insults to privacy are increasingly a daily occurrence. As research and experimentation move into long-term care with increasing demands, the informed consent and confidentiality protections will move into higher visibility, One very necessary daily need is to be sure that the re-release prevention codes are clear to all outside agencies.

Justice

We list justice last for a good reason. In many ways this principle is a basic assumption underlying the previous six. All persons are to be treated equally and fairly. That is a definition most would recognize. However, there is a second and equally important aspect to justice. It is that all healthcare resources are to be distributed equally or fairly among all. So, we speak initially of that which is fair, due, or owed to all. All persons shall be treated equally. To deny anyone what is rightfully theirs is an injustice. Like cases should be treated equally. There is, of course, to be no discrimination on the basis of any of the usual list of life states, whether it be income, race, age, and so on. Then there is to be a fair and equitable distribution of services and resources. In both instances above, our values and prejudices must be carefully examined. With the latter, though, we have more difficulty. Who receives access to available technologies? This involves decision making on the individual resident level. On a second level, what technologies should we as a society keep on developing and placing in long-term care facilities, even though all may not have access? Or, what technologies should a facility purchase in the name of remaining competitive in the marketplace when the cost must be distributed to all residents indirectly? Fair distribution at both individual and societal levels is a vexing issue, but one with which we are constantly confronted.

There are other principles that are not covered in this brief explanation. The above seven, however, are the assumptional basis for a majority of the decisions we must make. One final comment is necessary. It should be clear that we seldom have the luxury of operating from only a single principle at a time. Most often, the situations we work with involve an intertwining of the above seven principles with one or the other being predominant without being determinative of the decision. To quote an old cliche: "Would that life were that simple!"

As we conclude the ethical framework discussion, there are several general concerns that need to be addressed, Because the residents of long-term care facilities are often present for long periods of time, the need for ethical watchfulness is more difficult than in other health care settings, Patterns of behavior or ways of doing things by staff tend to erode overtime because of long-term proximity to residents and to the infinite variety of personality and behavior traits exhibited by everyone in the facility. A kind of "ethical slippage" mentioned earlier is common. Dehumanization of residents and staff can occur over time. A large long-term care facility this author has consulted for had very long corridors. On the first morning that I came in the door, at one end of each hallway I noticed that 48 patients were sitting in silence in wheelchairs outside their rooms facing the other end of the corridor. All had their backs to each other. When asked about the practice, the administration said the residents were waiting to be wheeled to breakfast. I suggested they be turned toward each other. The next visit, I entered the same door to the noise of conversation and laughter. A little thing? No, not at all.

A second concern is that of maintaining our sensitivity to the ethical issues.[7] The following are some questions being presently developed into an inventory that can be performed periodically in the facility. At present, it is only in a preliminary form.

The first pan of the inventory is an overall check on the philosophy of the institution and its "fit" in the health care delivery continuum, and to determine what progress the institution is making toward a true long-term care model. Many long-term facilities are a curious mix of the two models at present (see box).

This list is dualistic, but for our purposes puts the emphasis on the possibilities inherent in the long-term care mission. A second inventory part is much less developed as yet but contains the following questions to help us focus on more specific ethical problem areas:

1. What are the ethical issues and dilemmas that you typically encounter in your area of specialty? What are the ethical issues and dilemmas that your long-term care facility deals with? Are there areas in which information management should have more input?

2. What mechanisms or processes do you use to resolve the dilemmas? Are they effective? Is there someone outside your department and facility who also oversees your ethical process?

3. Does the ethics committee have a multi-disciplinary membership including an outside ethicist, lawyer, and community members acting as resident advocates?
4. Does the ethics committee review and develop policy for the institution where ethical questions are involved?
5. Are information management professionals members of the committee?
6. What is done with whistle blowers in your facility? Are they ostracized, isolated, rewarded? What is the message you are sending to the staff and residents?
7. What are the channels available to report unethical behavior? Do they work? How can they be improved? What does your facility do with issues of harassment, violence, and discrimination in any form?
8. Is there lack of congruence between stated mission and ideals of the facility and what is practiced? Is there a mechanism for addressing inconsistencies?
9. What is the power structure of the facility? Is it a power and control model with little participation by those on the bottom? Does the leadership model ethical integrity on a daily basis?
10. How do new employees learn about the ethical behavior required of them? Is there ongoing education for all staff on ethical standards?
11. If your facility is undergoing financial stress, does the ethical practice change? What do you justify now that you did not when the bottom line was positive?
12. What are short-, medium-, and long-term consequences to your department and to the institution of unethical organizational practices? Have some already occurred? Where do you go with your observations? Is the ethics committee available to you and others with complaints and does it provide confidentiality and job safety to those who bring the issues?
13. As a result of the above questions, what are the policies that need to be reviewed, revised, or developed because no policy presently covers the area of concern?

This is but the beginning of an ethics inventory procedure that is currently in development, but it provides some guidelines to help the facility develop its own procedure.[9]

There are a myriad of ethical issues confronting information management professionals. The number and complexity of those issues will be exploding among us in the next few years. Fundamental to our dealing with such issues is our ability to see the macropicture of our institutions and how information management impacts increasingly in

Medical Model

1. Characterized by reductionism, a looking at smaller and smaller "pieces" of the person
2. Focus on curing with caring as byproduct
3. Orientation on illness
4. Tending toward ignoring impact of psychosocial and spiritual on physical states
5. Focus: patient
6. Physician control of patient care

Long-Term Care Model

1. Characterized by holism, seeing the total person with the illness or disability as only part of the whole person
2. Focus on caring, with curing as fortunate by product if it happens at all
3. Orientation on health, as much as is possible; healthy management of illness or disability; symptom management
4. Moving toward maximization of awareness of the possible, of empowerment, of self care
5. Focus: patient, family unit, friends
6. Team approach emphasizing patient autonomy[8]

broader areas of ethical concern. Because of the special nature of long-term care facilities, the more relaxed atmosphere, the higher number of staff who have daily access to residents who have little education in ethical issues and ethical practice, and the longer term relationship these facilities have with families, the information specialist has a very important role. The specialist may well be one of few on the staff who has knowledge of the ethical concerns and is more of a "generalist" on the staff interacting with many more people than in an acute care situation. The information professional becomes watchdog, reviewer, educator, and record keeper.

References

1. Catholic Health Association. "Unraveling Ethical Issues: New Questions for Society." *Health Progress* 9 (1994).

2. Beauchamp, T. L., and Childress. J. F. *Principles of Biomedical Ethics.* 4th ed. New York: Oxford University Press, 1994.

3. Brown B. F. "Proxy Consent for Research On the Incompetent Elderly." in *Ethics and Aging! The Right to Live, The Right to Die.* J.E. Thorton and E.R.Winklerr, eds. Vancouver, British Columbia, Canada: The University of British Columbia Press, 1988, pp. 183–193.

4. Burnside, B. "Gerontology's Challenge from its Research Population." In *Ethics and Aging! The Right to Live, the Right to Die.* J.E. Thornton and E.R. Winkler, eds. Vancouver, British Columbia, Canada: Tho University of British Columbia Press, 1988, pp. 194–207.

5. Roberto, K.A. "Ethical Challenges Facing Family Caregivers of Persons with Alzheimer's Disease." In *Ethics and Values in Long Term Health Care.* P.J. Villani,ed. New York and London: The Haworth Press. Inc., 1994, pp. 49–64.

6. Haddock J. "Towards Further Clarification of the Concept 'Dignity.' " *Journal of Advanced Nursing* 24, no. 5 (1996): 924–931.

7. Mohr, W. "Ethics, Nursing, and Health Care in the Age of 'Re-form.' " *Nursing and Health Care: Perspectives on Community* 17 (January 1996): 16–21.

8. McWilliam, C.L., et al. "Creating Health and Chronic Illness." *Advances in Nursing Science* 1.8, no. 3 (1996): 1–15.

9. Kane, R., and Caplan, A L., eds. Everyday Ethics: Resolving Dilemmas in Nursing Home Life. New York: Springer Publishing Company, 1990.

DIRECTING THE FUTURE OF INFORMATION MANAGEMENT

NFORMATION TECHNOLOGY continues to develop rapidly. Its management, consequently, requires an eye to the future, not just to the present. As futurist Eckhard Pfeiffer (1998) advised: "Organisations that want to shape the future. . . . [must] learn to anticipate the possible directions the future may take and . . . encourage their people to challenge conventional thinking." This final chapter is intended to help in the effort to anticipate those new directions.

In her analysis of the new JCAHO information management standards, Bradley (1995) argued that these standards are radically different from former norms and that they substantially affect the future of information management in healthcare. They entail, Bradley suggested, a new understanding of the nature of health information and of information management activities. Global networking, managed care, and distance learning are additional factors that affect the future of information management in healthcare organizations. And, of course, technology for health information systems, developing apace, substantially drives this future (Kerr and Jelinek 1999). Furthermore, the recasting of incentives, strategies, and relationships in healthcare will have significant implications for the development and management of information systems. In effect Bradley, too, was stressing the need for a new way of thinking about information and health information systems.

Some informed observers note that the increased scrutiny of costs and competition that accompanies reform is changing the ground rules for technology management. Acquiring and managing the state of the art might no longer be the major concern. Rather, information management might focus on questions such as: Will the new technology advance the mission of the organization? Will the technology address client interests? Will it be attractive to the medical staff? Will it reduce operating costs? (Heinemann 1992).

With healthcare institutions increasingly at risk for the costs and outcomes of care rendered, healthcare executives will likely be under pressure to maintain an awareness and understanding of emerging information systems and the concomitant skills needed to manage the new and changing technology. They will need agility and proficiency in calculating the hows and whys of shifting information needs. Let's see what St. Serena's is up to in this regard.

CASE STUDY

Case Nine: The Jedi of St. Serena's

As the new millennium began, St. Serena's convened a seminar on emerging technologies in healthcare to help it plan for the future. Among those invited to participate were futurist Herb Gerjoy, technology guru Tim Tremble, and healthcare policy analyst Rory Philbin. At Samantha's direction, Stewart ensured that all department heads participated.

Herb opened the discussion with a wide-ranging view of organizations in the future. He emphasized the need to break away from former paradigms of healthcare information systems. "The rapid and massive extension of information technology is changing the whole informational and organizational environment," Herb suggested. "St. Serena's, as with all healthcare institutions, is no longer a stand-alone enterprise. Because of information technology, which eventually will be in the hands of nearly all individuals and groups connected with the institution, information needs, availability, and processing are radically different concepts in the 21st century than they were in the past." To engage successfully in this new reality, Herb maintained that "St. Serena's should develop new ways of thinking about the information it needs and about ways of accessing, processing, and managing that information."

Rory agreed and stated that the nature of the healthcare environment has already changed dramatically and that managed care initiatives, as well as sociological and demographic developments, will hasten further evolution of this healthcare environment. "Policy reforms will continue swiftly," he stressed, "which would result in major adjustments in the economics, politics, and organization of healthcare. Those organizations that are effective in the new alignment will be those that figure out what information they need, where they can best get it, and how they can harness it." Those organizations that cling to the former understanding of information needs and systems will have difficulty surviving.

Last to speak was Tim who predicted that major, new technological developments, in the near term, will alter the way information is accessed and processed. "The concept of integration will no longer mean intra-organization information arrangements. Enabled by new technology integration in the future will mean that information is accessed from external sources that are integrated with all technology-based organizations. Knowing what information you want and need will become even more the key to success because technology will enable easy access."

Samantha was excited. She had always envisioned a St. Serena's in the forefront of developments like these. Stewart, on the other hand, was apprehensive. "What does all this talk mean and how the heck do we proceed?" he mused to himself. Department heads present were mostly thinking about today's challenges.

Questions for Discussion

1. What key aspects of the future of health information management do you derive from the comments at the seminar?
2. Can you give Stewart some ideas on how to proceed to prepare for this emerging future?
3. What difficulties can you anticipate at St. Serena's in trying to fulfill Samantha's vision?

COMMENTARY

As Rory emphasized at the St. Serena's seminar, the paradigm shift in healthcare delivery has spawned a new and complex environment, which forces healthcare organizations to adapt to new information needs and priorities.

New Realities

The increasing presence of managed care arrangements is a major drive in the paradigm development. In the managed care world, understanding the cost of providing services and managing those costs is a prerequisite to viability. Of key importance is the organizational capacity to capture detailed cost information; the articulation and monitoring of standardized data definitions pertaining to outcomes and costs; and the inculcation of an organization-wide emphasis on quality control, cost containment, and customer satisfaction (Johnson 1993). This paradigm shift entails new and probably dynamic information needs.

Accompanying these structural finance and delivery changes is an increased insistence on new regulatory information standards and requirements. As a consequence, more robust information system requirements are emerging. New data needs are appearing as well as demands for more reporting frequency.

Changing medical staff relations are also appearing in this more intensely competitive environment as is pressure to acquire patients. This competition suggests a broadening of the focus of information systems in the future. Looking to technology to improve services, to capture a wider market share, or to enhance customer satisfaction is a likely consequence as healthcare institutions struggle for success and survival (Wachel 1992).

Healthcare reform and the managed care trend are also driving a demand for more information sharing within healthcare systems, among a wider healthcare networks, and even within a global reality. At the same time, autonomous departments within institutions will have to better understand the financial and administrative consequences of everyday decisions. Information access and exchange will be required for this "interoperability" within healthcare systems and networks (Ferguson 1993).

In brief, the emerging environment demands that managers be comfortable with information technology and the evolving growth of information system functions and capabilities, a fact which, undoubtedly, prompted the St. Serena's seminar. Among these fast emerging realities are e-health (Internet/intranet) services, decision support systems, and advanced clinical information technologies (Ball 2000).

While earlier information technology addressed relatively simple needs through automation of well-defined processes, the emerging era of rapidly developing technology and changing environments is reengineering the whole healthcare enterprise. Healthcare managers will need to continually adjust, anticipate, and respond to the resulting new realities.

Emerging Technologies

Past data-processing and telecommunication technologies have tremendously affected the development of healthcare information systems. Beginning with financial and administrative applications in the 1960s, most large healthcare organizations now have technology-based systems that also serve innumerous clinical areas such as patient scheduling, patient records management and diagnosis assistance. Now, widespread information sharing through more integrated networks appears to be the common future. Integration and open-system architecture will require more development of standards; that is, agreements on formats, procedures, and interfaces that permit designers of hardware, software, databases, and telecommunications to develop products and systems that will be compatible with any other product and system. This requirement for standards development may be one of the reasons that Stewart is a bit anxious about the future.

Separate islands of technologies that support information systems within healthcare organizations have typically been the norm. Recognizing the cost-efficiency emphasis, the huge capital expenditures for separate systems, and the limitations of systems based on a single technology, St. Serena's has moved in the integration direction. Developments in information technology, such as integrated office products, artificial intelligence systems, and telemedicine products, enable further movement in this direction.

Virtual reality systems are fast emerging as training tools for clinicians. These systems enable risky and costly surgical procedures, for example, to be tested ahead of time. Software models of patients are programmed using data from various electronic and computer-assisted diagnostic tests. By importing this outside data, physicians can operate in "virtual reality" to determine the most efficient and effective procedure.

One illustration of the benefits, and practicality, of emerging technology integration is Harvard Community Health Plans' use of interactive protocols to collect information directly from the patient. The Plan has patients in hundreds of households using personal computers to receive medical advice and general healthcare information. The system is designed to improve patient education, raise the quality of healthcare, and lower costs by reducing the number of unnecessary visits. This system is suggestive of future realities (Bergman 1993a).

These emerging technologies dovetail with rising user expectations of Internet "convenience." Abilities such as tracking patients throughout whole networks, accessing electronic medical records from all locations, and networking groups and facilities over a large area are likely to become common. The regional healthcare system of the future will have its internal clinical and administrative systems connected with each other and with an external healthcare information network. Samantha sees this and Stewart knows some of the challenges involved in getting there. In these settings, new approaches to patient care and efficient operations are clearly likely. For example, each patient encounter could be tracked from initial complaint through treatment to final outcome. Physicians could admit patients remotely and check inpatient status from their offices (Kasputys and Lazarus 1993).

Another example is set forth by the Milwaukee-based Wisconsin Health Information Network. This network has successfully combined software and telecommunications so that client users can transmit, receive, and store all forms of healthcare data using image and voice means. Physicians can send and receive clinical and administrative data from their offices to hospitals (Bergman 1993b). Of course, a major challenge that face St. Serena's and all visionary healthcare organizations in employing these new technologies is managing issues like security and privacy.

Managing Future Information Technologies

While healthcare executives, like Samantha, generally perceive the potential of emerging technologies, they may tend to underestimate the managerial challenges involved. Seasoned implementers like Stewart might have a more sober perspective. Analysts Boxerman and Gribbins (1991) offer useful advice. They caution that a major concern of executives should be the logic of the systems that the technology executes. They argue that healthcare executives should focus on the appropriateness of various models, the accuracy of databases, and the skill levels of functional specialists. Most importantly, they contend that executives should address four major aspects of new technology efforts: (1) time constraints in implementation, (2) institutional capabilities, (3) degree of employee acceptance of constant technological changes, and (4) the degree of collaboration among working departments affected by new technology. These aspects undoubtedly prompted Stewart's concerned musings at the St. Serena's seminar.

Moreover, technological innovation initiated by the paradigm shifts in the healthcare industry will further affect decision-making burdens on healthcare executives. Mindful of this, Pennsylvania University's Wharton School has developed a number of action guidelines specifically to assist in the task of managing emerging technology (Simpson 1993). These guidelines, listed below, provide some starting points for executives, like Samantha and Stewart, as they confront an accelerating pace of new priorities and information needs.

First, determine the "risk personality" of the organization. How averse to risk are the organization's key players? Do they generally cope well or poorly with shifts in strategies and adjustments to environmental changes? Perhaps some work in these areas is a prerequisite.

Second, assess business plans with a view toward existing and emerging technology. How can information system technologies be linked with the strategic direction of the organization?

Third, evaluate what significant developments in healthcare might affect the use of technology. How might, for example, the continued trend of managed care and competition create new information needs, and how might technology help?

Fourth, integrate technology plans and assessments into a business plan. How does, and could, the organization use current and emerging information technologies to attain long- and short-term goals and objectives?

Fifth, develop and employ leadership and rewards methods of inducing change. How does, and could, the organization, for example, communicate its comfort level with innovation through senior-level management attitudes and action?

I would add a sixth guideline—carefully evaluate the security, privacy, and social implications of employing new technologies.

The managerial challenges associated with emerging technology require an in-depth understanding of the ramifications for the organization as a whole, for the staff, and for the patients. As paradigmatic, financial, administrative, and other changes in healthcare delivery continue to evolve, information management is certainly a key to the viability of healthcare organizations. The concepts probed in this book are offered as aids in meeting those challenges.

References

Ball, M. 2000. "Forces and Trends: Opinions on the Future of Healthcare Information Technology." *Health Management Technology* 21 (1): 14.

Bergman, R. 1993a. "Computers Make 'House Calls' to Patients." *Hospitals* (20 May): 52.

———. 1993b. "Telecommunicators Making Their Way into the Healthcare Market." *Hospitals and Health Networks* (5 September): 60.

Boxerman, S., and R. Gribbins. 1991. "Technology Management in the 1990s." *Healthcare Executive* (January): 21–3.

———. 1996. "Changing Concepts of Health Information and Health Information Work." *Bulletin of the Medical Library Association* (84): 5.

Bradley, J. 1995. "Management of Information: Analysis of the Joint Commission's Standards for Information Management." *Topics in Health Information Management* 16 (2): 51.

Ferguson, J. 1993. "I/S Interoperability a Must in Tomorrow's Complex Healthcare Environment." *Computers in Healthcare* (November): 22–8.

Heinemann, C. 1992. *Healthcare Executive* (January/February): 32.

Johnson, D. 1993. "Hospitals Must Prepare for the Paradigm Shifts to Managed Care." *Health Care Strategic Management.* (December): 10–3.

Kasputys, J., and S. Lazarus. 1993. "Health Information Networks: Connecting Your Healthcare Organization to the Future." *Healthcare Executive* (November/December): 21–3.

Kerr, J., and R. Jelinek. 1999. "The Impact of Technology in Healthcare and Health Administration." *Journal of Health Administration Education* 8 (1): 5–10.

Pfeiffer, E. 1998. "Future Tilt: How and Why Companies Need a Culture of Continuous Renewal." In *Straight from the CEO.* London: Price Waterhouse, 2.

Simpson, R. 1993. "Managing Innovative Technology." *Nursing Management* 10 (4): 18–9.

Wachel, W. 1992. "CIO—Roles and Relationships." *Healthcare Executive* (January/February): 14–6.

READING

We conclude with a conceptually pace-setting article focused on the future of information management. First, Anand, Manz, and Glick bring us back to the basic concepts discussed in Chapter 2—information management is by no means synonymous with the management of information technology. Second, they clarify concepts of organizational development and use them to expand our understanding of the nature of information management in a way that may be better suited to future developments. Third, they suggest approaches to managing information in the environment of the 21st century. How might their approach be useful to St. Serena's and its effort to be in the vanguard of information management?

An Organizational Memory Approach to Information Management

Vikas Anand, Charles C. Manz, and William H. Glick

Abstract

We extend and adapt a model of group memory to organizations. Using this extended model, we identify information management challenges of the next century and suggest that organizations can address these challenges by locating a large portion of their information-processing activities outside their formal boundaries, by adopting novel socialization tactics, and by focusing on the management of soft knowledge forms (e.g., tacit knowledge, judgment, and intuitive abilities). Whereas current theories increasingly equate information management with the management of information technology, we argue that information technology needs to be complemented by organization-level processes related to organizational memory.

Scholars traditionally define information management as the process by which relevant information is provided to decision makers in a timely manner (Davis, 1997). It has become an important tool that helps build organizational competitive advantage in today's globalized and turbulent environments (Parker & Case, 1993). The importance of information management is reflected in the development of master's-level programs in information management (or related areas) by business schools and the increasing frequency of chief information officers (CIOs) in many large organizations (Caldwell, 1996; Machlis, 1997).

However, despite the importance of information management, organizational researchers are not taking the lead in developing conceptual and theoretical models of information management that can clarify the organizational implications of these trends. Instead, information management largely has been defined from an information systems perspective and equated with the management of information technology. For instance, Davis argues that information management and management information systems are "synonyms that refer to an organization system that employs information technology in providing information and communication services and the organization function that plans, develops, and manages the system" (1997: 138).

Organization researchers seeking insights into information management can use models and theories of organizational memory as starting points. Although organizations do not "remember" in the true sense of the word, organizational (or group) memory is a convenient metaphor that can be used to define the information and knowledge known by the organization and the processes by which such information is acquired, stored, and retrieved by organization members (Anand, Skilton, & Keats, 1996; Huber, 1991; Walsh & Ungson, 1991; Weick, 1979).

In this article we first describe a model of group memory—transactive memory—and then extend and adapt it to organizations. Using insights from this model, we identify ways in which organizations might

Reprinted with permission from the Academy of Management Review *23 (4) October 1998: 796–809.* Vikas Anand is a doctoral candidate at Arizona State University. Charles Manz is professor at the University of Massachusetts. William Glick is chair of the management department at Arizona State University.

approach information management challenges that arise from increasing environmental turbulence, globalization, and the advent of advanced communication technologies. We argue that organizations might adopt novel socialization practices and locate information-processing activities increasingly outside formal boundaries to meet future information requirements.

Information technology will, of course, continue to play an important role in information management. However, we argue that to achieve effective information management, organizations will need to pay greater attention to managing soft knowledge, such as tacit knowledge, judgment, and intuitive abilities. The development of advanced information and communication technologies has increased the need for adopting an organization-level approach to information management. Consequently, efforts to implement technically oriented management information systems can contribute to effective information processing only when accompanied by an appropriate set of organizational strategies.

For our purpose in this article, we define information in a manner similar to that used by Daft and Weick (1984), who argue that organizations scan their environments to obtain data. This data is then assigned meaning (through interpretation) and constitutes information. We also use the term information to refer to communicable forms of knowledge, such as explicit knowledge (Polanyi, 1966). In contrast, we use the term soft knowledge to refer to forms of knowledge (such as tacit knowledge, belief structures, intuition, and judgmental abilities) that are not easily communicated.

Transactive Memory in Groups

Wegner and his colleagues developed the model of group transactive memory (Wegner, 1986; Wegner, Erber, & Raymond, 1991; Wegner, Guiliano, & Hertel, 1985). They segregated the information held in a group's memory into two components: (1) the information stored by group members in their individual memories and (2) directories held by group members that identified the existence, location, and means of retrieval of information held by other individuals, Their model proposes that the encoding, storage, and retrieval of information in the group are facilitated by the various communication interactions or transactions (and, hence, the name transactive memory) between group members. We discuss these components briefly to provide a point of departure for the organizational model.

The information stored in the individual memories of group members can be segregated into internal and external components (Harris,

1980). The internal component consists of information known personally by group members. The external component consists of information that is not personally known by members but which can be retrieved when required. Such information may be stored in files, electronic storage devices, or other inanimate locations or in the minds of other individuals (Wegner, 1986). Thus, the memories of group members effectively include information held by other individuals, if the location of such information is known and easily retrievable by the members (Wegner, 1986).

Directories contain idiosyncratic information items that inform group members about the existence and location of external information, as well as the means of retrieving such information (Wegner, 1986). The contents of individual's external memories are determined by the informal lion held in their directories. Directories, however, can sometimes be faulty, because they may be based on biased or outdated perceptions of the expertise held by other individuals (Agnew, Ford, & Hayes, 1994; Stein, 1997; Wegner, 1986).

Directories generally are maintained with respect to chunks or classes of information and knowledge, rather than with respect to specific items. For instance, an individual is unlikely to hold information that a particular taxation manager is a specialist on a specific tax clause. Instead, the individual's directory likely informs him or her that the manager is a specialist in a broad category of tax issues.

Information in directories also includes the labels that group members attach to chunks of information. Labels are held idiosyncratically and play a critical role in facilitating information retrieval (Anand et al., 1996). When group members use the same labels to tag information, they can easily access information from each other.

The following example highlights the importance of directory information:

Managers at the propulsion systems division of a major aerospace company selected an engineer to become the in-house expert in a new technology. In a wave of management changes, the champions of the technology all moved out of the division. The expert engineer was reassigned to normal duties. After another wave of changes in management, it became apparent that the technology was critical, but no one remembered that there was an expert already on staff, and the process was repeated (Anand et al., 1996:16).

Clearly, the required expertise was available within the firm. However, the directories of the new management team were uninformed about it, leading them to waste organizational resources in duplicating existing expertise.

Externally held information can be used by group members only when they obtain it through communication. The communication process may be simple (one member asking for and receiving the desired information from another) or may involve a series of transactions.[1] For instance, a manager may ask her secretary for a piece of information. The secretary, not personally possessing the item, may recall that the manager relayed that information to another colleague. On being so informed, the manager may now retrieve the required information from her colleague.

Applying Transactive Memory to Organizations

The information available to an organization can be chunked into a variety of domains—for example, information related to a specific production technique represents an information domain that is distinct from information pertaining to a specific geographic market. Employees generally specialize in one or two domains but also maintain directories about the knowledgeable people in other domains. Information from individuals specializing in different domains is retrieved through communication and communicative transactions between employees who play a key role in the encoding, storage, and retrieval of of information (Corner, Kinicki, & Keats, 1994; Daft & Lengel, 1986; Shrivastava & Schneider, 1984; Walsh, 1995; Weick, 1979). Hence, organizations are likely to be apt settings for the application of transactive memory.

There are, however, significant differences between organizations and the small groups studied by Wegner et al. during their development of transactive memory models. First, unlike the well-defined groups studied by those authors, organizations possess multiple subgroups, with different degrees of overlap (e.g., product development teams, functional departments, and regional offices). Second, organizations increasingly possess advanced technologies that help locate information without utilizing individuals' directories. Third, when sharing information, organizational members can choose from a variety of communication media available to them: the media chosen often determines the effectiveness with which information is shared (Trevino, Daft, & Lengel, 1990). Finally, earlier transactive models ignore the role of soft knowledge in memory processes. When relevant soft knowledge is available

---

[1] *Externally held information also comprises data that are stored in such storage devices as computers. However, retrieval from such devices is relatively uncomplicated, and we use the term externally held information to refer primarily to information that is stored in the minds of other individuals.*

within a small group, it is easy to access. If, however, the relevant soft knowledge is available only in a distal part of the organization, then retrieval of that soft knowledge becomes a challenge. These factors significantly influence information-sharing and -retrieval processes within organizations. requiring us to adapt transactive memory models before we apply them to organizations. . . .

Multiple Organizational Groups

The simple groups Wegner et al. used to test the concepts related to transactive memory models were associated with a single memory. However, the situation is much more complex in large organizations, where multiple transactive memories may be discerned, depending on the focal unit of analysis. Given the possibility of multiple levels of analysis, we differentiate between the memories viewed from different levels. We used the term systemic memory to describe the memory discerned when we focus on the organization as the unit of analysis. The memories we discern when examining organizational subunits we term group memories.

Systemic and group memories represent the same construct at different levels of analysis. For instance, an organization's systemic memory may contain large amounts of knowledge and information (because it employs large amounts of knowledgeable employees), but key group memories may be deficient in knowledge and information because of poorly developed directories and/or barriers to communication encountered by group members. Alternately, an organization, on average, may have relatively low amounts of knowledge and information, but certain organizational groups-for example, a product development team-may possess very knowledgeable members with very well-developed directories relevant to designing a product for manufacture. Hence, assertions about an organization's systemic memory may not generalize to the group memories. . . .

The boundaries of group and systemic memories are complicated further by the possibility that the multiple, and often overlapping, groups may cross formal organizational boundaries—for instance, a top manager may participate in several decision-making groups. A typical manager also belongs to other formal and informal groups (such as the board of another firm, social acquaintances, ex-classmates, and so on) that transcend organizational boundaries. . . . Similarly, knowledge and information held by outsiders such as distributors, customers, and suppliers is included in the external memory of other managers. External information can be a source of competitive advantage, but if it is not used, then organizations can make avoidable errors as demonstrated by the following example:

A paper manufacturer changed the wood used to palletize (a form of packaging) its paper in an Asian country. Unfortunately the wood proved susceptible to attack by local insects that bored first through the wooden pallets and then through the paper packaged in them. Tons of paper were scrapped. During discussions with a distributor (renowned for his packaging knowledge), managers were told: "if only you had asked us. . . . One of your competitors used the same wood years ago and suffered the same fate" (confidential personal communication).

Locating Information

Members must first locate information before accessing it from organizational memory. Wegner (1986) suggests that information location is determined through two processes. The first occurs when organization members possess directories that identify the holders of required information. In this case the focus of retrieval shifts to communicating the information. The second occurs when members requiring information do not possess relevant directories and engage in a search process through a series of strong and weak ties. However, organizations may provide alternative ways of locating information. Consider the example below:

At Office Equipment, contributors of solutions send their ideas to an electronic library where they are reviewed. Those accepted are stored in the library. A potential adopter can gain access to the library, review an index cataloging classes of problems and solutions and then review a specific best practice. When an interesting solution is identified, the adopter can collect further information by consulting corporate staff or the contributor of the best practice (Goodman & Darr, 1996:9).

This example shows that organizational memories may be more efficient owing to the impact of networked computer systems. Critical documents are stored and organizational discussions conducted on computers that communicate with each other (Kovel, Quirk, & Gabin, 1996). Further, organizational intranets often maintain listings of employees, along with their areas of specialization (Zorn, Marshall, & Paned, 1997). This allows members to identify information or the likely holders of desired information using software search engines that search organizational computer networks for documents labeled with previously defined key words (Senna, 1997; Zorn et al., 1997). Search engines can substitute synonyms and translations of key words to cast a broader net using information technology. One can also direct them to search through the full text of all documents, looking for any character strings that are relevant for current search. Thus, search engines are not limited to the prospective labels assigned at the time of storage but can search at a much more detailed level when previously minor terms become important in future searches.

Alternately, employees may broadcast a request for desired information through the corporate intranet or through external internet sources, such as listservers supported by the Academy of Management. Thus, they may be able to locate information stored elsewhere in the organizational memory by using their directories, by using search engines, or by using email broadcasts. The latter two means of information location have not been considered in traditional transactive memory models. We use the term locators to inclusively refer to those mechanisms that perform the role of locating (within and outside the organization) information for organization members.

The locators available to organizational members determine the amount of outsider-held information and knowledge that is available in the systemic memory. Thus, analogous to human memory, information and knowledge in an organization's systemic memory may be differentiated into internal and external components. The internal component refers to knowledge and information personally known to employees (and has been the focus of traditional studies of organizational memory), whereas the external component consists of knowledge and information employees can access from outsiders. Similarly, while the internal group memory is determined by the internal memory contents of group members (and. hence, on the group composition), the group's external memory comprises additional information that its members can retrieve from the organization's systemic memory. Clearly, the amount of information transferred to a group's external memory depends on the locators available to the group members. . . .

Communication Media and Organizational Memory

Desired information is transferred to a group or organization through a series of transactive communications. Previous research on transactive memory has been limited to contexts with rich communication media, such as face-to-face or telephone conversations. However, with increased geographic dispersion of organization members and with the advent of new communication technologies, organization members can choose from a variety of communication media: face-to-face conversation, electronic communication, telephone and video conferencing, and so on. The use of multiple media by organization members creates challenges to traditional models of transactive memory.

Many of the transactive processes of group memory are dependent on the use of rich media, such as face-to-face communication. For instance, when group members jointly attempt to interpret newly encountered data, they assign to it common labels that assist in subsequent retrieval (Liang, Moreland, & Argote, 1995). Alternately, information retrieval in groups often requires a series of multiple communicative cues. which are best provided during face-to-face communication (Wegner, 1986). Further, it is essential to use rich media when the information being communicated is complex and equivocal in nature (Daft & Lengel, 1986).

However, it is neither practical nor desirable to use rich communication media all the time. Simple and unequivocal information can be communicated effectively and efficiently using such lean media as memos and e-mail (Daft & Lengel, 1986). Indeed, using rich media to transmit information that is traditionally communicated through lean media can lead to miscommunication (Trevino et al., 1990).

Trevino et al. (1998) term an entity that varies the media used to match the nature of the information being transmitted media sensitive. It follows, therefore, that the ability of groups (or individuals) to effectively access information (which occurs when the information means the same thing to the receiver as intended by the sender) from external sources depends on their media sensitivity. . . .

Organizational Memory and Soft Knowledge

Earlier models of transactive memory were developed based on simple information items and do not focus on noncommunicable forms of knowledge. However, organizational reality is more complex. Decision situations may be equivocal or ambiguous, and complete information is rarely available (Bazerman, 1997; Weick, 1995). Under such conditions decision makers need to rely on soft knowledge, such as belief structures, judgment, and intuition (Agor, 1988. 1991; Bazerman, 1997; Walsh, 1995). The importance of soft knowledge is highlighted by the following example:

A data driven individual was hired by McCown De Leeuw, a buyout partnership in Menlo Park, California. She was sent to check out a potential acquisition target. She returned with a recommendation to buy because the numbers said so. The co-founder George McCown then visited and what he saw shocked him. "I could tell in the first two minutes of talking to the CEO that he was experiencing serious burnout. The guy was overwhelmed with problems. On paper things looked great. But he knew what was coming down the line. Jane had missed those cues completely." She no longer works for the firm (paraphrased from Farnham, 1996).

Given differences among individuals' soft knowledge and given that some forms of soft knowledge may be more relevant to a specific decision than other forms of soft knowledge, our model of organizational memory departs from transactive memory by introducing four processes that complicate organizational information processing:

1. directories or locators may be used to expand the decision-making group to include experts who have the relevant soft knowledge;

2. reputational and perceptual processes may influence the recognition and evaluation of the relevance and quality of an individual's expertise for a given decision (Cicourel, 1990; Walsh & Ungson, 1991);

3. the experts identified through locators may be asked to interpret available data and communicate their interpretations and recommendations to the decision makers; and

4. locators/directories may be used to shift decision problems to experts likely to possess soft knowledge relevant for the decision context (Cohen, March, & Olson, 1972).

Each of these processes expands the potential of organizational memory beyond the original model of transactive memory, which focused on communicable forms of information. These processes also expand the definition of information management-from a focus on timely access to information for decision makers-to include the management of soft knowledge. . . .

Organizational Memory and Information Management

Organization theorists have emphasized that information and knowledge acquired by one part of an organization must be communicated speedily to other parts (Garvin, 1993; Nevis, DiBella, & Gould, 1995). However, organization members collectively acquire enormous quantities of information on an ongoing basis; if all such information were to be transmitted to all parts of the organization, its members would suffer from information overload (Daft & Huber, 1987).

Our model of organizational memory suggests an alternative method that involves the creation of recognized information domains and the development of directories and locators within the organization. This approach requires that employees be informed about the kind of information existing in various domains and be facilitated in their efforts to acquire required information. Such an approach involves

- incorporating relevant information and soft knowledge in an organization's systemic memory;
- ensuring that relevant information and soft knowledge in an organization's systemic memory are available to its various group memories;
- designing organization processes and norms that allow for the coming together of decisions, knowledge, and information; and
- disrupting and re-creating organizational memory when changes in an organization's environment have rendered the existing memory obsolete.

Incorporating Information and Knowledge in the Systemic Memory

An information or soft knowledge item is incorporated in an organization's systemic memory when at least one organization member either personally possesses the item or can retrieve it from an outsider. Ensuring that sufficient knowledge is available in their systemic memories may require organizations to locate information-processing activities outside organizational boundaries and to identify and link up with externally located knowledge sources. These activities, of course, complement activities that ensure continuous knowledge acquisition by organizational employees.

Externalization of information. A critical issue, with respect to the management of systemic memories, is the extent of externalization. By "externalization" we mean that the tasks of scanning and interpreting data from select environmental sectors are contracted to outside information providers and/or stocks of tacit knowledge are located outside organizational boundaries. Such external information and knowledge providers are linked to the organization through formal or informal ties.

Formal links may be contractual in nature. For instance, the business press has noted the emergence of specialized firms that provide organizations with information on such diverse issues as the future political climate in developing countries, the financial and business backgrounds of possible joint venture partners, and information on job candidates (Clark, 1997; McCafferty, 1997). Market research firms and research institutes are examples of other forms of formal information providers. Informal external information providers, however, provide information because of their relationships with the organization or its members. Thus, Caterpillar's worldwide distributors are charged with the responsibility of providing it with information about local customers and conditions (Fites, 1996). Alternately, researchers have cited instances where colleagues in other firms are the source of critical informational input into the firm (Leibiskind, Oliver, Zucker, & Brewer, 1996; Powell, Koput, & Smith-Doerr, 1996).

Globalization and increased turbulence in environments are likely to increase the extent of the externalization required of firms. Globalization requires firms to develop integrated strategies aimed at meeting the requirements of their various markets (Lovelock & Yip, 1996), which necessitates that they consider information from a larger number of markets. Globalization also has increased the number of competitors and the number of factors that managers must consider when making decisions (Huber & Glick, 1993). This further requires firms to acquire and process larger quantities of information. Simultaneously, surviving in competitive global markets creates the pressure on organizations to be lean, thus limiting their information-processing capacities (Cooper, Folta, & Woo, 1995).

The challenge of having larger information content in the systemic memory with reduced personnel may be met through extensive externalization, because it is unlikely that the fewer employees can effectively scan and process information from all relevant environmental sectors. Indeed. organizations may even need to depend on outsiders for the processing of information related to entire domains.

A second factor contributing to increased externalization of information is that of economics. Information in turbulent environments is subject to rapid obsolescence (Eisenhardt, 1989), so there is a need for frequent updating, leading to higher information costs. Externalization can help reduce costs in two ways: (1) specialist information providers are more likely to develop efficient routines for gathering information, since this will be their core business (Quinn, 1993), and (2) specialist information providers can distribute the information costs over several users (e.g., credit-reporting bureaus, economic forecasting services, and brokers), leading to reduced information costs per organization. Following Quinn (1993) and the resource-based theorists, we argue that organizations need to internally store only that information not possessed or easily acquired by competitors and which provides value to the firm (Barney, 1991); it is increasingly inefficient to internally retain other forms of information.

Externalization of soft knowledge. There is also increasing pressure for increased externalization of soft knowledge that may be required for constructing and structuring problems in the face of incomplete information (Daft & Weick, 1984; Huber, 1991). Under these circumstances access to the tacit knowledge of outsiders (e.g., consultants, distributors, and research professors) can be very helpful. In this context, Stewart (1997) describes an interesting firm-Teltech Resource Network-that markets a directory of academics, technical experts, and experts within the client organization. A search engine located with this directory is customized to first locate experts within the client organization and then identify relevant outsiders. With knowledge increasingly becoming a source of competitive advantage (Grant, 1996), differences in organizational abilities to tap soft knowledge from external sources can conceivably become significant determinants of organizational outcomes.

Organizations can achieve the externalization of information and soft knowledge through two primary means. First, they can develop formal relationships with information and expertise providers (e.g., Clark, 1997; Hargadon & Sutton. 1998). Second, they can learn from other organizations through strategic alliances or by involving such entities as key distributors and suppliers in key decision processes. Additionally, organizations need to ensure that their employees constantly interact with outsiders. Thus, instead of a few employees acting as boundary spanners (Tushman & Scanlon, 1981), all employees may need to assume this responsibility, to some extent.

Those with information technology-based approaches to information management generally assume the availability of information and soft knowledge somewhere in the organization and focus on making them more accessible throughout the organization. However, employees often obtain large amounts of information from outside sources. Because external information is often accepted at face value, the legitimacy and reliability of these external sources become important information management components. Thus, the ability of organizations to identify and link up with external information sources appropriate for current and future environments emerges as an important component of effective information management.

Ensuring Availability of Relevant Knowledge info Group Memories

Knowledge held in organizational systemic memories is useful when it is also available to the various group memories within the organization. This is achieved through the development of locators. Although search engines are gaining in importance, they will only supplement and not replace directories for several reasons. First, since interorganizational electronic linkages are uncommon (at least for the present), search engines cannot substitute directories pertaining to extraorganizational knowledge and information. Second, electronic broadcast messages assume that information holders use e-mail and are motivated to respond. Oftentimes, these assumptions are not well founded. Finally, since most organizations do not make conscious efforts to identify the holders of soft knowledge (Agor, 1991), search engines are unlikely to be helpful in identifying such individuals.

Another issue regarding the management of directories is the increasing cultural diversity among employees, resulting from the globalization of the workforce. Culturally diverse individuals tend to categorize and label information differently (Cox, 1993; Fine, 1996). Thus, in order to effectively retrieve information from other members, members' directories will need to inform them of the variety of labels applicable to given information domains. To some extent, this problem may be overcome by the use of smart search engines that translate the chosen key words into all possible equivalents, but members also will need to be made aware of the existence of multiple labels.

Organizations can ensure that employee directories contain information about external information holders, soft knowledge holders, and the probable labels used by them by adopting novel socialization techniques. Socialization processes could focus on introducing newcomers to external information and knowledge holders, and encourage them to maintain the contacts they bring into the organization. Additionally, there will be a need to continuously socialize longer-tenured employees about new sources of information. Other processes that acquaint members with the expertise of other individuals can benefit the development of directories (Nonaka & Takouchi, 1995), such as ceremonies, recognition events, the use of crossfunctional teams, and job rotation. Sfmultaneously, organizations will need to aggressively develop locators (especially those that rely on new technologies) that help identify information and knowledge sources within the organization.

Bringing Together Decisions, Information, and Soft Knowledge

Groups and individuals working on a given decision context likely possess only small portions of required information and knowledge in their internal memories (Huber, 1991). A large portion of required knowledge and information is stored in their external memories, and a primary challenge lies in ensuring that decisions, information, and soft knowledge are brought together in a timely manner.

Communication practices and information technology. Increasing complexity, uncertainty, and equivocality in business environments (Huber & Glick, 1993) require increased communication frequency and an increased use of rich communication media (Trevino et al., 1990). The new, emerging communication technologies will help to support these trends. For instance, video conferencing allows for the transmission of multiple communication cues (Fulk & DeSanctis, 1995). Newer group decision support systems (e.g., Boland, Tenkasi, & Te'eni, 1996) allow for richer communication in decision-making teams with geographically dispersed members.

Although some communication technologies have increased their media richness, it is unlikely they will be able to substitute for face-toface communication entirely. Thus, organizations need to create opportunities that increase face-to-face interactions among members. Typical means for accomplishing these involve the use of periodic conferences, project review meetings, and techniques that foster a culture encouraging frequent, informal, interpersonal contact.

Norms of participation in decisions. A primary challenge for information management involves the use of soft knowledge. This challenge can be met through the use of norms for participation in different decision contexts. When decision makers need to use tacit knowledge from the organization's memory, they can adopt several approaches.

One approach could involve reversing the traditional process: communicating the decision problem to the holder(s) of relevant soft knowledge, instead of trying to obtain relevant information for the original decision makers (Cohen et al., 1972). This approach could include complete delegation of the responsibility to make the decision. In a second approach, the problem or aspects of the problem could be communicated to the tacit knowledge holders so that they provide information in the form of opinions or suggested alternatives, or they identify additional information and knowledge domains that may facilitate the decision-making process. A third possible approach involves inviting the tacit knowledge holders (identified through locators) to the decision site and involving them in the decision process. This method is likely to be prohibitively expensive in global organizations, where tacit knowledge holders are geographically dispersed. However, it also offers some advantages. For instance, Tyre and von Hippel (1997) show that the visual cues present at a problem site elicit information and solutions that would not otherwise have been obtained. This approach may be used when the decision problem is of high importance to the organization.

Prior research has shown that managers may choose inappropriate communication media because of existing social norms (Fulk, Schmitz, & Steinfeld, 1990) or because of top management's espoused preference for a particular medium (Markus, 1994). It is also likely that similar factors may exclude individuals possessing relevant soft knowledge from the decision-making process. In effect, information management may be more effective if employees are made aware that their participation norms determine the availability of soft knowledge and that the use of information technology may be ineffective with respect to ensuring the availability of soft knowledge at critical decisions points.

Disrupting and Re-creating Organizational Memory

Effective information management may sometimes require the disruption and re-creation of organizational memories. This is likely when organization members have extensive access to locators, but the expertise and/or information domains located are faulty or outdated. Members may perceive individuals to be experts because their knowledge was relevant in earlier environmental conditions or because of longstanding relationships (Agnew et al., 1994; Stein, 1997).

However, the frequency with which organizations are exposed to radically altered environments is increasing (D'Aveni, 1994). During such changes, former expertise may be rendered irrelevant, and once-valuable social networks may cease to be a useful information source for decision making in the new environment. In such cases the existing organizational memory may be an obstruction, rather than an aid, to information management. Disruption and recreation of portions of the organization's memory may be required.

Implications and Future Research Directions

We have attempted to take a fresh look at information management in organizations. Specifically, we have used the concept of organizational memory to understand the manner in which organizations acquire, store, and utilize information in their various activities, and we have suggested that information management efforts may be more successful if their prime focus is on the individual and the organization, rather than on technology. Further, we have proposed that information management is enhanced by the adoption of organizational-level approaches that focus on such issues as organizational socialization processes, communication practices, and social networks. While most current research into information management has been conducted from an information technology perspective, our arguments suggest that organizational information environments cannot be understood completely until this perspective is viewed in conjunction with traditional organizational research. Here, we briefly outline some promising research directions.

Recently, scholars have shown significant interest in examining organizational information and soft knowledge as possible sources of competitive advantage. Researchers have examined an organization's knowledge by focusing on the expertise and skills of its employees. However, our model suggests that an organization's knowledge may be held by outsiders as well as employees. Consequently, focusing merely on employees may provide an incomplete assessment of organizational knowledge. A truer picture will likely emerge by focusing also on an organization's externally held knowledge, which suggests additional research opportunities.

For instance, how does externalization affect performance? What are the tradeoffs involved in externalizing information outside organizations? Further, is externalization contingent on environmental conditions? For example, in turbulent environments conditions change rapidly; thus, there is a need to update information constantly. In such environments, relying on external providers of information may be more beneficial, for they can specialize in specific environmental segments and distribute the costs over several users.

The proposed model also offers suggestions for adapting socialization processes and information technology to utilize information and soft knowledge more effectively. Future research is needed on the effects of socialization processes and information technology on the development of effective directories and the adoption of flexible norms of participation in decisions. In previous research scholars have examined the effects of socialization on newcomers' knowledge about organizational expectations, goals, and performance appraisal systems (Saks & Ashforth, 1997). Socialization will likely shape the directories and communication patterns of newcomers. How do organizations increase "know-who" among their members? Additionally, the literature does not address how organizations socialize their members to access outsiders to support increasing externalization.

Throughout this article our focus has been on what the organization can do to facilitate effective information management. However, successful information management is also critically dependent on the self-motivated efforts of members to develop their directories and on their willingness to use these directories to obtain required knowledge. Thus, information management is likely to be more effective in organizations with climates that encourage employee initiative and participation (Sims & Manz, 1996).

Our proposed approach to information management also places much greater reliance on a broader range of sources of information and soft knowledge. Future research on information management will need to address the effects of source credibility, perceived levels of expertise, reputation, status differentials, the internal and external legitimacy of decision processes, and trust within and between organizations. How, when, and from whom information and knowledge are solicited and utilized will become more important than who is initially assigned responsibility for a decision.

Finally, in developing an organizational memory model and then drawing implications for information management, we have viewed the organization as an information processor (Simon, 1976). This perspective assumes that information exists within and outside the organizational boundary and that the organization needs to process it. However, this approach often overlooks the role of organizations as knowledge creators. For instance, Nonaka and Takouchi (1995) identify a variety of organization processes that facilitate the creation of knowledge within organizations. Our model has not incorporated the dynamics of knowledge creation or disintegration; however, these dynamics are important for future studies of information management.

Conclusions

As we enter the new millennium, effective management of information increasingly will become central to achieving organizational effectiveness. We have argued that an organizational memory approach would go beyond the latest methods of managing information systems and state-of-the-art information technology. We have proposed an organizational memory approach to more accurately reflect the realities of competing and surviving in complex and dynamic organizational environments.

This approach proposes information management as a multilevel phenomenon, in which the use of information technology needs to be aligned with specific organizational processes. Our model can guide researchers in their search for effective organizational processes and techniques that will improve the utilization of information and knowledge in key decisions. Directories, locators, communication media, socialization, externalization of soft knowledge, norms of participation in decisions, processes for disrupting organizational knowledge, and similar concepts can guide future research on information management and should become part of the common vocabulary among information managers.

References

Agnew, N. M., Ford, K. M., & Hayes, P. J. 1994. Expertise in context: Personally constructed, socially selected or reality relevant? International Journal of Expert Systems: Research and Applications, 7: 65–88.

Agor, W. H. 1988. The logic of intuitive decision making: How top executives make important decisions. Organizational Dynamics, 14(3): 5–18.

Agor, W. H. 1991. How intuition can be used to enhance creativity in organizations. Journal of Creative Behavior. 25(1): 11–19.

Anand, V., Skilton, P. F., & Keats. B. W. 1996. Reconceptualizing organizational memory. Paper presented at the annual meeting of the Academy of Management, Cincinnati, OH.

Barney, J. B. 1991. Firm resources and sustained competitive advantage. Journal of Management. 17: 99–120.

Bazerman, M. H. 1997. Judgment in managerial decision making (4th ad.). New York: Wiley.

Boland, R. J., Tenkasi, R. V., & Te'eni, D. 1996. Designing information technology to support distributed cognition. In J. R. Meindl, C. Stubbard, & J. F. Porac (Eds.), Cognition within and between organizations: 245–290. Thousand Oaks, CA: Sage.

Caldwell. B. 1996. IS hiring drive is on at GM. Informationweek, December 23: 18.

Cicourel. A. V. 1990. The integration of distributed knowledge in collaborative medical diagnosis. In J. Galegher, R. E. Kraut. & C. Egido (Eds.), Intellectual teamwork: 214–242. Hillsdale, NJ: Lawrence Erlbaum Associates.

Clark, K. 1997. The detectives. Fortune, April 14: 122–126.

Cohen, M. D., March. J. G.. & Olson, J. P. 1972. A garbage can model of organizational choice. Administrative Science Quarterly. 17: 1–25

Cooper, A C., Folta, T. B., & Woo, C. 1995. Entrepreneurial information search. Journal of Business Venturing. 10: 107–120.

Corner, P. D., Kinicki, A. J., & Keats, B. W. 1994. Integrating organizational and individual perspectives on choice. Organization Science. 5: 294–308.

Cox, T. H. 1993. Cultural research in organizations: Theory, research and practice. San Francisco: Berrett-Koehler.

Daft, R. L., & Huber, G. P. 1987. How organizations learn: A communication perspective. Research in the Sociology of Organizations. 5: 1–36.

Daft, R. L., & Lengel, R. H. 1986. Organizational informational requirements, media richness and structural design. Management Science. 32: 554–571.

Daft, R. L., & Weick, K. E. 1984. Towards a model of organizations as interpretive systems. Academy of Management Review. 9: 284–295.

D'Aveni, R. A. 1994. Hypercompetition: Managing the dynamics of strategic maneuvering. New York: Free Press.

Davis. G. B. 1997. Management information systems. In G. B. Davis (Ed.), The Blackwell encyclopedic dictionary of management information systems: 139–145. Oxford, England: Blackwell.

Eisenhardt, K. M. 1989. Making fast strategic decisions in high-velocity environments. Academy of Management J,urnal. 32: 543–576.

Farnham, A. 1996. Are you smart enough to keep your job? Fortune, January 15: 34–59.

Fine, M. G. 1996. Cultural diversity in the workplace: The state of the field. Journal of Business Communication, 33: 495–502.

Fites, D. V. 1996. Make your dealers your partners. Harvard Business Review, 74(2): 84–97.

Fulk, J., & DeSanctis, G. 1995. Electronic communication and changing organizational forms. Organization Science, 6: 337–349.

Fulk, J., Schmitz, J., & Steinfeld, C. W. 1990. A social influence model of technology use. In J. Fulk & C. W. Steinfeld (Eds.), Organizations and communication technology: 117–140. Newbury Park, CA: Sage.

Garvin, D. A. 1993. Building a learning organization. Harvard Business Review, 71(4): 78–91.

Goodman, P. S., & Darr, E. D. 1996. Exchanging best practices through computer-aided systems. Academy of Management Executive, 10(2): 7–19.

Grant, R. M. 1996. Prospering in dynamically-competitive environments: Organizational capability as knowledge integration. Organization Science, 7: 375–387.

Hargadon, A., & Sutton, R. I. 1997. Technology brokering and innovation in a product development firm. Administrative Science Quarterly, 42: 716–749.

Harris, J. E. 1980. Memory aids people use: Two interview studies. Memory and Cognition, 9: 31–38.

Huber, G. P. 1991. Organizational learning: The contributing processes and the literatures. Organization Science, 2:88–115.

Huber, G. P., & Glick, W. H. 1993. Sources and forms of organizational change. In G. P. Huber & W. H. Glick (Eds.), Organizational change and redesign: Ideas and insights for improving performance: 3–15. New York: Oxford University Press.

Kovel, J., Quirk, K., & Gabin, J. 1996. The Lotus notes idea book. Reading, MA: Addison-Wesley.

Leibiskind, J. R., Oliver, A. L., Zucker, L., & Brewer, M. 1996. Social networks, learning and flexibility: Sourcing scientific knowledge in new bio-technology firms. Organization Science, 7: 428–443.

Liang, D. W., Moreland, R., & Argote, L. 1995. Group versus individual training and group performance: The mediating role of transactive memory. Personality and Social Psychology Bulletin, 21: 384–393.

Lovelock, C., & Yip, G. S. 1996. Developing global strategies for service businesses. California Management Review. 39(2): 64–86.

Machlis, S 1997. Still looking for a few good CIOs. Computerworld, 31(8): 28.

Markus, M. L. 1994. Electronic mail as the medium of managerial choice. Organization Science. 5: 502–527.

McCafferty. J. 1997. Deal detectives. CFO, 13(2): 16.

Nevis. E. C.. DiBella. A. J., & Gould, J. M. 1995. Understanding organizations as learning systems. Sloan Management Review 36(Winter): 73–95.

Nonaka, 1.. & Takeuchi, H. 1995. The knowledge creating company. New York: Oxford University Press.

Parker, C., & Case, T. 1993 Management information systems: Strategy and action (2nd ed). Watsonville, CA: Mitchell McGraw-Hill.

Polanyi, D. M. 1966. The tacit dimension, London: Routledge and Kegan Paul.

Powell, W. W., Koput. K. W. & Smith-Doerr, L. 1996. Interorganizational collaboration and the locus of innovation: Networks of learning in biotechnology. Administrative Science Quarterly, 41: 116–145.

Quinn, J. B. 1993. Intelligent enterprise. New York: Free Press.

Saks, A. M., & Ashforth, B E. 1997. Organizational socialization: Making sense of the past and the present as a prologue for the future. Journal of Vocational Behavior, 51: 234–279.

Senna, J. 1997. Phantom indexes your intranet. Infoworld, 19(23): 74.

Shrivastava, P., & Schneider, S. 1984. Organizational frames of reference. Human Relations. 37: 795–809.

Simon, H. A. 1976. Administrative behavior. New York: Free Press.

Sims, H. P., & Manz, C. C. 1996 Company of heroes: Unleashing the power of self-leadership. New York: Wiley.

Stein. E. 1997. A look at expertise from a social perspective. In P. J. Feltovitch, K. M. Ford. & R. R. Hoffman (Eds.). Expertise in context: Human and machine: 181–194. Menlo Park, CA: AAAI Press.

Stewart, T. A. 1997. Does anyone around here know . . . ? Fortune. 136(6): 279–280.

Trevino, L. K., Daft, R. L., & Lengel. R. H. 1990. Understanding managers' media choices: A symbolic interactionist perspective. In J. Fulk & C. Steinfeld (Eds.), Organizations and communication technology: 71–94. Newbury Park, CA: Sage.

Tushman, M. L., & Scanlon, T. J. 1981. Boundary spanning individuals: Their role in information transfer and their antecedents. Academy of Management Journal 24: 83–98.

Tyre, M. J., & von Hippel, E. 1997. The situated nature of adaptive learning in organizations. Organization Science. 9: 71–83.

Walsh, J. P. 1988. Selectivity and selective perception: An investigation of managers' belief structures and information processing. Academy of Management Review. 13:873–896.

Walsh, J. P. 1995. Managerial and organizational cognition: A trip down memory lane. Organization Science. 6: 280–321.

Walsh, J. P., & Ungson, G. R. 1991. Organizational memory. Academy of Management Review, 16: 57–91.

Wegner, D. M. 1986. Transactive memory: A contemporary analysis of the group mind. In B. Mullen & G. R. Goethals (Eds.), Theories of group behavior: 185–208. New York: Springer-Verlag.

Wegner, D. M., Erber, R. & Raymond, P. 1991. Transactive memory in close relationships. Journal of Personality and Social Behavior. 61:923–929.

Wegner, D. M.. Guiliano, T.. & Hertel, P. 1985. Cognitive interdependence in close relationships. In W. J. Ickes (Ed.), Compatible and incompatible relationships: 253–276. New York: Springer-Verlag.

Weick, K. E. 1979. The social psychology of organizing. Reading, MA: Addison-Wesley.

Weick, K. E. 1995. Sensemaking in organizations. Thousand Oaks, CA: Sage.

Zorn, P., Marshall, L., & Paned. M. 1997. Surfing corporate intranets: Search tools that control the undertow. Online. 21(3): 30–51.

INDEX

AAMC. *See* Association of American Medical Colleges

Access: codes, 213–14; controls, 223, 249; issues, 250; principles, 247; safeguarding, 230

Accuracy, 39

Acquisition, 107, 109

Adaptability, 153

Administration benefits, 8

Advance directives, 269

Affordability, 92–93

Agency for Healthcare Research and Quality, 228

Alternatives, 79

American Civil Liberties Union, 228

American Society for Testing and Materials (ASTM), 243

Analysts, 53–54

Appropriate technology, 93–96, 100, 101

Architecture, 132–50

Asset management, 107, 112–13

Association of American Medical Colleges (AAMC), 243, 246

ASTM. *See* American Society for Testing and Materials

Attitudes, 175

Audit trail, 222, 248, 249

Automated clinical decisions, 28

Automated intelligence, 28–29

Autonomy, 266–67

Badmouthing, 169

Batch system, 46–48

Behringer vs. Princeton Medical Center, 228

Beneficence, 267–68

Best principles, 101

BPR. *See* Business process redesign

Brigham and Women's Hospital, 8

British Medical Association, 218, 219–20, 222

Bureaucrats, 185

Business: plans, 283; practices, 101; process, 105; strategy, 89, 90

Business process redesign (BPR), 105

Bystanders, 183

Calculation, 43, 44

Care Management Institute, 22

Center for Democracy and Technology, 243, 251

Centralization, 125, 153, 155, 161–62
Change: agents, 158–59, 160, 179–80; commitment, 179–80; emotional response, 179; monitor, 182; preparation principles, 180; responses, 182–85; rewards, 182, 283
Charting system, 7–8, 20–21, 25–26
Chief information officer (CIO), 134–35, 143–44, 285
CHIN. *See* Community health information networks
Chowa, 100
CIO. *See* Chief information officer
Clinical information system, 19–23, 28–29
Clinical repository, 26–27
Code of connection, 221–22
Code of Fair Information Practices, 251
Codes, 212
Collection, 42
Co-location, 97
COM. *See* Computer output microfilm
Commitment, 179–81
Communication: corporate level, 126; media, 291–92; practices, 297–98; system analysis, 44–45
Community health information networks (CHIN), 30
Competitive advantage, 89, 289–90
Competitive strategy, 91–92, 101
Completeness, 40
Complexity, 153
Computer: anxiety, 194, 195–96, 196, 197; applications, 187–88; busters, 216; crime, 206; downloads, 210; downtime, 11, 15; error, 11, 14, 36; intensity, 197; literacy, 174; output, 55; usage, 5; viruses, 206, 210–11
Computer-based Patient Record Institute (CPRI), 243, 245, 246

Computerese, 36
Computerized access, 210–11
Computerized data system, 51
Computerized information system, 45
Computer ouput microfilm (COM), 55
Computer Professionals for Social Responsibility (CPSR), 14
Computer Security Act, 213
Concessions, 44
Conciseness, 40
Confidentiality, 235; conceptual distinction, 229; definition, 227–28, 242; ethical issues, 270–71; guidelines, 219; guiding principles, 240–52, 244–45; manager's role, 218–23
Confirmatory factor analysis, 198
Contract fulfillment, 107, 109–10
Control, 53–55
Corporate structure, 125–26
Covert acts, 169
CPRI. *See* Computer-based Patient Record Institute
Critics, 185
Crozer-Keystone Health System, 10–11
Cyberpunks, 213
Cynics, 184, 185–86

Data: automation, 7; calculation, 43; classification, 214; collection, 42, 53, 63; definition, 38–39; encryption, 222, 223; identification, 42; information versus, 38–41; loss, 209; manipulation, 209–10; organization, 214; pollution, 11–12; privacy restrictions, 235; proliferation, 36; protection legislation, 222; qualitative, 199; reporting, 43; security, 218–23, 242, 252; sharing, 7; sorting, 43; storage, 237; systems, 41; tampering, 170; trespass, 234

Database systems, 49
Data Privacy Directive, 241
Decentralization, 125, 130
Decision making, 98; assistance, 8; informed judgments, 51; intuition, 51; participation, 298–99; rational, 51
Decision support systems (DSS), 28–29, 46, 95–96, 187–88
Dehumanization, 272
Democratic government, 52
Denial of reciprocity stage, 158
Department of Health and Human Services (DHHS), 241, 243, 246, 251
Depersonalization, 259, 261
Deployment process: acquisition, 107, 109; contract fulfillment, 107, 109–10; requirements determination, 106–7, 108–9
Design phase, 82
DHHS. *See* Department of Health and Human Services
Dignity issue, 269
Directories, 287, 293, 297
Disclosure, 247, 248
Disposal, 54
Distributed system, 48

Economic factors, 170, 252
EDI. *See* Electronic data interchange
EDP. *See* Electronic data processing
Education, 181, 252
Efficiency, 153
Efficiency syndrome, 214
Electronic data interchange (EDI), 95
Electronic data processing, (EDP), 46
Electronic medical records (EMR), 7, 8, 177–78; end-user acceptance, 189; implementation study, 193–97, 195, 196; model, 192–93; national link-up, 31–32; perceived usefulness, 189–97, 193, 196,

203; potential, 18–23, 25–27; practitioner application, 202–203; productivity, 188–89; project evaluation, 198–99; project management, 197–98; push toward, 188–89
Electronic superhighway, 258
Employers, 247
EMR. *See* Electronic medical records
Encryption, 222, 223
End-user, 32, 189, 196–97
Enterprise data netowrk, 7, 10–11, 48
Environment, 62, 147–48
Equipment protection, 209
Ergonomics, 174
Error-detection, 174
Errors, 232
Ethics, 263–74
European Union, 240
Evaluation phase, 83
Evidence-based medicine, 29
Executive information systems, 95–96
Expenditures, 1, 6, 10, 19
Experts, 293
Explicit knowledge, 98
External information, 287–90
Externalization, 294–96
Extranet, 28, 30

Facilitators, 143
Feedback mechanisms, 173, 199
Fence-sitters, 183
Filtering, 55
Firebrands, 184
Firewalls, 31, 211, 215
Fiscal issues, 10–11, 79
Floor-ceiling pre-emption, 246
Floor pre-emption, 246
Forced disclosure, 248
Formalization, 153–55, 162
Freedom of information laws, 14, 233
Fully integrated system, 48–49

Gemba, 93
General Medical Council, 219
Generic information needs, 39
Globalization, 295, 297
Golub's Law of Computerdom, 74
Grapevine structure, 127, 181
Group memory model, 284–301

Hacker Associates, 3
Hackers, 206, 216, 220
Happy campers, 182–83
Hardware trap, 76
Harmonization, 100
Harvard Community Health Plan, 7, 281
HBO & Co., 25, 26, 29
Healthcare Financial Management Association, 6
Healthcare reform, 280
Health Insurance Portability and Accountability Act (HIPAA), 241, 251
Health maintenance organization (HMO), 19
Health plan, 23
High-tech hermits, 260
HIPAA. *See* Health Insurance Portability and Accountability Act
Historical factors, 171
HMO. *See* Health maintenance organization
Hospital information system (HIS), 150–51; acceptance, 157–59; functional characteristics, 151–52; means/objectives, 152–57; selection, 160–63; socialization models, 158–60
Human design, 98–100
Human judgment, 98, 99
Human life, 269
Hybrid managers, 97

IAIMS. *See* Integrated Advanced Information Management Systems
Identifiable information, 246–48

Identification, 42, 44
Impact analysis, 78, 79–80
Individual characteristics, 189–90, 194–97, 196
Individualism, 101
Individual tasks, 127–29
Information: accuracy, 232; acquisition process, 102–19, 104; bound, 261; characteristics, 39–41; collection, 230–31; context, 62, 64; corrections, 248; costs, 52–53; definition, 38–39, 286; disposal, 54; environment, 62; increase, 52; integration, 2–5; maintenance, 54; needs, 39, 44; power, 235–36; processing, 58, 64, 65, 66; purges, 231–32; reproduction, 54–55; retrieval, 62–63; secrecy, 232; security policy, 222; sharing, 48, 96, 280; sources, 300–301; structure, 66–67; theory, 69–70; updates, 231; usage, 53, 76–78, 231; value, 99; withholding, 248
Information management, 58–62; components, 60–61, 61; definition, 285; emerging technologies, 281–82; framework, 56–70, 63; future directions, 277–83; group memory model, 284–301; guiding principles, 87, 90–102; impact, 50–56; improvements, 53–56; knowledge creation, 67–69; levels, 66; mind-set, 87, 88–102; myths, 35–36; new realities, 280; organizational memory, 293–96; policies/procedures, 238; research directions, 299–301; tasks, 36–37
Information overload syndrome, 11–12
Information system, 62–64; analysis, 41–45, 42, 76, 77; design, 98–100; development, 80, 82; implementation plan, 80; life

cycle, 73–74, 104–5; misuse, 211; problem solving, 45; project phases, 82–86; security, 242–43; study, 81–86; successful, 76

Information technology: attitude toward, 9–10; benefits, 8; business usage, 5; challenges, 2–5, 282–83; communication practices, 297–98; expenditures, 1, 6, 10, 19; glitches, 8–9; healthcare implications, 15–16; management model, 87; performance improvements, 1–2; potential, 6–8, 18–23; problems, 8–14, 88; procurement process, 87, 102–19; public agency usage, 6; software, 32-33

Informed consent, 247, 251

Informed judgment, 51

Initiation phase, 82

Installation, 82

Integrated Advanced Information Management System (IAIMS), 134; concept, 144–45; interorganizational, 146–47; scope, 145–46

Integrated database system, 48

Integration, 97–98, 100, 212, 236, 281

Intellectual factors, 171

Interactive protocols, 281

Internal information, 287

Internet, 1, 30–31, 258

Interoperability, 280

Intranet, 28

Intuition, 51, 56

Invisible property, 211–12

Isolation, 260–61

Jargon, 36

JCAHO. *See* Joint Commission on Accreditation of Healthcare Organizations

JMMC. *See* Muir (John) Medical Center

Job: displacement, 170; enrichment,

98; rotation, 97; standardization, 161

Joint Commission on Accreditation of Healthcare Organizations (JCAHO), 3, 5, 39–41, 40, 228, 234, 277

Just-in-time system, 90–91

Justice, 271–72

Kaiser-Permanente, 18–23, 28

Killer app, 25, 31

Knowledge, 98–99; creation, 67–69; explicit, 98; management, 57; soft, 286, 288–89, 292–96, 298–301; tacit, 98–99, 298–99

Koop Foundation, 243, 246

Labels, 287

Lakeland Regional Medical Center, 7–8

Legal issues, 14, 80

Locators, 290–91, 293, 296–97

Logic bomb, 210

Longitudinal study, 198

Long-term care, 263–74

Lutheran General Hospital System, 7

Macroinformatics, 65

Maintenance, 54

Managed care, 280

Management: function, 54; involvement, 77; perspective, 15–16; process, 107, 108, 111–14

Management information system (MIS), 35, 45–49

Manager, 59–60, 65, 74, 76–78, 218–23

Mandates, 175

Manipulation, 259

Market forces, 30

Match-up system, 35–36

Medical Information Protection Act, 243, 245, 246, 251, 252

Medical Privacy and Security Protection Act, 243, 246, 251, 252

Medical records, 18. *See also*
    Electronic medical records: federal
    confidentiality proposals, 234–35;
    flaws, 41; real-time system, 47
Medical staff relations, 280
Medline, 21
Meta Group, 9
Microfilm, 51
Microinformatics, 57, 65
Middle management, 168
Model Privacy Law, 243
Modernity, 52
Moses Cone Health System, 26–27
MU-HSC. *See* University of Missouri-
    Columbia Health Sciences Center
Muir (John) Medical Center
    (JMMC), 25–29
Muskegon (Michigan) General
    Hospital, 15

National Association of Insurance
    Commissioners (NAIC), 243,
    245, 246
National Clinical Information System,
    28–29
National Committee for Quality
    Assurance (NCQA), 23, 31–32
National Health Service Wide Area
    Network, 219
National Research Council (NRC),
    243, 246
Needs assessment, 198
Network navigating, 206
New York Telephone Company, 7
Nomura Research Institute, 97
Nonuse, 169
Notice of information practices, 252

Objectives, 78
Office/clinic conditions, 191, 194–
    95, 197, 203
Office of Management and Budget
    (OMB), 55–56
Offline, 47
Online system, 46–48

Open-system architecture, 281
Operating functions, 126
Operational factors, 171–72
Operational goals, 90, 92–95, 101
Operational issues, 11–12
Oracle Corp., 29
Organizational bonding, 96–98, 100
Organizational culture, 124
Organizational factors, 171
Organizational impact, 79, 121–24;
    control guidelines, 130; degree,
    130; framework, 124–29, 129,
    133, 150–63; interrelationships,
    129–30; managerial implications,
    129–31; principles, 132–50
Organizational issues, 12–13
Organizational matrix, 140–41
Organizational memory: communi-
    cation media, 291–92; disruption,
    299; information management,
    293–96; recreation, 299; soft
    knowledge, 292–93
Organizational model: programming
    support, 139; role-based, 136–41,
    139; shared-services hybrid, 137,
    138; structural hybrid, 135–36
Organizational practices, 191
Organizational support, 191, 195–
    97, 196, 203
Organizational variables, 153–54
Outsourcing relationships, 103, 104
Oxford Health Plans, 19

Particular information needs, 39
Patient accounting system, 36
Patient care values, 190–91, 194
Patient records network, 7
People value, 100–101
Perceived usefulness, 189–97, 193,
    196
Performance goals, 89
Performance improvement, 1–2,
    92–93, 100
Performance rewards, 158
Permanente Co., 28

Permissiveness stage, 158
Personal impact, 80
Personal information, 229–34
Personal security strategy, 215
Personal usefulness, 203
Personnel turnover, 128
Pharmacy: benefits, 175–76; information system, 207–8, 257; prescriptions, 22
Physician–patient relationship, 190–91, 197, 250, 252
Planning, 144–45
Power shifts, 126
Power users, 88
Preliminary study phase, 82
Privacy: computer issues, 236–37; conceptual distinction, 229; consciousness, 238; definition, 242; fiscal factors, 235; guiding principles, 240–52, 244–45; inferential factors, 235–36; issues, 225–232; laws, 14; legal factors, 233–34; management issues, 237–38; operational factors, 235; political factors, 234–35; protection measures, 237–38
Privacy Act, 233, 235
Problem solving, 78
Procedural changes, 125–26
Procedural requirements, 154–55
Processing benefits, 8
Procurement process: benchmarks, 117; efficiency issues, 115; evolution of, 103–5, 104; framework, 105–14, 107, 118; management agenda, 116–19; management issues, 115–16, 116; performance assessment, 115–16, 117; role clarification, 117–18; working relationships, 116, 117–18
Productivity, 153, 188–89, 262
Professional Property Management, 9–10
PROMIS, 190

Propaganda, 55
Providence Health System, 30–31
Provider organizations, 220
Psychological factors, 170–71
Psychological issues, 13
Purchasing organizations, 220
Push technology, 28, 29, 31

Qualitative data, 199
Quality management, 108, 113–14

Rational arguments, 185
Real-time system, 47, 48
Reasonably identifiable information, 246
Recording methods, 43, 47
Records, 51–52, 54
Regression equations, 196
Relevance, 41, 44
Remote access, 212
Reorganization, 125
Reproduction, 43, 44, 54–55
Requirements determination, 106–7, 108–9
Research, 67–69, 118, 249
Resistance, 165–69, 184–85; causes, 170–72, 173; forms, 169–70; management, 172–76; physician, 20–23, 168; prevention strategies, 177, 178–86; responses, 185–86
Resisters, 185
Resource management, 50–56
Respect, 99
Retention/recruitment efforts, 130
Retrieval, 43, 44, 62–63
Return on investment, 92–93
Reward system, 182
Risk assessment, 214–15
Risk personality, 283

Sabotage, 169, 184
Safety issues, 174
St. Alphonsus Medical Center, 7
Saint Joseph's Hospital and Medical Center, 7

St. Serena's Healthcare System (case study), 2–7; future planning issues, 278–80; information management, 37–49; organizational survey, 122–24; privacy issues, 225–29; security problems, 207–8; social impact issues, 256–59; staff resistance, 165–69; steering committee, 74–77
SDLC. *See* System development life cycle
Secrecy, 232
Secret database, 248, 251
Secure image principle, 213
Security, 205–8; administrative measures, 215–16; audit, 216, 222; budget, 223; challenges, 211–14; conceptual distinction, 229; consciousness, 215; guiding principles, 240–52, 244–45; issues, 12, 23, 80, 228; management, 214–16; manager's role, 218–23; measures, 221–23, 238; mechanisms, 249; policy, 222; problems, 209–11; social/psychological resistance, 213–14; technical measures, 215
Seven-Eleven Japan, 90–91, 97, 99
SIM. *See* Society for Information Management
Slates, 25
Social factors, 171
Social group, 127
Social impact, 80, 255–59; intellectual dimension, 260; managerial action, 261–62; political aspects, 259; psychological aspects, 259; sociological dimension, 260–61
Socialization, 300
Socialization models, 158–60
Society for Information Management (SIM), 102–119
Socio-political issues, 14

Soft knowledge, 286, 288–89, 292–96, 298–301
Software, 32–33
Sorting, 43, 44
Specialization, 153, 156
Special purpose systems, 46–48
Staff involvement, 173–74
Standards, 281
Storage, 43, 51
Strategic alignment, 90–92
Strategic instinct, 90–92
Stratification, 153, 156–57, 161–62
Structural equation modeling, 198
Structural hybrid organization, 135–36
Stylized writing, 24, 25
Sunquest Data Systems, 27
Sunshine laws, 14, 233
Supplier management, 107, 110–11
Support stage, 158
Survey, 199
System development life cycle (SDLC), 104–5
Systematic thinking, 78–86
Systemic memory, 289, 294–96

Tacit knowledge, 98–99, 298–99
Techies, 212
Technical impact, 79
Technician, 74, 75, 77
Technician trap, 76
Technological change, 148–49
Technological solutions, 93–96, 98
Technophobia, 13
Techno stress, 166
Telemedicine, 7, 257
Test phase, 82, 83
Timeliness, 39–40, 44
Times–Mirror Center for the People and the Press, 5
Total quality management (TQM), 99–100
Training, 99, 118, 130–31, 173, 181, 238
Transactive memory, 285, 286–301

Treatment guidelines, 22
Trojan horse, 210
Truth telling, 269–70

Uniform Health Care Information
	Act, 239
United HealthCare, 23
U.S. Census Bureau, 6
United States Privacy Protection
	Commission, 228
UNIVAC-I, 5–6
Universal language, 27, 30–31
University of Chicago Hospital, 11
University of Missouri-Columbia
	Health Sciences Center (MU-
	HSC), 136–41

User friendliness, 100–101
User resistance. *See* Resistance
User satisfaction, 172
Utility, 262–69

Vendors, 97, 149–50
Vendor trap, 76
Virtual reality, 281

Warrant requirement, 246–47
Western New York Health Science
	Consortium, 7
Wisconsin Health Information
	Network, 282
Work group structure, 126–27

ABOUT THE AUTHOR

An educator and public service professional with extensive experience in healthcare, higher education, government, and ministry, John Abbott Worthley holds professorships in the United States and Asia.

Author of eight books, his prolific writings on various aspects of public service management and policy span nearly three decades. Consultant to hospitals and various healthcare enterprises, he has lectured on the subject of information management in settings that range from Wuhan University in China to the Computer Congress of Berlin, Germany. His book, *Managing Computers in Healthcare*, was a popular three-edition text.

Dr. Worthley is a retired Navy commander and has been active in New York state politics. He serves in hospital chaplaincies as well as performs other pastoral work. A graduate of the College of the Holy Cross, he holds master's degrees in foreign affairs from the University of Virginia and in theology from the Seton Hall Seminary as well as a management doctorate from the State University of New York at Albany.